Genital and Perianal Diseases
A Color Handbook

Tomasz F. Mroczkowski, MD
Professor of Dermatology
Tulane University School of Medicine and Associate Professor of Research
Louisiana State University School of Medicine
New Orleans, Louisiana, USA

Larry E. Millikan, MD
Emeritus Professor and Chairman of Dermatology
Tulane University School of Medicine
New Orleans, Louisiana, USA

Lawrence Charles Parish, MD, MD(Hon)
Clinical Professor of Dermatology and Cutaneous Biology
Director of the Jefferson Center for International Dermatology
Jefferson Medical College of Thomas Jefferson University
Philadelphia, Pennsylvania, USA

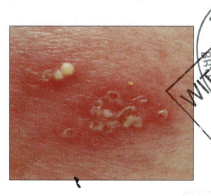

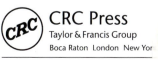

CRC Press
Taylor & Francis Group
Boca Raton London New York

CRC Press is an imprint of the
Taylor & Francis Group, an **informa** business

CRC Press
Taylor & Francis Group
6000 Broken Sound Parkway NW, Suite 300
Boca Raton, FL 33487-2742

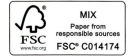

Printed on acid-free paper
Version Date: 20130801

International Standard Book Number-13: 978-1-84076-190-0 (Paperback)

Visit the Taylor & Francis Web site at
http://www.taylorandfrancis.com

and the CRC Press Web site at
http://www.crcpress.com

Contents

Preface

When penicillin was introduced in 1943 as the *magic bullet*[1] outshining Paul Ehrlich's discovery of arsphenamine[2], the world began to think that venereal disease (VD), as sexually transmitted diseases (STDs) were known, would be something of the past. By the 1950s, such venerable institutions as the *Archives of Dermatology* (recently renamed *JAMA Dermatology*) and the American Academy of Dermatology had disposed of any mention of the great pox or, for that matter, VD in their titles. Syphilis had been conquered, or so many experts thought. As the Editor-in-Chief of the *Archives of Dermatology* wrote:

'The diagnosis and treatment of patients with syphilis is no longer an important part of dermatologic practice. The papers on syphilis that are now submitted to the Archives (sic) are few and far between. Few dermatologists now have patients with syphilis; in fact, there are decidedly fewer patients with syphilis, and so continuance of the old label, "Syphilology", on this publication seems no longer warranted.'[3]

Fast-forward to the next generation that had benefits never before conceived. Birth control pills made pregnancy from chance sexual encounters much less likely, and a multitude of antimicrobials could tame even gonorrhea. Alas, carelessness entered the scene, bacterial resistance exploded, and the human immunodeficiency virus (HIV) was no longer an unwanted effect of sexual activity that was not considered the norm but an actual infection.

STDs have not disappeared. The incidence of syphilis is on the rise, not only in men who have sex with men (MSM), but also in the heterosexual population. Resistant organisms are evident, and diseases such as genital warts or even molluscum contagiosum, have caught the public's attention. Not so long ago, there was hysteria about herpes simplex infection. This anxiety has been transferred to the human papilloma virus (HPV) and with some justification. Let's also take into account that poison ivy dermatitis may be sexually transmitted, just as life is!

HIV infection still runs rampant in many parts of the world. The advent of multiple drugs for control of this scourge has made progression to the acquired immunodeficiency syndrome (AIDS) less likely, but there are still far too many people, even children, with this dreadful disease. With HIV infection, many diseases that had standard presentations now can show exaggerated signs and symptoms, making their recognition all the more necessary for rapid initiation of appropriate therapy.

Whereas STDS were once a limiting speciality of medicine, they now extend to all disciplines. Although syphilis has been recognized as involving every organ system, many patients are taken aback when they are informed that poison ivy dermatitis may be considered an STD. Similarly, many other conditions may involve the genitalia, and we have included chapters to cover this focus. Because a malignancy is on the penis or the vulva, the cause may not even be remotely an STD; rather, the cause might remain elusive. Additional chapters have also been included to cover genital adornment and genital mutilation, conditions that are increasingly seen.

With these factors in mind, we thought it appropriate to bring to health care professionals a current publication on diseases considered to be STDs, as well as other entities that afflict the anogenital region. We have previously created books on the subject[4-7], which have provided the basis for this manual, but the subject could not be so ably handled if it were not for our excellent contributors, who have labored long and hard to create what we hope will be a worthwhile endeavor.

Dr Tomasz F. Mroczkowski would like to thank 'Czelej Publishers' from Lublin, Poland, for permission to use images in this book.

Tomasz F. Mroczkowski, MD
Larry E. Millikan, MD
Lawrence Charles Parish, MD, MD(Hon)

Contributors

Zeena Aldujali, MD
Department of Dermatology
Tulane University School of
Medicine
New Orleans, LA, USA

Olubukola Babalola, BS
Department of Dermatology
University of Connecticut
Health Center
Farmington, CT, USA

Juliana L. Basko-Plluska,
MD
Section on Dermatology
University of Chicago Pritzker
School of Medicine
Chicago, IL, USA

Anthony V. Benedetto, DO,
FACP
Clinical Professor of
Dermatology
University of Pennsylvania
School of Medicine and
Dermatologic SurgiCenter
Philadelphia, PA, USA

Jack M. Bernstein, MD
Coordinator, Research and
Development
VA Medical Center
Dayton, OH
Professor of Medicine and
Pathology
Boonshoft School of
Medicine, Wright State
University
Dayton, OH, USA

Erin Boh, MD, PhD
Professor and Chairman of
Dermatology
Tulane University School of
Medicine
New Orleans, LA, USA

Nicole A. Carreau, MD
Department of Medicine
Icahn School of Medicine at
Mount Sinai
New York, NY, USA

Laila M. Castellino, MD
Chief, Infectious Diseases
Veterans Affairs Medical
Center
Dayton, OH
Assistant Professor of
Medicine
Boonshoft School of
Medicine, Wright State
University
Dayton, OH, USA

Osamah J. Choudhry, MD
Department of Neurosurgery
New York University Langone
School of Medicine
New York, NY, USA

Tunisia Finch, MD
Section on Dermatology
University of Chicago Pritzker
School of Medicine
Chicago, IL, USA

Greta Forster, MBChB
FRCOG, FRCP
Lead Clinician, Haven
Whitechapel London
Consultant in Genito-urinary
Medicine, Barts and The
London NHS Trust
London, UK

Jane M. Grant-Kels, MD
Professor and Chairman of
Dermatology
University of Connecticut
Health Center
Farmington, CT, USA

Rim Ishak, MD
Department of Dermatology
American University of Beirut
Medical Center
Beirut, Lebanon

Andreas D. Katsambas, MD
Professor of Dermatology
University of Athens
Athens, Greece

Abdul-Ghani Kibbi, MD
Professor and Chairman of
Dermatology
Director of Faculty Affairs
Faculty of Medicine
American University of Beirut
Beirut, Lebanon

Ngianga-Bakwin Kandala,
PhD Cstat Csci
Principal Research/Associate
Professor
University of Oxford and
University of Warwick
Warwick Medical School
Division of Health Sciences
Populations, Evidence, and
Technologies Group, Warwick
Evidence
Coventry, UK

Nikita R. Lakdawala, MD
Department of Dermatology
University of Connecticut
Health Center
Farmington, CT, USA

W. Clark Lambert,
MD, PhD
Professor of Dermatology
Professor of Pathology
Rutgers University – New
Jersey Medical School
Newark, NJ, USA

Danielle Marcoux, MD
Division of Dermatology
Department of Pediatrics
Sainte-Justine Hospital
University Hospital Center
University of Montreal School
of Medicine
Montreal, Quebec, Canada

Edward C. Monk, MD
Dermatologic SurgiCenter
Philadelphia, PA, USA.

Radhika Nakrani, BS
Department of Dermatology
University of Connecticut
Health Center
Farmington, CT, USA

Helen Nicks, MBBS, BSc,
MRCOG
Research Fellow in
Gynecology, University
College Hospital
Sexual Offences Examiner
The Haven Whitechapel
London, UK

Electra Nicolaidou,
MD, PhD
Assistant Professor
1st Dept. of Dermatology and
Venereology
National and Kapodistrian
University of Athens
School of Medicine
Andreas Sygros Hospital
Athens, Greece

Roman J. Nowicki, MD
Professor and Chairman
Department of Dermatology
Venereology and Allergology
Medical University of Gdansk
Gdansk, Poland

Shaily Patel, MD
Section on Dermatology
University of Chicago Pritzker
School of Medicine
Chicago, IL, USA

Vesna Petronic-Rosic, MD,
MSc
Associate Professor of
Dermatology and Clinic
Director
Section on Dermatology
University of Chicago Pritzker
School of Medicine
Chicago, IL, USA

Maryam Piram, MD
Department of Pediatrics
CHU de Bicêtre
Université Paris-Sud, Le
Kremlin, Bicêtre, France

Bobby Y. Reddy, MD
Department of Dermatology
Columbia-Presbyterian
Medical Center
New York, NY, USA

Adam Reich, MD
Department of Dermatology,
Venereology, and Allergology
Wroclaw Medical University
Wroclaw, Poland

Arlene Ruiz de Luzuriaga,
MD
Section on Dermatology
University of Chicago Pritzker
School of Medicine
Chicago, IL, USA

Joya Sahu, MD
Assistant Professor of
Dermatology and Cutaneous
Biology
Jefferson Medical College of
Thomas Jefferson University
Philadelphia, PA, USA

Freda Sansaricq, MD
University of Chicago Pritzker
School of Medicine
Chicago, IL, USA

Erin Santa, MD
Department of Dermatology
and Cutaneous Biology
Jefferson Medical College of
Thomas Jefferson University
Philadelphia, PA, USA

Virendra N. Sehgal, MD
Consultant/Practicing
Dermato-Venereologist
Dermato-Venereology (Skin/
VD) Centre
Sehgal Nursing Home
Panchwati, Delhi, India
Visiting Professor, Skin
Institute and School of
Dermatology
Greater Kailash, New Delhi,
India

Jie Song, MD
Section on Dermatology
University of Chicago Pritzker
School of Medicine
Chicago, IL, USA

Christina Stefanaki, MD
Research Fellow
Dermatology Department
Andreas Sygros Hospital
Athens, Greece

Jacek C. Szepietowski, MD
Department of Dermatology,
Venereology, and Allergology
Wroclaw Medical University
Wroclaw, Poland

Stephanie N. Taylor, MD
Professor of Medicine and
Microbiology
Louisiana State University
School of Medicine
New Orleans, LA, USA

Prashant Verma, MD
Senior Resident, Department
of Dermatology and STD
University College of Medical
Sciences, and Associated
Guru Teg Bahadur Hospital
Shahdara, Delhi, India

Michael Waugh, MB, FRCP,
FRCPI
Nuffield Hospital, Leeds, UK
Emeritus Consultant
Genitourinary Physician
General Infirmary, Leeds, UK
Honorary Professor of
Venereology
Guglielmo Marconi University
of Rome
Rome, Italy

Abbreviations

ACD allergic contact dermatitis
AD atopic dermatitis
AGW anogenital wart
AIDS acquired immunodeficiency syndrome
ANA antinuclear antibody

BCC basal cell skin cancer
BP bullous pemphigoid
BUN blood urea nitrogen
BV bacterial vaginosis

CDC USA Centers for Disease Control and
    Prevention
CEA carcinoembryonic antigen
CF complement fixation (test)
CICD chemical irritant contact dermatitis
CK cytokeratin
CMV cytomegalovirus
CNS central nervous system
CP cicatricial pemphigoid

CRP C-reactive protein
CSF cerebrospinal fluid

DD diaper dermatitis
DEJ dermal–epidermal junction
DGI disseminated gonococcal infection
DH dermatitis herpetiformis
DHT dihydrotestosterone
DIF direct immunofluorescence
DNA deoxyribonucleic acid

EBA epidermolysis bullosa acquisita
EBV Epstein–Barr virus
ECM extracellular matrix protein
EIA enzyme immunoassay
EM erythema multiforme
EMPD extramammary Paget's disease
ESR erythrocyte sedimentation rate

FBL Fabry–Buschke–Lowenstein (tumor)

FDA Food and Drug Administration
FDE fixed drug eruption
FF fist fornication
FGM female genital mutilation
FTA-Abs fluorescent treponemal antibody
    absorbtion test

G6PD glucose-6-phosphate dehydrogenase
GLUT glucose transporter protein
GUD genital ulcer disease

H & E hematoxylin and eosin
HAART highly active antiretroviral therapy
HAEM herpes-associated erythema
    multiforme
HBV hepatitis B
HCMV human cytomegalovirus
HHV human herpes virus
HIV human immunodeficiency virus
HPV human papillomavirus
HSV herpes simplex virus

ICD irritant contact dermatitis
IDD irritant diaper dermatitis
Ig immunoglobulin
IH infantile hemangioma
IHC immunohistochemical
IIF indirect immunofluorescence
IN intraepithelial neoplasia
IVIG intravenous immunoglobulin

KS Kaposi's sarcoma

LABD linear IgA bullous dermatosis
LGV lymphogranuloma venereum
LPS lipopolysaccharide
LS lichen sclerosus
LSA lichen sclerosus et atrophicus

MC molluscum contagiosum
MCV molluscum contagiosum virus
MHC major histocompatibility complex
MIF microimmunofluorescence (test)
MRI magnetic resonance imaging
MRSA methicillin-resistant *Staphylococcus
    aureus*
MSM men who have sex with men

NAAT nucleic acid amplification test
NGU nongonococcal urethritis
NSAID nonsteroidal anti-inflammatory drug

PCR polymerase chain reaction
PEP postexposure prophylaxis
PET-CT positron emission tomography-
    computed tomography
PF pemphigus foliaceus
PG pemphigoid gestationis
PICD physical irritant contact dermatitis
PID pelvic inflammatory disease
PIN penile intraepithelial neoplasia
PNP paraneoplastic pemphigus
PPD paraphenylene diamine
PPP pearly penile papules
PUPPP pruritic urticarial papules and plaques
    of pregnancy
PUVA psoralen + ultraviolet A
PV pemphigus vulgaris

RA reactive arthritis
RFLP restriction fragment length
    polymorphism
RHA reverse hybridization assay
RLB reverse line blot
RNA ribonucleic acid
RPR rapid plasma reagin

SCC squamous cell cancer
SCCIS squamous cell cancer in situ
SJS Stevens–Johnson syndrome
SSSS staphylococcal scalded skin syndrome
STD sexually transmitted disease
STI sexually transmitted infection

TCS topical corticosteroids
TEN toxic epidermal necrolysis
TEWL transepidermal water loss
TNF tumor necrosis factor
TV trichomoniasis

VCA viral capsid antigen
VC-GCBL verrucous carcinoma giant
    condyloma of Buschke and Lowenstein
VD venereal disease
VDRL Venereal Disease Research Laboratory
    (test)
VEGF vascular endothelial growth factor
VIN vulvar intraepithelial neoplasia

WBC white blood cell
WHO World Health Organization

SECTION 1

SEXUALLY TRANSMITTED DISEASES

CHAPTER 1

Syphilis

Erin Santa, MD, and Joya Sahu, MD

- **Definition and epidemiology**
- **Primary syphilis**
- **Secondary syphilis**
- **Early latent syphilis**
- **Tertiary syphilis**
- **Congenital syphilis**
- **Treatment**

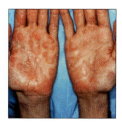
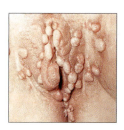
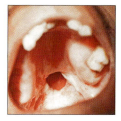
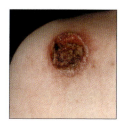

Definition and epidemiology

Syphilis (Lues) is a chronic sexually transmitted infection caused by the spirochete *Treponema pallidum*. The disease is defined by primary, secondary, and tertiary stages, with intervening periods of latency. If left untreated, it may be either self limiting or progress, causing serious complications several years after acquisition. Pregnant women, if untreated, may pass infection to their infants transplacentally – congenital syphilis[1,2].

In the USA, rates of syphilis fell by 95% between 1945 and 2000 with the advent of penicillin therapy[3]. Unfortunately, in more recent years, there has been a steady increase in rates of the disease, specifically in men who have sex with men (MSM). In the early 2000s, rates of syphilis were reported to be highest in MSM aged in their 30s; however, a recent study has shown that syphilis is increasingly affecting younger MSM, those between the ages of 15 and 29, in addition to black and Hispanic MSM[4,5].

Primary syphilis

CLINICAL FEATURES

The primary infection usually appears after an incubation period, ranging from 10 to 90 days, with an average of 3 weeks. The initial lesion or 'primary chancre' appears at the point of inoculation, which is most commonly the genitals or anus. The first sign may be a dusky, red macule, which quickly develops into a pinkish papule and then a painless chancre with an ulcerated center (**1.1**). The classical chancre is usually solitary, regular in shape, round or oval, with clearly defined, raised, smooth borders, surrounded by a dull red areola or even normal skin (**1.2**). The base is finely granular, glistening, and clean (**1.3**), unless secondarily infected. On palpation, the base of the ulcer has hard button-like or cartilaginous induration. Squeezing or abrading the ulcer produces a serous or yellowish exudate containing spirochetes. The chancre of syphilis is painless, unless secondarily infected. In heterosexual men it

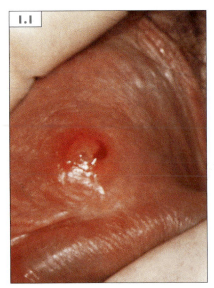

1.1 Primary lesion in the early stage of development.

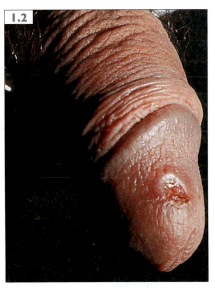

1.2 Classical primary chancre on the glans of penis.

is most commonly found on the penis (**1.4**), while in homosexual men, the anus (**1.5**), rectum, or mouth, and in women the labia and the cervix (**1.6**). Extragenital lesions are most commonly found in the oral cavity and on fingers. Multiple or erosive primary lesions are rare but do occur in men with concurrent HIV infections and in chronic alcoholics. Without treatment, the lesion usually heals spontaneously in 2–6 weeks, leaving a thin atrophic scar which, in many instances, becomes barely visible.

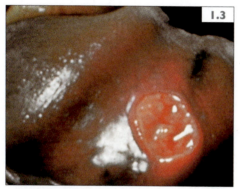

1.3 Classical primary chancre.

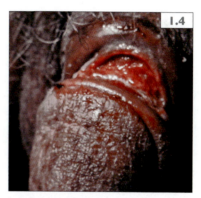

1.4 Primary chancre on the penis.

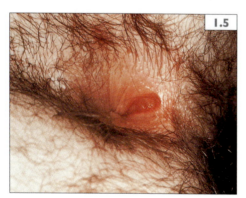

1.5 Primary chancre in the anus.

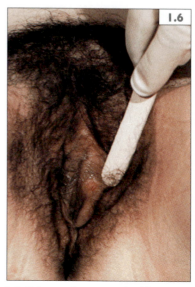

1.6 Primary chancre on the labium.

Unilateral or bilateral inguinal lymph-adenopathy follows the primary chancre on the genitalia within a few days (**1.7**). The enlarged nodes are firm on palpation, movable, and separate from one another, and the skin over them is not reddened. Such nodes are usually painless and do not suppurate. In women, the femoral nodes may also be involved.

COMPLICATIONS

In uncircumcised men, the most common complication is phimosis, when as a result of edema, the foreskin cannot be retracted behind the coronal sulcus. The other frequent complication is paraphimosis, when the retracted foreskin cannot be returned to its normal position. In circumcised patients, secondary infection may cause painful edema of the penile shaft and tender lymphadenopathy. Rare complications include Follman's balanitis, a superficial infection of the glans of penis, caused by *T. pallidum* itself.

In women, the most common complication is edema of the labium, at the site of the primary chancre.

DIAGNOSIS

The diagnosis of primary syphilis is based upon the clinical features (painless ulcer with regional lymphadenopathy), supported by the presence of *T. pallidum* on dark-field microscopic examination. Venereal Disease Research Laboratory (VDRL) and rapid plasma reagin (RPR) serologic tests are reactive in primary syphilis approximately 60–90% of the time, and the fluorescent treponemal antibody absorbtion test (FTA-Abs) or the new immunoassays, e.g. TREP-SURE, 86–100%. Serologic tests are more likely to be nonreactive if the chancre has been present shorter than a week.

DIFFERENTIAL DIAGNOSIS

The primary chancre in the genitals should be distinguished from: genital herpes, chancroid, lymphogranuloma venereum (LGV), Donovanosis (see *Table 3.1*, p. 34), Behçet's syndrome, carcinoma, traumatic lesions, or other infection, either bacterial or fungal in origin.

An extragenital chancre may be mistaken on the lips for herpes labialis (**1.8**), carcinoma, aphthous ulcer, or angular cheilitis; on the tongue for aphthous ulcer, squamous cell carcinoma, or tuberculosis; on the fingers for herpetic whitlow, paronychia, or traumatic abrasion; and in the anorectal region for hemorrhoids, anal fissure, carcinoma, rectal warts, and Bowen's disease.

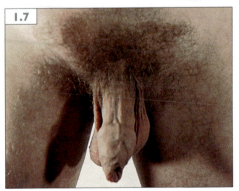

I.7 Unilateral inguinal lymphadenopathy due to primary syphilis.

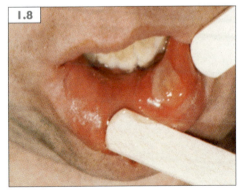

I.8 Primary chancre on the inner site of the lower lip. (Courtesy of Dr. Tomasz F. Mroczkowski.)

Secondary syphilis

Signs and symptoms of secondary syphilis commonly appear 6 weeks to 6 months after the initial infection; however, the eruption may follow the primary lesion as early as several days or with a delay of several months. At this stage, there may be multiple skin findings and/or a wide range of systemic involvement. In addition to cutaneous manifestations (the hallmark of secondary syphilis), patients may develop constitutional, flu-like symptoms which precede or accompany the first skin signs, with complaints of malaise, headache, muscular and joint aches, sore throat, hoarseness, and a low-grade fever. With these symptoms, generalized lymphadenopathy is frequently present. Some patients may have an enlarged liver and/or spleen.

Although constitutional and other signs may be present, the diagnosis of secondary syphilis is suspected primarily on the basis of the skin and mucous membrane lesions, which have certain common characteristics, allowing the physician to distinguish them from other skin diseases. One must always remember that the diagnosis of secondary syphilis must not be made on clinical grounds only and should be confirmed by serologic tests[6].

TYPES OF SKIN LESIONS
Macular eruption (roseola syphilitica)
The earliest cutaneous expression of secondary syphilis is a macular (roseolar) eruption, which usually appears 5–8 weeks after the primary chancre. It is first seen on the side of the trunk and later involves the chest, abdomen, and shoulders (**1.9**). The arms and legs are frequently affected, with the flexor surfaces being the sites of predilection. The macular eruption may be limited to the trunk or be generalized, but the palms, soles, and the face are usually spared except for a few lesions around the mouth. Because the macular eruption may be very discrete, it is best seen in natural daylight or with oblique artificial illumination. It usually disappears within a few days, but in rare instances it may persist and develop into a papular eruption. In pigmented patients, the roseolar eruption may leave slight postinflammatory pigmentation resembling tinea versicolor, which lasts for only a few days.

Maculopapular eruption
The maculopapular eruption is the hallmark finding of early secondary syphilis. It usually appears 2–4 months after infection. The eruption is generalized, involving the face, trunk, flexor surfaces of arms, and to a

1.9 Discrete macular eruption in secondary syphilis.

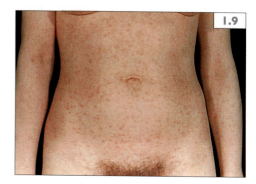

1.9

lesser extent, the extremities. The symmetric involvement of the palms and soles is characteristic (**1.10–1.12**). In this location, the papular lesions remain flat or may be only slightly elevated due to the pressure and the horny characteristics of the epithelium. Slight scaling may be present.

Papular eruption

This type of eruption, along with maculopapular eruptions, is the most common and characteristic for secondary syphilis. Papular lesions are usually fewer in number, larger, and in contrast to the rose-pink color of the macular eruption, tend to be darker (**1.13**). The papules may be widely distributed over the trunk, arms, legs, palms, and soles, as well as the face. The lesions may be isolated or grouped, forming arcuate or annular lesions. The latter are called 'nickle and dime' and frequently occur on the face of black patients (**1.14**). They can also be found in the scrotum, the vulva, and on the hands. Papules that develop along the hairline are called 'corona veneris'. Papular eruptions of secondary syphilis may resemble other skin diseases, and they are named depending on what they resemble, e.g. lichenoid, psoriasiform, pityriasiform, and so on. Although skin eruptions of secondary syphilis are generally nonpruritic and follicular, they uncommonly may produce mild itching[6].

In moist and warm areas of the body where skin surfaces are opposed, maceration of papules may occur. Moist papules may become eroded or fissured, called 'split papules', or may become elevated and condylomatous.

Condylomata lata are characteristic features of secondary syphilis. They are hypertrophic broad-based, exuberant papules with flat, moist tops, whitish to grayish in color (**1.15**). They may remain separate or may form round fleshy masses, covered by a thick mucoid secretion teeming with spirochetes. They are considered the most contagious lesions of secondary syphilis. Typically, they appear on the labia in women, around the anus and between the buttocks in men and women (**1.16**), and on the lateral surfaces of the scrotum in men. They have also been found on the inner aspect of the thigh, in the groin, and around the mouth, but rarely on other parts of the body.

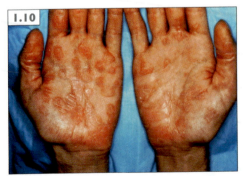

1.10 Maculopapular eruption on the palms in secondary syphilis.

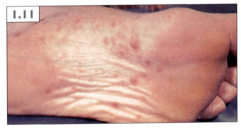

1.11 Maculopapular eruption on the sole of the foot in secondary syphilis.

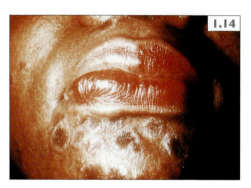

1.12 Secondary syphilis. Maculopapular rash on the palms and penis. (Courtesy of Dr. Tomasz F. Mroczkowski.)

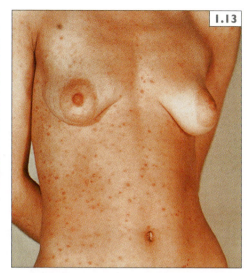

1.13 Papular eruption in secondary syphilis.

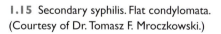

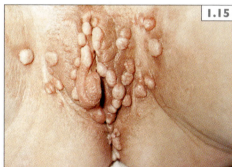

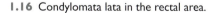

1.14 Secondary syphilis. 'Nickle and dime'. CDC's slide set (authors: Drs. Tomasz F. Mroczkowski and Sumner E. Thompson).

1.15 Secondary syphilis. Flat condylomata. (Courtesy of Dr. Tomasz F. Mroczkowski.)

1.16 Condylomata lata in the rectal area.

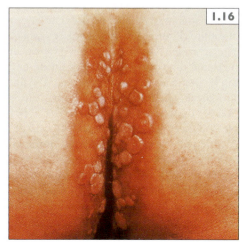

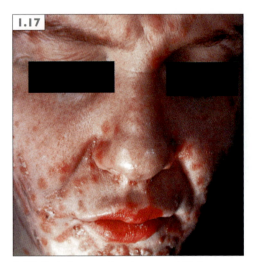

1.17 Pustular eruption due to syphilis in an HIV-positive patient.

Pustular eruption

Pustular eruption is much less common, comprising about 2% of all eruptions of secondary syphilis, usually being maculopapular or papular lesions. It is most common on the face and scalp but can be seen elsewhere on the body. Pustular eruptions have been observed in patients with AIDS or those who are malnourished and have other debilitating diseases[7] (**1.17**).

MUCOUS MEMBRANE LESIONS

Mucous membrane lesions occur in about one-third of patients with secondary syphilis. The so-called 'mucous patches' appear at the same time as the papular eruption and can be found on the inner aspects of the lips and cheek, the tongue, the fauces, tonsils (**1.18**), the pharynx, and the larynx. They are usually round, flat or slightly raised, grayish white or glistening lesions, bordered by a dull-red areola. On the soft palate and fauces, the lesions may be grouped, forming an elongated ulceration called 'snail-tract' ulcer. Mucous patches in the nose and larynx may be responsible for the husky voice, characteristic of secondary syphilis.

Mucous patches may also appear on the genitals, where the vulva, penile glans, and the inner side of the prepuce are commonly affected. All mucous patches, regardless of location, are nonpruritic and painless, unless secondarily infected. They are highly infectious, because their exudates contain large numbers of spirochetes.

SYPHILITIC ALOPECIA

This is present later during the course of secondary syphilis, usually after 6 months. The hair loss is almost invariably patchy, giving rise to a characteristic 'moth-eaten' appearance (**1.19**). Hair loss occurs mainly on the sides and back of the head. At times, a diffuse thinning of the scalp hair may occur. In secondary syphilis, alopecia may also affect the eyelashes, eyebrows (**1.20**), and rarely the body hair. The hair loss is temporary, and regrowth of hair occurs regardless of whether the patient has been treated or not.

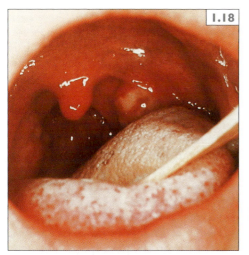

1.18 'Mucous patches' on the soft palate (fauces and tonsils).

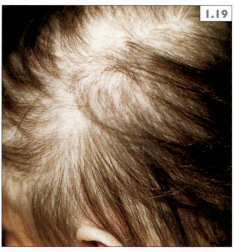

1.19 Scalp syphilitic alopecia ('moth eaten').

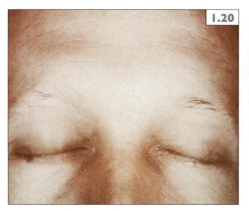

1.20 Facial syphilitic alopecia.

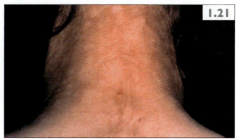

1.21 Secondary syphilis. Leukoderma. (Courtesy of Dr. Tomasz F. Mroczkowski.)

SYPHILITIC LEUKODERMA (COLLAR OF VENUS)

As the eruptions of secondary syphilis fade, small, numerous, patchy areas of hypopigmentation may persist. This is more frequently seen in women, especially those of dark complexion. It is best seen on the neck and back, giving rise to the term 'collar of Venus' (**1.21**). The duration of this hypopigmentation is variable.

DIAGNOSIS

The diagnosis of secondary syphilis can be made with certainty if the patient presents with characteristic skin or mucosal lesion; however, it should always be supported by reactive cardiolipin (RPR or VDRL), treponemal, or other tests. The FDA has recently approved the use of TREP-SURE to screen and diagnose syphilis infection. TREP-SURE, a qualitative enzyme immunoassay for *in vitro* detection for antibodies to *T. pallidum*, is the initial screening test or diagnostic confirmatory test of choice owing to its high sensitivity and specificity. It may be falsely nonreactive in early incubating cases of syphilis, and if clinical suspicion is present, retesting is recommended in 2–4 weeks. A reactive TREP-SURE result should be followed by a confirmatory, reactive nontreponemal test result.

Diagnosis of syphilis now begins with TREP-SURE, rather than a nontreponemal test, which was recommended in the past. If this test is reactive, it should be confirmed with a nontreponemal test, such as an RPR. If RPR is reactive, this confirms the diagnosis of syphilis. If it is nonreactive, a second treponemal test should be ordered, such as an FTA-ABS. If the second treponemal test is reactive, this confirms the diagnosis of syphilis. If it is nonreactive, syphilis is unlikely. If the TREP-SURE is nonreactive and there is still clinical suspicion of syphilis, one should have the test repeated in 2–4 weeks. If the TREP-SURE is equivocal or reactive, it may be repeated in this case, as well[8].

DIFFERENTIAL DIAGNOSIS

Macular eruptions can be mistaken for: measles, rubella, tinea versicolor, drug reactions, erythema multiforme, typhoid fever, and mononucleosis[9].

Papular eruptions should be distinguished from: pityriasis rosea, lichen planus, psoriasis, parapsoriasis, and urticaria pigmentosa.

Annular lesions may mimic: erythema multiforme, granuloma annulare, annular lichen planus, and dermatophytoses.

Palmar lesions may be mistaken for: contact dermatitis, pustular psoriasis, dyshydrosis, and erythema multiforme.

Plantar lesions may be mistaken for: tinea pedis, dyshydrosis, pustular psoriasis, and keratoderma blennorrhagica associated with Reiter's syndrome.

Pustular eruptions can be mistaken for: acne, rosacea, chickenpox, and drug eruptions due to bromides and iodides.

Condylomata lata should be distinguished from: hemorrhoids, genital warts, and squamous cell carcinoma.

Mucous membrane lesions in the mouth can be mistaken for: aphthous ulcers, labial herpes, viral exanthemas, 'strep throat', Stevens–Johnson syndrome, leukoplakia, and pemphigus.

Mucous membrane lesions on the genitalia can be mistaken for: genital herpes, balanitis and balanoposthitis, genital warts, erythroplasia of Querat, lichen planus, psoriasis, and Behçet's syndrome.

Alopecia syphilitica can be mistaken for: alopecia areata, traumatic alopecia, and ringworm of the scalp.

Early latent syphilis

The USA Centers for Disease Control and Prevention (CDC) classifies syphilis of less than 1 year's duration as 'early latent syphilis'. Latent infection may be interrupted one or more times by the appearance of symptoms and signs of secondary syphilis. At times, patients with very discrete skin eruptions or inapparent mucous membrane lesions may be misclassified as having latent infection. Patients with this diagnosis are considered to be potentially contagious due to the possibility of recurrence of infectious and inapparent lesions of secondary syphilis[8].

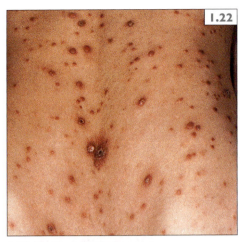

1.22 Tertiary syphilis (gumma).

Tertiary syphilis

Tertiary syphilis may develop as early as 3–4 years after the primary stage or as late as 20 years. It is rare in developed countries owing to the adequate treatment of syphilis in the early stages or common use of antibiotics for other reasons.

Tertiary syphilis is characterized by the presence of mucocutaneous and bony lesions, cardiovascular, ophthalmic, and auditory manifestations, and neurosyphilis. At this point, the disease is usually no longer contagious.

The defining lesion of late syphilis is the gumma, a nontender nodular or ulcerative lesion that varies in size from a few millimeters to centimeters (**1.22, 1.23**). Initially, such lesions are firm, but with further tissue destruction they develop a 'gummy' consistency, secondary to the accumulation of necrotic tissue. Gummas have a predilection for skin, bone, mucous membranes, or any area of previous trauma, although they may appear in any organ system of the body. Their behavior is varied: they may be indolent and heal with scarring, or they may expand rapidly, causing extensive tissue damage (**1.24**). Gummas heal with proper treatment of syphilis, although extensive scarring is common.

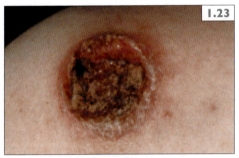

1.23 Tertiary syphilis (gumma). (Courtesy of Dr. Tomasz F. Mroczkowski.)

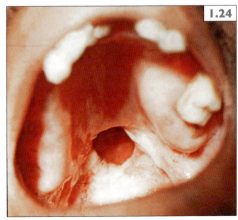

1.24 Tertiary syphilis. Perforation of the hard palate.

Cardiovascular syphilis presents later, with a latency of 15–30 years. Organisms invade vessel walls, most notably the vasa vasorum of the proximal aorta. They cause an inflammatory reaction in the vessel walls, leading to asymptomatic aortitis, aortic regurgitation, or saccular aneurysm formation in the descending aorta.

Neurosyphilis can be divided into symptomatic and asymptomatic kinds, and may occur at any point in the disease process. Approximately 10–20% of patients with primary syphilis display cerebrospinal fluid (CSF) pleocytosis[10]. Asymptomatic neurosyphilis occurs earlier than symptomatic neurosyphilis, appearing months to years after infection. Asymptomatic neurosyphilis occurs in 25% of patients with untreated latent syphilis and consists of CSF abnormalities in the absence of clinical neurologic manifestations. On CSF examination, there is pleocytosis, increased protein, or a reactive VDRL. Within 10 years of the onset of asymptomatic neurosyphilis, 20% of patients will develop symptomatic neurosyphilis.

Symptomatic neurosyphilis is divided into meningeal disease, meningovascular disease, and parenchymatous disease. Meningeal syphilis usually occurs within the first year of infection. Symptomatic meningeal involvement takes place usually several years after infection. During the first year there might be transient meningeal involvement(irritation), not the syphilis of the CNS. It presents similarly to aseptic meningitis, with symptoms such as fever, stiff neck, photophobia, confusion, nausea, and/or vomiting. Cranial nerve palsies and mental status changes are also common. Meningovascular disease typically occurs 5–10 years after initial infection. Symptoms are largely due to inflammation of the pia and arachnoid maters, as well as the arteries. The most common presentation of meningovascular syphilis is a stroke-like syndrome with focal neurologic deficits, most often involving the middle cerebral artery. Lastly, parenchymatous syphilis includes general paresis and tabes dorsalis, which appear >20 years after initial infection (25–30 years for tabes dorsalis). With general paresis, patients present with changes in sensorium, personality, and affect. In addition, they will have hyper-reactive reflexes and Argyll Robertson pupils, which react to accommodation but not to light. Tabes dorsalis occurs secondary to demyelination of the posterior columns of the spinal cord and presents with a foot drop, plus an ataxic, wide-based gait, along with loss of vibration sense and proprioception.

DIFFERENTIAL DIAGNOSIS

The differential for the lesions of tertiary syphilis might include cutaneous tuberculosis, cutaneous atypical mycobacterial infection, invasive fungal infection, or a neoplastic process such as lymphoma or metastatic carcinoma/sarcoma[2,9]. In addition, the gummas may resemble granulomatous diseases such as sarcoidosis or Wegener's granulomatosis; however, pulmonary involvement in syphilis is extremely rare, which helps to distinguish it from the aforementioned diseases[10].

Congenital syphilis

Congenital syphilis transmission is transplacental from mother to fetus or intrapartum, if the infant comes in contact with an active lesion during birth. Manifestations of the disease are classified as early, late (depending upon whether they appear before or after the first 2 years of life, respectively), and residual stigmata. Early manifestations resemble late secondary syphilis in the adult. Cutaneous findings include bullae and/or vesicles on the palms and soles (**1.25, 1.26**), superficial desquamation, and papulosquamous lesions. Rhinitis, or 'snuffles' is present in 23% of cases. There may also be hepatosplenomegaly, jaundice, or lymphadenopathy, in addition to thrombocytopenia and anemia. Late manifestations are more like tertiary syphilis in the adult, and include cardiovascular syphilis, eighth nerve deafness, recurrent arthropathy, and asymptomatic neurosyphilis. Residual manifestations, or classic stigmata, are saber shins, 'mulberry' molars, Hutchinson's teeth, and a saddle nose (**1.27**).

Treatment

The preferred treatment of syphilis at any stage is penicillin. The CDC recommends benzathine penicillin G 2.4 million units given in a single intramuscular dose for the treatment of primary, secondary, and early latent syphilis. Penicillin-allergic patients may be given oral doxycycline 100 mg twice a day for 14 days or oral tetracycline 500 mg four times a day for 14 days. Azithromycin may be used to treat early disease, given as a single 2 g oral dose, although there is evidence of resistant *T. pallidum* strains in certain areas of the USA. Ceftriaxone is another treatment option, for which optimal dosing and duration of therapy have not yet been defined. Pregnant women who are allergic to penicillin should undergo penicillin desensitization for treatment with benzathine

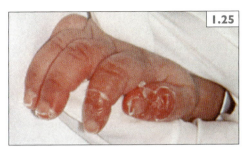

1.25 Congenital syphilis. Bullous lesions on the fingers. (Courtesy of Dr. David H. Martin, New Orleans, LA.)

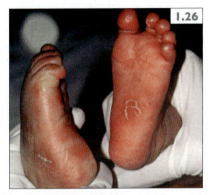

1.26 Congenital syphilis. Maculobullous rash on the feet. (Courtesy of Dr. David H. Martin, New Orleans, LA.)

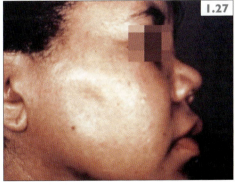

1.27 Congenital syphilis. Saddle nose. (Courtesy of Dr. Larry E. Millikan.)

penicillin. Late latent syphilis, latent syphilis of unknown duration, and tertiary syphilis are each treated with three doses of benzathine penicillin 2.4 million units intramuscularly, with doses spread 1 week apart[11,12].

Neurosyphilis requires additional diagnostic testing and a longer treatment period. CSF analysis on all patients is not necessary, as CSF abnormalities are common even in early syphilis; however, if a patient shows any signs of neurologic involvement, including cognitive dysfunction, cranial nerve deficits, ophthalmic or auditory symptoms, or motor/sensory deficits, CSF examination should be ordered. The standard test for neurosyphilis is CSF-VDRL. These patients should also receive an ocular slit-lamp ophthalmic examination and otologic testing. Recommended therapy for neurosyphilis is aqueous crystalline penicillin G, 18–24 million units per day, given as 3–4 million units IV either every 4 hours or by continuous infusion for 10–14 days[7]. Other treatment is possible with procaine penicillin, 2.4 million units IM once daily, plus probenecid, 500 mg orally four times a day, both for 10–14 days.

Treatment may be complicated by the Jarisch–Herxheimer reaction, which results from massive destruction of the infectious organisms. This reaction is characterized by a flu-like illness, with fever and worsening of the clinical picture, but it is usually self-limited and resolves within 24 hours[13,14]. In patients with cardiovascular syphilis or neurosyphilis, this reaction can be quite severe but it can be lessened with pretreatment with corticosteroids. Patients should receive 10–20 g of prednisone three times a day for 3 days, beginning 24 hours before treatment for syphilis.

SYPHILIS IN HIV-POSITIVE PATIENTS

For patients with HIV, diagnosis and treatment of syphilis are essentially the same as for patients who do not have HIV. There are reports of HIV-positive patients with syphilis having unusual serologic titers. These abnormalities include higher-than-normal values or delayed appearance of seroreactivity; however, these tests can be interpreted as usual. If syphilis is suspected in an HIV patient, and serologic results are unclear, one should use alternative tests for diagnosis, such as dark-field microscopy, if available. Follow-up testing should be performed at 3, 6, 9, 12, and 24 months. If serologic titers do not decrease fourfold within 12–24 months of treatment, CSF examination should be considered. According to the CDC, treatment of syphilis at any stage, including neurosyphilis, in HIV-positive patients is the same as for HIV-negative patients. CSF examination is not necessary unless neurologic symptoms are present[13].

All patients being tested for syphilis should also be offered testing for HIV. The chancres caused by syphilis make transmission of HIV much easier. It is estimated that the risk of acquiring HIV is 2–5 times higher if exposed while syphilis is present. In addition, these lesions, which can cause disruptions of mucosal membranes, may bleed easily, also making transmission of infection more likely. In areas of high HIV prevalence, the CDC recommends that patients with primary syphilis be retested for HIV 3 months after initial testing, if the first test was negative[14].

Gonorrhea

Jack M. Bernstein, MD

DEFINITION

Gonorrhea is a sexually transmitted disease which predominantly involves the urogenital areas. The primary site of infection in men is the urethra, while in women the cervix of the uterus. In persons practicing oral or anal sex, the oropharynx or rectum can be infected. A newborn may acquire infection from their mother during passage through the infected birth canal. The most common complication of gonorrhea in women is pelvic inflammatory disease (PID), and in men, epididymitis. In rare instances disseminated gonococcal infection (DGI) may occur.

Slang terms used to indicate gonorrhea include: 'clap', 'gleet', 'morning drip', and 'running rage'.

ETIOLOGY AND EPIDEMIOLOGY

Gonorrhea is a disease caused by the bacterium *Neisseria gonorrhoeae*, a gram-negative diplococcus (**2.1**). It is the second most commonly reported communicable disease in the USA, with a prevalence rate peaking at 421 per 100,000 population in men in their 20s and 570 per 100,000 population in women between the ages of 15 and 24[1]. Gonorrhea is transmitted by intimate physical contact and exposure of a susceptible mucosal surface, usually in the urogenital region, anus, or even the oropharynx. A common urban legend states that gonorrhea may be contracted by contact with a contaminated toilet seat, but this is unfounded[2].

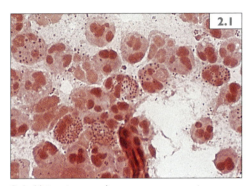

2.1 *Neisseria gonorrhoeae*, a gram-negative diplococcus.

CLINICAL PRESENTATION

In men, the usual presenting complaint is one of urethritis and dysuria, accompanied by a copious purulent discharge from the penis (**2.2**). The incubation period ranges from 2 to more than 8 days. Nongonococcal urethritis usually presents with a mucopurulent discharge; however, the two syndromes may overlap, and treatment for urethritis must be targeted at both gonococcus and chlamydia. Epididymitis is also seen in men with gonorrhea. Proctitis is usually not a sequela of penile infection in men but is acquired by anoreceptive intercourse, usually in men who have sex with men (MSM)[3]. Clinical manifestations of proctitis may include a mucopurulent discharge, tenesmus, and anorectal pain.

In women, the most common site of infection is the cervix. In almost 50% of women, infection may be asymptomatic. Vaginal pruritus may be reported and/or a mucopurulent discharge may be observed. In contradistinction to what is seen in men, anorectal infection and proctitis may be seen concurrently with cervical or urethral gonorrhea. Gonococcal infection may progress to PID in a minority of cases. PID occurs in 10–40% of cases in women and may be the presenting manifestation of disease[4–6].

Oropharyngeal infection may occur in both sexes as a result of orogenital contact. Clinically, patients may be asymptomatic or may have pharyngitis. Similarly, gonococcal conjunctivitis may be seen in adults as a result of contact with infectious secretions[7] (**2.3**). In a minority of cases, visceral dissemination may ensue, as is seen in gonococcal arthritis (**2.4**) and in the cutaneous manifestations of DGI.

Infection of newborn infants with *N. gonorrhoeae* is a result of acquisition by passage through the birth canal of an infected mother. Transmission may occur from mother to child in 30–40% of pregnant mothers with cervical infection. The most common manifestation of disease in the newborn infant is ophthalmia neonatorum (**2.5**). Newborn infants may also develop disseminated disease with gonococcal arthritis, bacteremia, and meningitis[8].

Primary cutaneous gonorrhea is uncommon. The clinical features are nonspecific, and it is rarely recognized in the absence of clinically evident genital disease. Because *N. gonorrhoeae* usually binds to mucosal surfaces, extragenital manifestations may be associated with trauma, along with disruption of the cutaneous barrier. Primary cutaneous gonorrhea may be seen in the absence of clinically evident urogenital disease[9,10]. Manifestations of both genital and extragenital disease include herpetiform lesions, papules, pustules (**2.6**), and ulcers.

Disseminated gonococcal disease occurs in 0.5–3% of patients with gonorrhea. Risk factors include recent menstruation or pregnancy in women, systemic lupus erythematosus, and complement deficiency states. Clinical manifestations include tenosynovitis, dermatitis, and polyarthralgias. The dermatitis is manifested by pustular or pustulovesicular lesions (**2.7**). Only a small number of lesions may be present, and they may be evanescent, persisting for only 3–4 days[11–15].

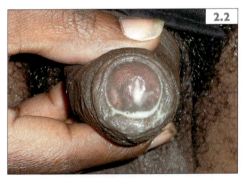

2.2 Typical presentation of gonorrhea in a male. Purulent urethral discharge. (Courtesy of Dr. Tomasz F. Mroczkowski.)

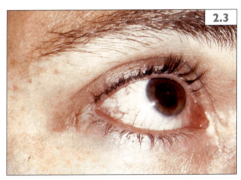

2.3 Gonococcal conjunctivitis.

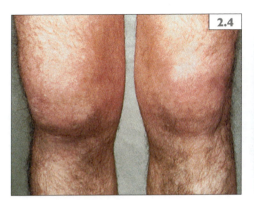

2.4 Gonococcal arthritis.

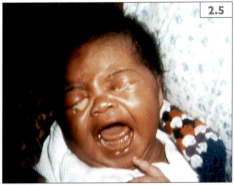

2.5 Ophthalmia neonatorum.

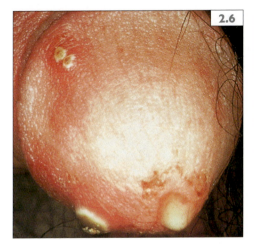

2.6 Gonococcal pustules.

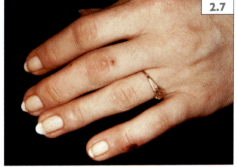

2.7 Pustulovesicular dermatitis due to *Neisseria gonorrhoeae*.

LABORATORY STUDIES

In men, symptomatic gonococcal urethritis may be diagnosed by a Gram stain of urethral discharge. Copious white cells may be seen with associated gram-negative intracellular diplococci. In women, or in extragenital infection, a Gram stain of vaginal secretions has very low sensitivity. Nucleic acid amplification techniques are extremely sensitive and specific (>95%)[16]. In men, a urethral swab should be obtained and, in women, vaginal swabs are optimal.

COURSE, PROGNOSIS, AND COMPLICATIONS

After the incubation period, men present with urethritis and dysuria. In the absence of treatment, the purulent discharge may continue for a prolonged period.

In women, asymptomatic disease is common. Estimating the true risk of the progression of cervical/ urethral gonorrhea progressing to PID is difficult given the significant rate of coinfection with *Chlamydia trachomatis*[17].

A subset in both men and women may progress to disseminated gonococcal infection with both rheumatologic and cutaneous manifestations. Gonococcal endocarditis is an extremely rare complication of the disease.

DIAGNOSIS

The clinical recognition of uncomplicated genital gonococcal infection can be quite simple with an attendant good history, physical exam, and Gram stain of the penile exudate. Culture on chocolate agar may confirm infection. In women, there may be no external manifestations of disease, and diagnosis might best be approached utilizing nucleic acid technology such as polymerase chain reaction (PCR). In the disseminated disease state, classical microbiological techniques, such as Gram stain and culture, may be utilized as with aspirated synovial fluid from suspected gonococcal arthritis. Blood cultures may also be useful, as well as skin biopsy and cultures of the cutaneous lesions.

TREATMENT

Table 2.1 presents the USA 2010 Centers for Disease Control and Prevention Guidelines.

Table 2.1 USA Centers for Disease Control and Prevention recommended regimens for the treatment of gonococcal infection

Uncomplicated gonococcal infections of the cervix, urethra, and rectum
Ceftriaxone 250 mg IM in a single dose
OR, IF NOT AN OPTION
Cefixime 400 mg orally in a single dose
OR
Single-dose injectable cephalosporin regimens
PLUS
Azithromycin 1 g orally in a single dose
OR
Doxycycline 100 mg orally twice a day for 7 days

Uncomplicated gonococcal infections of the oropharynx
Ceftriaxone 250 mg IM in a single dose
PLUS
Azithromycin 1 g orally in a single dose
OR
Doxycycline 100 mg orally twice a day for 7 days

Disseminated gonococcal infection
Ceftriaxone 1 g IM or IV every 24 hours

Alternative regimens
Cefotaxime 1 g IV every 8 hours
OR
Ceftizoxime 1 g IV every 8 hours

Gonococcal meningitis and endocarditis
Ceftriaxone 1–2 g IV every 12 hours

Ophthalmia neonatorum
Treatment: Ceftriaxone 25–50 mg/kg, not to exceed 125 mg ONCE
Prophylaxis: Erythromycin (0.5%) ophthalmic ointment

From: Workowski KA, Berman SM; Centers for Disease Control and Prevention (2010). Sexually transmitted diseases treatment guidelines. *MMWR Recomm Rep* **59**(RR-12):49–55.

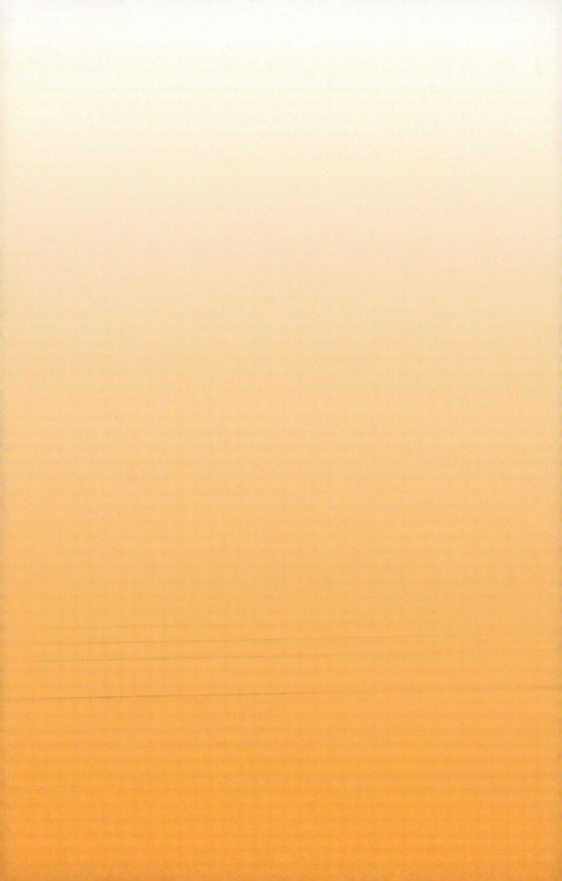

Chancroid

Stephanie N. Taylor, MD

DEFINITION, ETIOLOGY AND EPIDEMIOLOGY

Chancroid is a sexually transmitted genital ulcer disease, caused by *Haemophilus ducreyi*, a small, fastidious, gram-negative rod. The World Health Organization estimated that the annual global prevalence of chancroid was 7 million cases in 1995[1]. Although uncommon in North America and declining worldwide, chancroid incidence once exceeded that of syphilis worldwide[2,3]. Endemic areas include Africa, Asia, and Latin America and there is a strong association with prostitution[4]. In the USA, episodic outbreaks have been known to occur in the inner cities with the number of cases peaking at a high of 5,001 in 1988[5]. These outbreaks were associated with crack cocaine use and sex in exchange for drugs or money. Since 1988, the numbers have sharply declined to an all-time low of 8 cases reported in the USA in 2011[5]. These data should be interpreted with caution, however, because *H. ducreyi* is difficult to culture, and as a result, may be underdiagnosed and under-reported[5].

The male-to-female ratio among patients with proven chancroid ranges from 3:1 in areas where it is endemic to as high as 25:1 in outbreak situations[6]. This difference is noted in both naturally occurring infection and in experimental disease in humans and macaques. It has also been suggested that women may be asymptomatic carriers or reservoirs of the infection. In addition, chancroid is also associated with human immunodeficiency virus (HIV) transmission and acquisition[7]. The ulcers serve as both a portal of entry and an exit for the virus.

H. ducreyi enters the skin during sexual intercourse through microabrasions in the skin. A papule develops into a pustule that goes on to ulcerate. This has been demonstrated in both animal and human challenge models, and multiple virulence factors have been identified[8,9]. Evaluation of histopathology reveals deep, necrotic ulcers surrounded by an infiltrate of neutrophils, macrophages, Langerhans cells, and CD4 and CD8 cells. Viable organism is also found within the ulcers.

CLINICAL PRESENTATION

After an incubation period of 4–7 days, chancroid begins as a papule that evolves into a pustule. The classic nonindurated, painful, and purulent ulcer with undermined borders occurs after the pustule erodes[10] (**3.1**). Single and multiple ulcers have been identified and they are usually limited to the genital area (**3.2**, **3.3**). Rarely ulcers secondary to autoinoculation or local contact have been reported on the breast, thighs (**3.4**), anus, hands, mouth, abdomen, and feet. These do not represent hematogenous dissemination from the primary genital site. Even in HIV-infected patients, there have been no cases of opportunistic, disseminated, or systemic infection; however, multiple ulcers, longer duration of ulceration, and treatment failure have been recognized.

In women most ulcers are found at the vaginal entrance including the labia minora and majora, vestibule, and clitoris. In men ulcers are most often seen on the external or internal surface of the prepuce, the frenulum, or the coronal sulcus. Lesions can also be seen on the urethral meatus or the shaft of the penis. Ulcers are more likely to be multiple in women and singular in men. Coalescence of smaller ulcers can also occur and leads to the formation of a single giant ulcer or a serpiginous ulcer. Another characteristic finding is unilateral, tender inguinal lymphadenopathy in up to 50% of patients (**3.1**, **3.5**). This can form fluctuant nodes that can rupture spontaneously or require incision and drainage (**3.4**).

The differential diagnosis of genital ulcer diseases (GUDs) includes syphilis, herpes, granuloma inguinale, bacterial infections (i.e. carbuncle, furuncle), squamous cell carcinoma, and post-traumatic injury (*Table 3.1,* see pages 34, 35 used with permission). There are also several clinical variants of chancroid such as serpiginous chancroid, characterized by multiple ulcers that coalesce to form a serpiginous pattern. Another example is phagedenic chancroid, in which the ulcers cause extensive destruction of the genitalia following secondary or superinfection of the ulcers by anaerobes such as *Fusobacterium* spp. or *Bacteroides* spp. Other types include dwarf, giant, follicular, and transient, and mixed chancroid where the ulcer occurs in conjunction with a syphilitic ulcer.

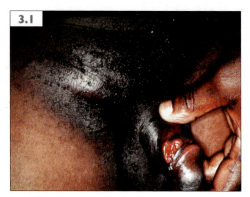

3.1

3.1 Chancroid ulcer with inguinal adenopathy. (From Martin DH, Mroczkowski TF [1994]. Dermatologic manifestations of STDs other than HIV. *Infect Dis Clin North Am* **8**:550, with permission.)

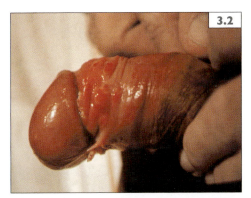

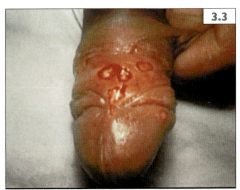

3.2 Multiple chancroid ulcers. (Courtesy of Dr. Tomasz F. Mroczkowski.)

3.3 Multiple chancroid ulcers. (Centers for Disease Control STD slide file.)

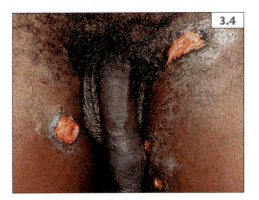

3.4 Ulcers secondary to autoinoculation or local contact onto thighs and suppurative inguinal node. (Courtesy of Dr. Tomasz F. Mroczkowski.)

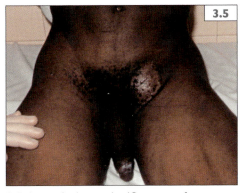

3.5 Inguinal adenopathy. (Courtesy of Dr. Tomasz F. Mroczkowski.)

Table 3.1 Helpful diagnostic features in the differential diagnosis of genital ulcer disease caused by sexually transmitted diseases

Feature	Primary syphilis	Genital herpes	Chancroid	Lymphogranuloma venereum	Donovanosis
Incubation period	9–90 days, avg. 2–4 weeks	2–7 days	Range 1–35 days, avg. 3–7 days	3 days to 3 weeks, avg. 10–14 days	Precise data unavailable; probably from a few days to several months
Number of lesions	Usually one, may be multiple	Multiple; may coalesce, more with primary episodes than with recurrences	Usually 1–3, may be multiple	Usually single	Single or multiple
Description of genital ulcers	Sharply demarcated round or oval ulcer with slightly elevated edges; may be irregular, symmetrical 'kissing chancre'	Small, superficial, grouped vesicles, erosions, or both; lesions may coalesce, forming bullae or large areas of ulcerations; lesions have irregular borders	Superficial, shallow, sharply demarcated ulcer; irregular, ragged, undermined edge; size from a few millimeters to 2 cm in diameter	Papule, pustule, vesicle, or ulcer discrete and transient; frequently overlooked	Sharply defined, irregular ulcerations or hypertrophic, verrucous, necrotic or cicatricial granulomas
Base	Red, smooth, and shiny or crusty; oozing serous exudate when squeezed	Bright, red, and smooth	Rough, uneven, yellow to gray color	Variable	Usually friable; rough, beefy granulations; can be necrotic, verrucous, or cicatricial
Induration	Firm; does not change shape with pressure	None	Soft; changes shape with pressure	None	Firm granulation tissue
Pain	Painless; may become tender if secondarily infected	Common; more prominent with initial infection than recurrences	Common	Variable	Rare

Feature	Primary syphilis	Genital herpes	Chancroid	Lymphogranuloma venereum	Donovanosis
Inguinal lymphadenopathy	Unilateral or bilateral, firm, movable, and nontender; does not suppurate	Usually bilateral, firm, and tender; more common in primary episodes than in recurrences	Unilateral, bilateral rarely occurs; overlying erythema: matted, fixed, and tender; suppuration may occur	Unilateral or bilateral; initially movable, firm, and tender; later indolent; fixed and matted; 'sign of groove' may suppurate; fistulae	Pseudobuboes; subcutaneous perilymphatic granulomatous lesions that produce inguinal swellings
Constitutional symptoms	Rare	Common in primary episode; less likely in recurrences	Rare	Frequent	Rare
Course of untreated disease	Slowly (2–6 weeks) resolves to latency	Recurrence is the rule	May progress to erosive lesions	Local lesions heal; systemic disease may progress; disfiguring; late complications	Worsens slowly
Diagnostic tests	Darkfield examination, direct immuno-fluorescence, FTA-ABS, VDRL	Tzanck smear, culture, Pap smear, direct immunofluorescence, electron microscopy, direct immuno-peroxidase staining, serology	Culture, biopsy (rarely used), Gram-stained smears have low specificity	LGV complement fixation test, isolation of the microorganism by culture	'Donovan bodies' in tissue smears; biopsy

(From Mroczkowski TF, Martin DH [1994]. Genital ulcer disease. *Dermatologic Clinics* **12**(4):761, with permission.)

LABORATORY STUDIES AND DIAGNOSIS

Gram stain of ulcer secretions or lymph node pus can be performed but these stains lack specificity and sensitivity. Ulcer bases can also be contaminated with other organisms so the stains may be misleading. Stains reveal gram-negative, pleomorphic coccobacilli in a 'school of fish' or 'fingerprint' pattern.

H. ducreyi is a very fastidious organism and even though culture was the gold standard for many years, isolation of the organism is difficult. Special medium is required and even under the best conditions and in highly experienced laboratories, the sensitivity of culture is only about 75%. The laboratory diagnosis of chancroid was reviewed in detail by Lewis[11]. The new gold standard

Table 3.2 USA Centers for Disease Control and Prevention recommended regimens for the treatment of chancroid

Azithromycin, 1 g PO in a single dose
OR
Ceftriaxone 250 mg IM in a single dose
OR
Ciprofloxacin 500 mg PO twice daily for 3 days
OR
Erythromycin base 500 mg PO 3 times daily for 7 days

From: Workowski KA, Berman SM; Centers for Disease Control and Prevention (2010). Sexually transmitted diseases treatment guidelines. *MMWR Recomm Rep* **59**(RR-12):1–110.

however, is polymerase chain reaction (PCR) methods that improve sensitivity. The Roche M-PCR, a multiplex PCR assay, is available at, for instance, the USA Centers for Disease Control and Prevention (CDC), and simultaneously identifies *H. ducreyi*, *Treponema pallidum*, and herpes simplex virus types 1 and 2[12].

Monoclonal antibodies have been developed and used to identify *H. ducreyi* in ulcer secretions. Antigen detection methods are inexpensive, sensitive, and rapid, but are not commercially available[13].

Serologic methods have been developed that detect antibody to *H. ducreyi*. These assays are not able to distinguish between recent and past infections, but they do provide screening tools for epidemiologic studies[14].

COURSE, PROGNOSIS, AND COMPLICATIONS

Tender, suppurative lymphadenopathy can be seen in up to 50% of patients. Some develop extensive adenitis and large inguinal abscesses. Nodes larger than 5 cm should be aspirated or incised and drained to prevent draining sinus or giant ulcer formation.

Another complication of chancroid is the development of phimosis. This is a late complication and results from thickening and scarring of the foreskin. Therapeutic circumcision may be necessary.

The development of superinfected ulcers has also been noted. These ulcers are coinfected with mixed aerobic and anaerobic organisms such as *Fusobacterium* and *Bacteroides* species. These ulcers may become very large and destructive and may even result in extensive scarring.

TREATMENT

Table 3.2 presents the recommended treatment regimens for chancroid[15].

CHAPTER 4

Lymphogranuloma Venereum

Virendra N. Sehgal, MD, and Prashant Verma, MD

DEFINITION

Lymphogranuloma venereum (LGV) is one of the eminent sexually transmitted diseases (STDs), manifesting either cutaneous or systemic features. It primarily affects the lymphatic system of the anogenital region. *Chlamydia trachomatis*, serotypes L1, L2, and L3 is its causative organism[1]. Microtrauma to the skin/mucous membranes may predispose the entry of the organism into the lymphatic vessels and lymph nodes of the genitalia, resulting in lymphangitis and/or lymphadenitis[2].

EPIDEMIOLOGY

LGV is of worldwide importance. It is most prevalent in the tropics, notably in some parts of India, Africa, and South East Asia[3]. In 2003, an outbreak of LGV proctitis was detected in men who have sex with men (MSM) in Rotterdam, The Netherlands. It was caused by LGV serovar 2, identified by nested polymerase chain reaction (PCR) and restriction fragment length polymorphism (RFLP) analysis; however, its clinical features were in contrast to the classic bubonic form, characterized by genital ulcer and inguinal lymphadenopathy. The latter is endemic in some developing countries, and it is speculated that the serovar 2 causing the atypical clinical features in The Netherlands was introduced by a traveler who acquired the infection in one of the developing countries[4].

It is difficult to assess the epidemiology with the available data; nonetheless, it is worthwhile to take stock of the information from 2003 to 2008. It appears that the incidence of LGV has increased in different countries in Europe, with the largest numbers reported in the United Kingdom, France, The Netherlands, and Germany. Italy, Austria, Denmark, Portugal, and Spain have also witnessed an increase in the incidence of LGV since 2006. The profile of infected individuals, MSM with proctitis over 25 years of age and predominantly coinfected with human immunodeficiency virus (HIV), has remained largely unchanged throughout the epidemic[5]. In the United Kingdom, where over 800 cases were detected, 13 presented with unusual clinical features: five cases of urethral LGV, three cases of inguinal buboes, one case of a solitary penile ulcer, and another case with a penile ulcer and bubonulus[6].

CLINICAL PRESENTATION

The clinical course of LGV can be divided into three stages.

Primary stage

After a requisite incubation period (3–30 days), a tiny, painless papule, vesicle, or ulcer, appears at the site of inoculation. The prepuce and glans in men, and the vulva, vaginal wall, and occasionally, cervix in women are the usual sites of affliction. The primary lesion is invariably self-limiting. It may not always occur and may pass unnoticed by the patient[1].

Secondary stage

It occurs some weeks after the primary lesion. It may primarily involve the inguinal lymph nodes, the anus, and rectum. The inguinal form is more common in men than in women, because the lymphatic drainage of the vagina and cervix is to the retroperitoneal rather than the inguinal lymph nodes. Proctitis is more common in those who practice receptive anal intercourse and is considered to be due to direct inoculation. The presence of unilateral, painful inguinal, and/or femoral lymphadenopathy are its cardinal features.

Enlarged lymph nodes are usually firm, and a biopsy reveals small discrete areas of necrosis, surrounded by proliferating epithelioid and endothelial cells. These areas of necrosis may enlarge to form stellate abscesses, which may coalesce and break down to form discharging sinuses (**4.1**), although this phenomenon occurs in less than one-third of patients and is more common in chancroid. The 'Groove sign', characterized as linear fibrotic depressions parallel to the inguinal ligament, bordered above and below by enlarged and matted lymph nodes and covered by adherent, erythematous skin[1,7] is seen in 10–20% of cases (**4.2**).

Extragenital inoculation may give rise to lymphadenopathy outside the inguinal region. Cervical lymphadenopathy following oral sex, mediastinal and supraclavicular lymphadenopathy due to pneumonitis subsequent to accidental inhalation of the LGV strains of *C. trachomatis*, and preauricular lymphadenopathy resulting from a follicular conjunctivitis in the wake of ocular inoculation are the usual extragenital manifestations[1]. Constitutional symptoms, fever, malaise, myalgias, and headaches are its usual accompaniment.

Anorectal involvement in early LGV was described many years ago, predominantly in women and homosexual men, presenting with an acute hemorrhagic proctitis. Patients present with rectal pain and bleeding, often with pronounced systemic features (fever, chills, and weight loss). Proctoscopy may reveal a granular or ulcerative proctitis, resembling ulcerative colitis, confined to the distal 10 cm of the anorectal canal[8].

Tertiary stage

Chronic inflammatory lesions often lead to scarring (**4.3**) in both the eye and genital tract. Lymphatic obstruction, causing elephantiasis of the genitalia in both sexes plus strictures and fistulae of the rectum, are its usual sequelae. They are more common in women and may give rise to the syndrome of esthiomene (**4.4**) (Greek: 'eating away'), with widespread destruction of the external genitalia[1,7]. Enlargement and distortion in consequence to chronic edema may alter the morphology of the penis, likened to that of a saxophone, yet another remarkable outcome of lymphatic obstruction (**4.5**).

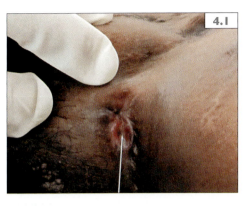

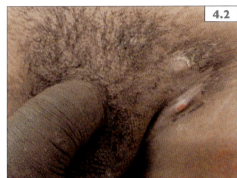

4.1 Areas of necrosis enlarging to form stellate abscesses, coalescing and breaking down to form discharging sinuses, indicated by the probe.

4.2 'Groove sign', linear fibrotic depressions parallel to the inguinal ligament, bordered above and below by enlarged and matted lymph nodes.

4.3 Chronic inflammatory lesions resulting in scarring on the genitals.

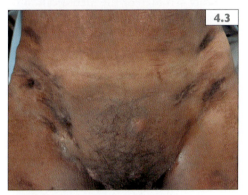

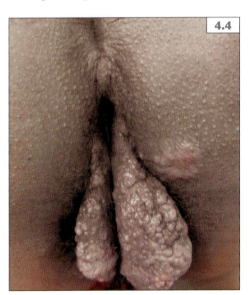

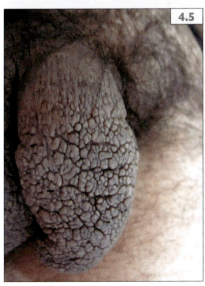

4.4 Esthiomene.

4.5 Enlargement and distortion of the penis ('saxophone').

DIAGNOSIS

The Frei skin test, a delayed-type hypersensitivity to chlamydial antigens, similar to the tuberculin test, was the mainstay for the diagnosis of LGV in the past. It is not as sensitive as a serologic test and probably resulted in many false positives due to genital chlamydial infection with serovars D–K, the prevalence of which has only been appreciated since the 1960s. Currently, the Frei test antigen is difficult to procure; hence, the diagnosis of LGV now depends on either serology or the identification of *C. trachomatis*. Histopathologic examination of biopsy specimens may also support the diagnosis[1].

Serology

The complement fixation (CF) test has been used for many years to diagnose chlamydial infections. It is genus specific and, therefore, does not distinguish between infections with *C. trachomatis, C. psittaci*, and the common respiratory pathogen *C. pneumoniae*. In view of the fact that serovars L1, L2, and L3 are invasive, this may lead to higher titers of serum antibody than uncomplicated genital infections with *C. trachomatis* serovars D–K. A titer of >1:256 is affirmative of the diagnosis, a titer of <1:32 rules it out, while in the very early stages it is difficult to exclude the diagnosis[9].

The microimmunofluorescence (MIF) test can distinguish between infections with different chlamydial species, but it has not been used very often in routine clinical practice because it requires a fluorescent microscope and a skilled technologist. An MIF immunoglobulin (Ig) G titre of >1:128 strongly suggests LGV, although invasive genital infection with *C. trachomatis* serovars D–K (for example, pelvic inflammatory disease) can also give rise to high serum titers of antichlamydial antibody[10].

Commercially available enzyme immunoassays, which detect chlamydial antigens (usually lipopolysaccharide, LPS), are widely used to diagnose urethral and cervical infection with *C. trachomatis* serovars D–K. These have not so far been evaluated for the diagnosis of LGV.

Culture

Culture may establish a specific diagnosis of LGV by isolation of *C. trachomatis* from bubo pus in 30% of cases, occasionally from the cervix in women or the urethra in men, and rarely from systemic sites[10]. *C. trachomatis* can be isolated in tissue culture, using HeLa-229 or McCoy cell lines, but this technique is not widely available[1]. Isolation of this pathogen remains difficult, and it can only be done in laboratories with specially equipped biohazard facilities and personnel experienced in cell culture. Only a few isolates have been recovered in the last 20 years, especially in the USA and in Europe[11]. Alternatively, *C. trachomatis* can be identified by direct fluorescent microscopy using a commercially available conjugated monoclonal antibody on a smear of bubo or ulcer material. This method is less demanding, but it still requires a fluorescent microscope and a skilled technologist[1].

Molecular diagnosis

The discrimination of LGV-serotypes from the other serovars of *C. trachomatis* is of major clinical importance, as different antibiotic treatment regimens are required. Detection is often based upon amplification of the well-known *omp-1* gene, which encodes the major outer membrane protein, whereas other nucleic acid-based applications have used the *pmp-H* gene, in which the unique deletion in the LGV-serovars facilitates the design of an LGV-specific PCR, or the species-specific cryptic plasmid of *C. trachomatis*. Considering the disadvantages of post-PCR amplicon handling, as well as the costs of these assays, these methods seem, at the moment, to be more suitable for epidemiological studies rather than the routine diagnostic laboratory[12].

PCR-based reverse line blot (RLB) hybridization tests, PCR-based microplate reverse hybridization assay (RHA), and two-step nested real-time PCR are highly specific and suitable for the detection of mixed *C. trachomatis* serovars in a specimen. These methods require handling of the PCR products for subsequent analysis, which is a possible source of contamination and therefore to be used with caution.

Single-tube nested amplification would create a rapid, safe and sensitive method for genotyping *C. trachomatis*. An *omp-1*-based real-time PCR assay may help to discriminate between the LGV-serovars L1, L2, and L3 and to subtype them. Detection of more than one gene of *C. trachomatis* may be necessary to avoid false-negative results due to mutation or recombination within the target sequences[13].

At present there is an epidemic of LGV proctitis in the Western world among MSM. HIV seropositivity and other sexually transmitted infections are the main risk factors. The approach to a patient with proctocolitis as recommended by the USA Centers for Disease Control and Prevention (CDC) is shown in **4.6**[13](*overleaf*).

The primary lesion and inguinal buboes should be distinguished from other diseases causing genital ulcers (*see Table 3.1* p. 34).

Pelvic or lumbar lymphadenitis should be distinguished from appendicitis, pelvic inflammatory disease, tubo-ovarian abscess, and anogenital lesions, such as hemorrhoids, plyposis, and pyogenic granuloma.

Proctitis, especially in MSM, should be distinguished from proctocolitis of other etiology (bacterial, protozoal, viral), carcinomas, and Crohn's disease.

TREATMENT[14]

Treatment is directed towards eliminating the infection and preventing ongoing tissue damage, although tissue reaction to the infection can result in scarring. Buboes may require aspiration through intact skin or incision and drainage to prevent the formation of inguinal/femoral ulcerations. However, doxycycline is the preferred antimicrobial to be used as the mainstay of therapy (*Table 4.1*).

Follow-up

Patients should be followed clinically until signs and symptoms have resolved.

Management of sex partners

Persons who have had sexual contact with a patient who has LGV within the 60 days before onset of the patient's clinical manifestations should be examined, tested for urethral or cervical chlamydial infection, and treated with a standard chlamydia regimen (azithromycin 1 g orally × 1 or doxycycline 100 mg orally twice a day for 7 days). The optimum contact interval is unknown; some specialists use longer contact intervals.

Special considerations
Pregnancy

Pregnant and lactating women should be treated with erythromycin. Azithromycin might prove useful for the treatment of LGV in pregnancy, but no published data are available regarding its safety and efficacy. Doxycycline is contraindicated in pregnant women.

Table 4.1 Recommended regimen for treatment of lymphogranuloma venereum

Doxycycline 100 mg orally twice a day for 21 days
Alternative regimen: Erythromycin base 500 mg orally four times a day for 21 days

(Some STD specialists believe that azithromycin 1.0 g orally once weekly for 3 weeks is probably effective, although clinical data are lacking)

HIV infection

Persons with both LGV and HIV infection should receive the same regimens as those who are HIV negative. Prolonged therapy may be required and delay in resolution of the clinical manifestations might occur.

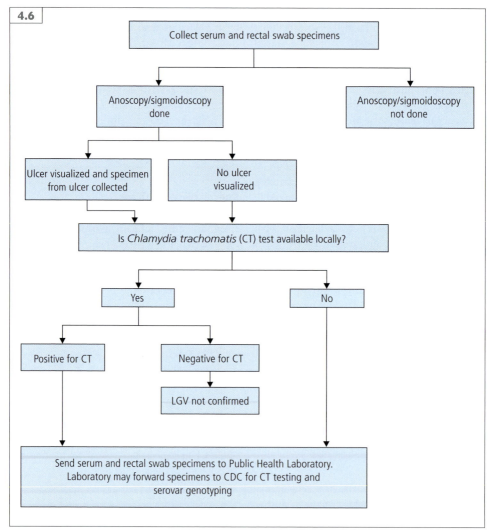

4.6 Centers for Disease Control and Prevention (CDC) guidelines for laboratory confirmation of lymphogranuloma venereum (LGV) proctocolitis. For patients with classic LGV symptoms (e.g. genital papule or ulcer and inguinal lymphadenopathy) and for patients who are asymptomatic sex partners of LGV case patients, collect urethral (or urine) specimens and test locally for CT. If positive for CT, urethral/urine specimen and serum specimen may be sent to CDC for typing.

CHAPTER 5

Donovanosis

Virendra N. Sehgal, MD, and Prashant Vermla, MD

INTRODUCTION

Donovanosis/granuloma inguinale is one of the distinct genital ulcerative diseases. It is also known as granuloma inguinale as it frequently affects the inguinal region.

The credit for its initial description as a pre-eminent clinical condition goes to McLeod, who in the year 1882 called attention to its morphological characteristics in India. Donovan in 1905, also working in India, described its causal agent[1-3]. In 1913, Aragão and Vianna from Brazil introduced the use of emetic tartar, the first effective medication used for the treatment of this disease[4].

ETIOLOGY AND EPIDEMIOLOGY

Donovanosis is caused by infection with *Donovania granulomatis/Calymmato-bacterium granulomatis*[4], recently renamed as *Klebsiella granulomatis* following comparative deoxyribonucleic acid (DNA) sequencing studies.

Although the entity has prevailed for more than a century, it remains largely unrecognized for it occurs in unspecified geographical locations and with sporadic incidence. Its pathogenesis and epidemiology are not understood in their entirety and they are subjects of continual investigation[5]. This entity is frequently encountered in African-Americans, in individuals with a lower socioeconomic status, and among those with poor hygiene. It is endemic in the tropics and subtropics; Papua New Guinea, South Africa (provinces of KwaZulu/Natal and East Transvaal), parts of India and Indonesia, and among the aborigines of Australia; Central America and the Caribbean, Peru (where the first cause of chronic genital ulcers in patients with immune deficiency disorder have been found), Argentina, French Guiana, and Brazil[6]. In addition, it appears that the disease is underestimated in various places where it is prevalent[6]. It has been suggested that a lack of experience in tropical diseases might be a cause of difficulty in identifying cases[7]. A contributing factor may be the widespread use of over-the-counter antibiotics, which can mask its clear-cut clinical features[8].

Adults between the ages of 20 and 40 years are most commonly afflicted[1,2] with no gender distinction. Transmission may occur during vaginal delivery, and careful cleansing of neonates born to infected mothers is recommended. The disease in children is often associated with contact with infected adults and/or through sexual abuse[8]. Only since the middle of the 20th century has there been a consensus that donovanosis can be transmitted sexually. In spite of the occurrence in sexually inactive children and adults, and the disease being proportionately rare in sex workers, the argument is based on the fact that in the majority of cases, those with this illness have a history of sexual activity. In a subcategory of those who are sexually active, there is a greater incidence of exclusively cervical lesions, anal lesions associated with the practice of sodomy,

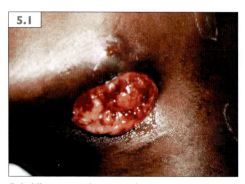

5.1 Ulcerogranulomatous lesion.

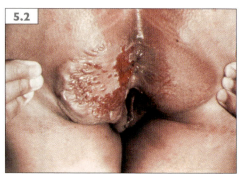

5.2 Hypertrophic perianal lesion.

genital lesions in the majority of cases (80–100%), concomitant sexually transmitted infections (STIs), sexual contact with sex professionals, and a high prevalence in the sexual partners of the cases studied[1,2,5,7,8]. It is supposed that the natural habitat of *K. granulomatis* could be the intestine and that the skin is affected by direct contact, anal coitus, or indirectly, through contamination of the genitals by fecal organisms.

CLINICAL PRESENTATION

The initial lesion is a hard papule, which appears 3–90 days after contact, with an average interval of 17.5 days after contact. The lesion erodes as it enlarges, resulting in several variants such as:

- Ulcerogranulomatous lesion: presents as a single, well-defined, friable, beefy-red, nontender, nonindurated ulcer with exorbitant granulation tissue. It bleeds on touch (**5.1**).
- Hypertrophic lesion: characterized by an irregular, friable, raised growth, which bleeds on touch. An ulcer with a well-defined, raised edge and an elevated, granulomatous base may also be seen (**5.2**).

- Necrotic lesion: presents as a large, foul-smelling, tender, nonindurated, irregular ulcer. Sometimes satellite ulcers are also found in the inguinal area; these are equally rapidly progressive and destructive (**5.3**).
- Sclerotic lesion: presents as a firm band-like scar without granulation.

Although lymphadenopathy is not characteristic, the inguinal subcutaneous tissue may become edematous. This is the pseudobubo (**5.4**) and may break, leaving behind an elevated, granulomatous ulcer. In homosexual men, anal lesions can be found. If the point of entry is the mouth, oral lesions can appear. In fact, no part of the body seems to be spared. Chronicity may result in osteolytic bone lesions, pseudoepitheliomatous hyperplasia of the genitalia (**5.5**), and eventually squamous cell cancer. Late complications include stenosis of the anal, urethtral, or vaginal orifices.

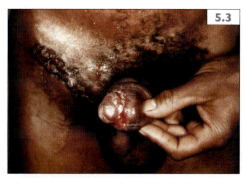

5.3 Necrotic lesion.

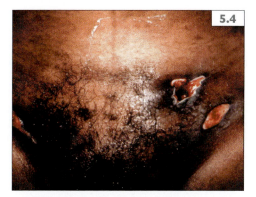

5.4 Pseudobubo breaking up to form sinuses.

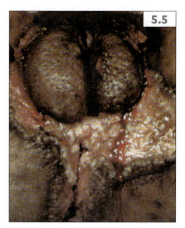

5.5 Pseudoepitheliomatous hyperplasia.

DIFFERENTIAL DIAGNOSIS

The ulcers may sometimes be difficult to differentiate from primary syphilitic chancres, condylomata lata, chancroid, and large human immunodeficiency (HIV)-associated herpes ulcers (see *Table 3.1*, p. 34). Amebiasis and carcinoma of the penis should be considered, if lesions are destructive or necrotic. Donovanosis-associated pseudoelephantiasis may mimic lymphogranuloma venereum (LGV). Donovanosis is often long standing and the possibility of dual infection with one or other of the classic causes of genital ulcer disease (GUD) should always be considered. Cervical donovanosis may mimic both carcinoma and tuberculosis of the cervix. Extragenital lesions may present atypically, often leading to protracted delay in the diagnosis[9,10].

LABORATORY DIAGNOSIS

Direct microscopy

Originally described by Donovan in 1905[3], the direct microscopy method has been the most widely used since then. Donovan bodies (**5.6**) appear with Giemsa, Wright, and Leishman stains. 'Rapid diff' is a useful quick version of the Giemsa stain[11]. This approach to diagnosis has been recommended consistently as a simple and reliable method. Surface debris from purulent ulcers should be removed gently with a cotton swab. Material may then be collected by rolling a swab over the lesion and pressing it directly onto a glass slide. The slide should be air dried and either stained immediately or, where this is not possible, fixed in 95% ethanol for 5 minutes and stained later. This approach to diagnosis works well in patients whose lesions have plentiful Donovan bodies. Additional methods listed below are more suitable for cases with low numbers of Donovan bodies.

Biopsy

Biopsy may be considered for smear-negative lesions, large lesions with easily removed friable tissue, any lesion where malignancy is suspected, and less common lesions of the mouth, anus, cervix, and uterus. Examination of biopsy material is more time consuming and may involve greater discomfort for the patient. Good results may be obtained by taking up to three 3–5-mm punch or snip biopsies and placing them in 10% formalin/saline solution. Smears for more rapid diagnosis may be made by smearing the inferior surface of one of the biopsy specimens onto a glass slide, avoiding respreading of any area and stopping when the specimen becomes dry. Biopsy tissue may be examined with the stains recommended for smears and also with silver stains or slow Giemsa.

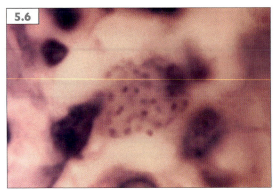

5.6 Donovan bodies (Courtesy of CDC/Susan Lindsley).

Culture
Successful culture techniques have been reported in human peripheral blood mononuclear cells[12] and in Hep2 cells[13]. So far, these techniques have only been successfully utilized by two research laboratories outside the United Kingdom (Darwin and Durban). Pretreatment of specimens with antimicrobials, such as vancomycin and metronidazole, is necessary to remove contaminants.

Polymerise chain reaction (PCR) (EURO GUIDE)
PCR methods have been used, including a colorimetric detection method[14,15]. A genital ulcer disease multiplex PCR test has been developed using an in-house nucleic acid amplification technique with *K. granulomatis* primers[16]. However, no commercial PCR tests for donovanosis are currently available.

Serology
Serologic tests have been developed but are not reliable.

TREATMENT
Several antimicrobial regimens have been effective, but only a limited number of controlled trials have been published. Treatment has been shown to halt the progression of lesions, and healing typically proceeds inward from the ulcer margins; prolonged therapy is usually required to permit granulation and re-epithelialization of the ulcers (*Table 5.1*). Relapse can occur 6–18 months after apparently effective therapy.

Follow-up
Patients should be followed clinically until signs and symptoms have resolved.

Table 5.1 USA Centers for Disease Control and Prevention (CDC) recommended regimens for the treatment of donovanosis

Doxycycline 100 mg orally twice a day for at least 3 weeks and until all lesions have completely healed

Alternative regimens
Azithromycin 1 g orally once per week for at least 3 weeks and until all lesions have completely healed
OR
Ciprofloxacin 750 mg orally twice a day for at least 3 weeks and until all lesions have completely healed
OR
Erythromycin base 500 mg orally four times a day for at least 3 weeks and until all lesions have completely healed
OR
Trimethoprim–sulfamethoxazole one double-strength (160 mg/800 mg) tablet orally twice a day

(The addition of an aminoglycoside (e.g. gentamicin 1 mg/kg IV every 8 hours) to these regimens can be considered if improvement is not evident within the first few days of therapy)

Management of sex partners
Persons who have had sexual contact with a patient who has granuloma inguinale within the 60 days before onset of the patient's symptoms and signs should be examined and offered therapy; however, the value of empiric therapy in the absence of clinical manifestations has not been established.

Special considerations

Pregnancy

Pregnancy is a relative contraindication to the use of sulfonamides. Pregnant and lactating women should be treated with the erythromycin regimen, and consideration should be given to the addition of a parenteral aminoglycoside (e.g. gentamicin). Azithromycin might prove useful for treating granuloma inguinale during pregnancy, but published data are lacking. Doxycycline and ciprofloxacin are contraindicated in pregnant women.

HIV infection

Persons with both granuloma inguinale and HIV infection should receive the same regimens as those who are HIV negative; however, the addition of a parenteral aminoglycoside (e.g. gentamicin) should also be considered.

Information, explanation, and advice for the patient

Patients with donovanosis are often embarrassed or ashamed and reassurance that they have a treatable condition is important, making it important to complete the antimicrobial regimen. Testing for HIV and syphilis should be performed.

Partner notification

Donovanosis is uncommon in partners of index cases but sexual contacts in the last 6 months should still be checked for possible lesions by clinical examination.

Nongonoccocal Urethritis

Nikita R. Lakdawala, MD, Nicole A. Carreau, MD, and Jane M. Grant-Kels, MD

DEFINITION

Nongonoccocal urethritis (NGU) is defined by the presence of leukorrhea and inflammation of the urethra and/or cervix not caused by gonorrhea[1]. It can result from both infectious and noninfectious causes.

Most cases of NGU are acute and resolve after treatment; however, a proportion of cases progress to chronic NGU, defined as the presence of recurrent or persistent urethritis 6 weeks after dispensing appropriate antibiotic treatment[2].

ETIOLOGY AND EPIDEMIOLOGY

Acute NGU is one of the most common sexually transmitted infections (STIs) among men[2]. In the USA, it has been estimated that there are 2 million cases per year[3]. Various etiologies of nongonoccocal urethritis have been recognized, but to date, no pathogen is identified in 20–50% of cases[4]. When a pathogen is isolated, it is most commonly *Chlamydia trachomatis* or *Mycoplasma genitalium*[4,5]. The next frequent cause of NGU is *Trichomonas vaginalis*, but its prevalence in urethritis depends on the population studied. Other bacteria and viruses have been found in association with NGU, but they are rather rare causes of the disease. They include: *Ureaplasma urealyticum*, *Haemophilus* spp., *Streptococcus* spp., *Gardnerella vaginalis*, herpes simplex virus, and adenoviruses[4].

C. trachomatis, an intracellular bacterium with an affinity for epithelial cells, is the most well established cause of NGU. Chlamydia is the most common sexually transmitted infection (STI) in the USA, with a prevalence of approximately 4% in young adults; annually, 2.8 million cases are estimated[6]; however, a certain group of infected men may remain asymptomatic. Studies from the 1970s and 1980s estimated cases of NGU resulting from chlamydia to range between 35 and 50%[2]; however, its overall prevalence has been declining, and newer studies predict that chlamydia may now account for as low as 15% of NGU cases[7,8]. Previously thought to be the most common pathogen in NGU, its prevalence is now thought to be equivalent to or less than that of mycoplasma-associated NGU; moreover, the prevalence of chlamydial NGU varies per age group and is higher among young men[1]. Complications of chlamydial NGU in men, can include epididymitis, prostatitis, and Reiter's syndrome, but are identified in only a small group of patients[1].

Mycoplasma genitalium, a motile organism, also has the ability to invade epithelial cells. Its incidence, ranging from 15% to 25% of NGU cases, has been found to be much higher than previously recognized, with data showing rates paralleling that of chlamydia[4]. Case reports also suggest that men infected with *M. genitalium* have more symptomatic urethritis compared to those infected with *Chlamydia trachomatis*[9].

Ureaplasma urealyticum has also been identified in association with NGU. While conflicting data exist on whether it plays a causative role, there is growing evidence that it is involved in the pathogenesis of urethritis[9]. The proportion of cases associated with this pathogen is uncertain, but some studies have identified the bacteria in 5–10% of NGU cases[9].

Trichomonas vaginalis is also associated with urethritis in men and can be either symptomatic or asymptomatic in nature[2]. The isolation of *Trichomonas vaginalis* is dependent upon the prevalence of the organism in the community and has been reported in 1–17% of cases of NGU[2,5]; however, background rates in control populations are reported to be as high as 8%[5].

Other bacterial pathogens including *Haemophilus* species, *Streptococcus* species, *Gardnerella vaginalis*, as well as *Staphylococcus saprophyticus*, and *Bacteroides ureolyticus* have been isolated in cases of NGU. There is no clear indication of whether these bacteria are commensal to the urethra or have implications in the pathogenesis of NGU[2].

Viral agents have also been linked to NGU. Certain subtypes of adenovirus have a particular affinity for both the eyes and genital tract. For this reason, many cases of adenovirus-associated NGU present simultaneously with conjunctivitis[4]. Complementing the seasonal pattern of adenovirus, predominance of these cases is noted in the autumn and spring[4]. Men with primary herpes simplex virus (HSV) infection may also have urethritis; however, recurrent HSV episodes have not been associated with NGU[10].

Behavioral patterns play a role in NGU. HSV-1 and adenovirus are isolated more frequently in men who have sex with men (MSM), whereas cases of *C. trachomatis* and *M. genitalium* are associated with heterosexual activity[4].

The remainder of the 20–50% of cases where no pathogen is isolated may be due to bacterial etiologies not yet identified[2]. Noninfectious etiologies are also possible. These can involve immune or chemical-mediated urethritis. Examples include Reiter's syndrome, which presents with sterile urethritis that is thought to be immunologically mediated[2]. Chemical urethritis can also occur secondary to latex exposure from urethral catheters, but data substantiating this are inconclusive[11].

A proportion of these cases will progress to chronic NGU. In both chlamydial and nonchlamydial NGU, the etiology of chronic NGU is uncertain. In the vast majority of cases, no pathogen is isolated[2]. While a difficult clinical entity to treat, complications from chronic NGU, such as urethral stricture and infertility, are uncommon[2].

CLINICAL PRESENTATION

Nongonoccocal urethritis presents with discharge of a mucopurulent, leukocytic exudate (**6.1**)[12]. The patient may experience dysuria or urethral pruritis[12]. In women, sustained endocervical bleeding is easily induced by passing a cotton swab through the cervical os, while men often have penile irritation[5,12]. Not all of these signs need to be present for diagnosis; in fact, the patient may have a completely normal examination[5,12]. Patients with *Chlamydia trachomatis*-related urethritis more commonly remain asymptomatic[12].

LABORATORY STUDIES

Several laboratory studies are employed in identifying urethritis and its associated pathogens. If a discharge is present, samples can be obtained approximately 0.5 cm into the urethra with a 5-mm plastic loop or cotton-tipped swab[5]. No data exist comparing the use of the plastic loop with the cotton-tipped swab[5].

Of the various tests available, Gram stain of the urethral smear is the preferred method of diagnosis due to its ability to diagnose urethritis and to assess for the presence of gram-negative diplococci, indicating infection with *N. gonorrhoeae* (**6.2, 6.3**)[1]. In patients where no overt discharge is present, the first-void morning urine specimen should be obtained and tested for leukocyte esterase followed by centrifugation and Gram stain of the sediment to assess for urethritis and to rule out gonorrhea[1].

A number of variables complicate Gram staining and microscopy in the diagnosis of NGU. They include inconsistency in sampling techniques and preparation of urethral smears, in addition to interobserver and intraobserver subjectivity in reading urethral smears[13]. For the first-void urine specimen, time since last passing urine can also affect results[13]. While Gram staining is widely used for making the diagnosis, owing to inconsistent results its validity has come into question, especially in light of new diagnostic tests available to isolate specific pathogens[7]. Employment of the nucleic acid amplification test (NAAT) has improved both

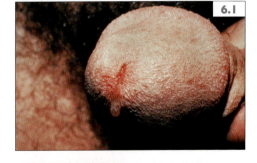

6.1 Nongonococcal urethritis (mucoid discharge). (Courtesy of Seattle STD/HIV Prevention Training Center, University of Washington, Seattle, WA.)

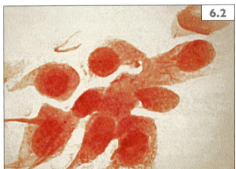

6.2 Normal urethral cells on Gram stain. (Courtesy of Seattle STD/HIV Prevention Training Center, University of Washington, Seattle, WA.)

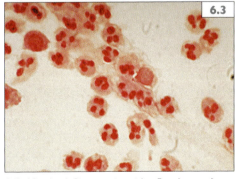

6.3 Urethral Gram stain with >5 polymorpho-nuclear leukocytes per high-power field (nongonococcal urethritis). (Courtesy of Seattle STD/HIV Prevention Training Center, University of Washington, Seattle, WA.)

sensitivity and specificity in the diagnosis of chlamydial NGU. Unfortunately, even this test can miss up to 3% of men with chlamydial NGU[14].

Laboratory studies to identify specific pathogens in nonchlamydial NGU are limited and diagnosis is more challenging. For *T. vaginalis*, a wet mount preparation is the most effective method of detection[2]. *Mycoplasma genitalium* does not grow well in culture. While polymerase chain reaction (PCR) is available in the research setting, it is not available in clinical practice. *Ureaplasma urealyticum* is more easily and cost-effectively cultured, but culture sensitivity is thought to be low[9]. At this time, isolating pathogens associated with nonchlamydial acute NGU is not necessary or recommended in clinical practice, because treatment remains unchanged. In patients with chronic NGU, isolating pathogens, if present, may be of benefit in developing a treatment plan[9].

COURSE, PROGNOSIS, AND COMPLICATIONS

NGU can be eliminated if the patient is compliant with appropriate treatment[15]; however, it is estimated that 20% of patients with chlamydial NGU have recurrent or persistent urethritis. The rate is even higher in cases of nonchlamydial acute NGU, where approximately 30–50% of men will subsequently develop a chronic NGU[2]. Symptoms such as chronic prostatitis, penile and pelvic pain, dysuria, and the development of premature ejaculation after treatment for acute NGU are suggestive of chronic NGU[12].

Reactive arthritis (RA, Reiter's syndrome) can follow chlamydial infection[5]. It is characterized by peripheral arthritis, ocular lesions (conjunctivities, uveitis, or iritis), and urethritis. Diagnostic criteria require arthritis of longer than 1 month duration and aseptic joint aspiration. RA can result from STI or after gastrointestinal infection, most commonly secondary to *Shigella*, *Salmonella*, *Yersinia*, and *Campylobacter* infection.

C. trachomatis is the pathogen most commonly associated with NGU. Alone, the bacterium accounts for 16–44% of cases of RA[16]. Many episodes of RA, found in patients with gonococcal urethritis, are thought to result from concomitant and unidentified *C. trachomatis* infection. *M. genitalium* is hypothesized to account for a small percentage of RA cases, but the association is not as well established. Almost all cases of RA due to STIs occur in men; only 10% of postgastroenteritis forms occur in women[16].

Two important dermatologic manifestions of RA are keratoderma blennorrhagicum and balanitis circinata[16]. The former, occurring in 10–25% of RA patients, presents with papulosquamous lesions primarily on the palms and soles which can progress to psoriasiform plaques (**6.4, 6.5**)[16]. Balanitis circinata is an inflammatory lesion on the glans or shaft of the penis that occurs in up to 69% of men with RA (**6.6**)[16]. The lesions are erythematous with shallow, somewhat circular and slightly raised, gray-white borders in circumcised men[16,17]. In uncircumcised men, they present as dry, hyperkeratotic plaques that resemble psoriasis[16]. HLA-B27 is strongly associated with both balanitis circinata and RA, suggesting that balanitis circinata may represent an early form of RA, even when presenting alone[16,17].

Because the urethral endothelial lining is a protective barrier, men with urethritis, or inflammation of the lining, have increased susceptibility to infection with human immunodeficiency virus (HIV) and a greater tendency to shed HIV if already infected[5]. Epididymo-orchitis, with impaired fertility in men, and chronic prostatitis have also been reported[5].

In women, some organisms causing NGU, such as *C. trachomatis, M. genitalium, M. hominis*, and *Gardnerella vaginalis* may cause pelvic inflammatory disease, which may lead to infertility and/or ectopic pregnancy. Pregnant women who are infected may have premature delivery and/or postpartum infection[15].

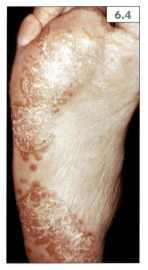

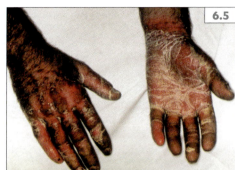

6.4 Keratoderma blennorrhagicum. (Courtesy of Dr. Jeffrey Callen, Louisville, KY.)

6.5 Psoriasiform changes in reactive arthritis. (Courtesy of Dr. Jeffrey Callen, Louisville, KY.)

6.6 Reactive arthritis: balanitis circinata. (Courtesy of Dr. Jeffrey Callen, Louisville, KY.)

DIAGNOSIS

Nongonococcal urethritis is a diagnosis of exclusion; it includes men with urethritis, asymptomatic or symptomatic, and an absence of gram-negative diplococci on Gram stain or a negative culture.

The diagnosis of urethritis is confirmed microscopically by detection of white blood cells (WBCs) on the Gram stain of urethral secretions taken from the anterior urethra[1]. Diagnosis involves evidence of at least one of the following: 1) mucopurulent or purulent discharge (**6.1**); 2) Gram stain of urethral smear demonstrating ≥5 WBCs per high-power field (**6.2**, **6.3**); 3) first-void urine specimen testing positive for leukocyte esterase test or microscopic examination of first-void urine sediment Gram stain demonstrating ≥10 WBCs per high-power field[1]. Detection of WBCs per high power (×1000) field is averaged over five fields with the greatest concentration of WBCs[5].

The USA Centers for Disease Control and Prevention (CDC) also recommends that if the patient does not meet the above criteria and is symptomatic, testing via NAAT for *N. gonorrhoeae* and *C. trachomatis* should be undertaken[1].

Gram stain of urethral smear is subject to interpretation error. Error in diagnosis correlates to the grade of urethritis, with a greater proportion of cases with low-grade urethritis diagnosed, falsely, as negative. The current diagnostic criterion, necessitating

≥5 WBCs, lowers overall sensitivity, because nearly one-third of men with *C. trachomatis* or *M. genitalium* NGU will demonstrate fewer than five WBCs on urethral smear[8]. Gram stain is more sensitive when an overt discharge is present; for these reasons, the use of microscopy in patients who are asymptomatic or present without discharge remains controversial[8]. Chronic NGU should be confirmed by microscopy with the same criteria used for acute NGU[2].

TREATMENT

The CDC treatment recommendations are presented in *Table 6.1*. For acute NGU, single dose regimens are recommended to improve compliance[12]. Also, to minimize transmission, intercourse should not be resumed until 7 days after completion of a treatment regimen and until all sexual partners have been treated[12]. Prevention of future infection involves testing and treatment of all sex partners encountered in the previous 60 days[12].

For recurrent and persistent infection, the CDC recommends treatment with the original antibiotic regimen if the patient did not receive the full course or if they sustained a repeated exposure to an untreated sex partner. If the patient completed the initial antibiotic regimen and no repeated exposures were present, they can be treated with one of the following: metronidazole, 2 g orally in a single dose or tinidazole, 2 g orally in a single dose. Azithromycin, 1 g orally in a single dose, should be added in combination if the antibiotic was not used as part of the initial treatment regimen.

Table 6.1 USA Centers for Disease Control and Prevention recommended regimens for the treatment of nongonococcal urethritis

Azithromycin, 1 g, in a single dose
OR
Doxycycline, 100 mg orally, twice a day for 7 days

Alternative regimens
Erythromycin base, 500 mg orally, four times a day for 7 days
OR
Erythromycin ethylsuccinate, 800 mg orally, four times a day for 7 days
OR
Levofloxacin, 500 mg orally, once daily for 7 days
OR
Ofloxacin, 300 mg orally, twice a day for 7 days

CHAPTER 7

Genital Herpes

**Radhika Nakrani, BS, Olubukola Babalola, BS, and
Jane M. Grant-Kels, MD**

DEFINITION

Genital herpes is a chronic recurring sexually
transmitted infection of the genital region
caused by the herpes simplex virus (HSV).
It is among the most common sexually
transmitted diseases, affecting both men and
women.

Clinical manifestations include pain,
itching, and one or more vesicles, although
many patients may even be unaware of the
infection. Synonyms include herpes genitalis,
herpes progenitalis, and genital herpes
simplex.

ETIOLOGY

HSVs are double stranded human
deoxyribonucleic acid (DNA) viruses that
intermittently reactivate[1]. There are two
types of HSV known to cause genital herpes:
HSV-1 and HSV-2.

Inoculation of the virus at susceptible
sites results in lesions of the epidermis
with occasional involvement of adnexal
epithelium. Often, lesions involve mucosal
surfaces (**7.1**). The virus can then spread to
the nervous system and establish latency in
neurons[1].

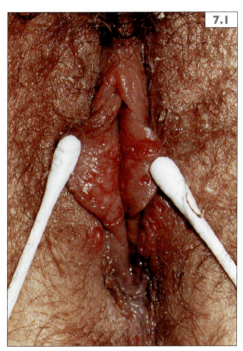

7.1 Genital herpes in a woman. (Courtesy of
Dr. Tomasz F. Mroczkowski.)

The majority of genital herpes cases are associated with HSV-2. HSV-2 is predominantly responsible for causing perigenital infections, affecting more than 50 million people in the USA[2]. More often, HSV-2 is associated with sexual transmission[2].

HSV-1 has traditionally been associated with oropharyngeal infections; however, recently HSV-1 is becoming increasingly common in genital infections, especially seen in college students, heterosexual women, and young men who have sex with men (MSM)[3,4]. Typically, HSV-1 is associated with childhood transmission and nonsexual skin-to-skin contact, most commonly involving the mouth and lips, and from contact sports[2].

Both types are capable of causing either genital or oropharyngeal infection and can produce mucosal lesions that are clinically indistinguishable[5].

Transmission of the virus is most common when patients are asymptomatic (i.e. subclinical reactivation and shedding of the virus in the genital tract)[1]. Reactivation of genital infections is 16 times more frequent with HSV-2 than HSV-1. The average recurrence is 3–4 times per year, but it is possible for the infection to reappear more frequently[1]. Shedding is also more frequent with HSV-2 than HSV-1 and is estimated to be responsible for 70% of the transmission of HSV-2[6]. For patients with a prior HSV-1 infection, acquisition of HSV-2 is common, while acquisition of HSV-1 by patients with prior HSV-2 is unusual[1]. Characteristics of HSV-1 and HSV-2 infection are presented in *Table 7.1*.

Table 7.1 Characteristics of herpes simplex (HSV)-1 and HSV-2 infection

	HSV-1	HSV-2
Site of infection	Skin above the waist	Skin below the waist
Site of latency	Trigeminal ganglia	Sacral ganglia
Age of primary infection	Children	Young adults
Transmission	Skin-to-skin contact, saliva	Sexual
Risk of acquiring HIV		Increased

HIV: human immunodeficiency virus.

EPIDEMIOLOGY

Serologic methods identifying the presence of HSV-2 antibodies have been the best way of studying the epidemiology of HSV-2[5]. In the most recent study of populations, 2005–2008, seroprevalence of HSV-2 among participants aged 14–49 years was 16.2%[7]. The prevalence of HSV-2 in women was almost double that of men (20.9% compared to 11.5%)[7] (**7.2**). In non-Hispanic blacks, the prevalence was triple that of non-Hispanic whites (39.2% compared to 12.3%)[7] (**7.3**). Seroprevalence of coinfection with HSV-1 and HSV-2 is 10.5%[5].

With adulthood, the overall prevalence rises rapidly in younger age groups and remains stable among people older than 30 years[5]. Prevalence is higher among persons who are divorced, separated, or widowed; those living below the poverty level; those who have ever used cocaine; those who have sex for the first time at the age of 17 years or younger; and those who have a larger number of lifetime sexual partners[2,5].

Geographically, the prevalence of genital herpes is highest in areas of Africa and parts of the Americas, and lowest in Asia[8].

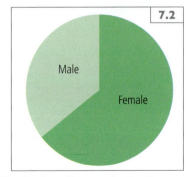

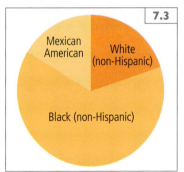

7.2, 7.3 Distribution of herpes simplex-2 seropositivity in USA by sex (left) and race (right). (Adapted from: Centers for Disease Control and Prevention [2010]. Seroprevalence of herpes simplex virus type 2 among persons aged 14–49 years, USA, 2005–2008. *MMWR* **59**:456–9.)

CLINICAL PRESENTATION

There are various stages of presentation for genital herpes.

Primary first episode

This pertains to an individual with no previous history of HSV infection who becomes infected. This phase may escape notice in healthy individuals[9]. Following infection, the virus incubates for a period of time ranging from 1 to 20 days, with an average of 4–6 days[8,9].

After incubating, a small macule or papule appears, rapidly progressing to a vesicle in 1 day[9]. Lesions may then progress to grouped vesicles (**7.4, 7.5**), pustules (**7.6**), or painful erythematous ulcers (**7.7**).

Typically, bilateral 'kissing' lesions of the external genitalia are observed; however, lesions may be anywhere in the perigenital, perianal, buttocks (**7.8**), or thigh region[10,11]. Pain, dysuria, vaginal and urethral discharge, pruritis, pelvic tenderness, and lymphadenopathy present locally[8,9].

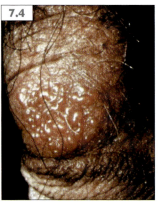

7.4 Clustered herpes simplex virus vesicles on the penile shaft.

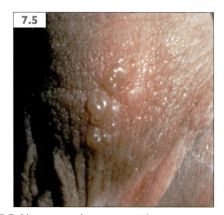

7.5 Herpes simplex virus vesicles.

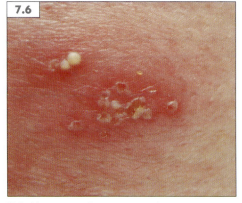

7.6 Herpes simplex virus pustules.

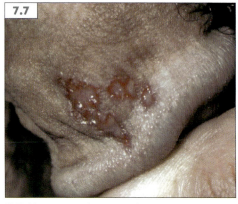

7.7 Herpes simplex virus ulcerations.

Occasionally, HSV genital tract disease is manifested by endometritis and salpingitis in women and by prostatitis in men[10]. About 15% of cases of acquired HSV-2 are associated with nonlesional clinical syndromes, such as aseptic meningitis, cervicitis, urethritis, and pharyngitis[10]. Atypical lesions can simulate fissures, furuncles, patchy erythema, linear ulcerations, or excoriations. These might be attributed to other causes such as candidal vaginitis or trauma from intercourse[11].

Constitutionally, fever, headache, malaise, and myalgia may appear within the first few days of appearance of lesions. Approximately two-thirds of women and 40% of men present with these symptoms during a clinically apparent first episode[12]. The presentation of symptoms is varied, with some being unaware of the infection and others requiring hospital stay[8].

Nonprimary first episode

This refers to infection in persons with a previous HSV-1 or HSV-2 infection. This tends to be less severe due to previous immunologic stimulation with antibody build-up, and may be mistaken for a recurrent episode[9].

Recurrent episode

This stage involves old infections presenting with new symptoms and signs, typically due to HSV-2[8].

Within 12 months after diagnosis, 90% of patients with a documented first episode of genital HSV-2 infection have at least one recurrence (**7.9**), 38% have six or more recurrences, and 20% have 10 or more recurrences[12]. Recurrent episodes tend to localize to the glans penis or penile shaft in men, the labia or vaginal introitus in women, and the anal area and buttocks in both men and women[9]. Itching, burning, fissure, irritation, and redness may precede vesicular eruption[8].

Approximately one-half of patients who recognize recurrences have prodromal symptoms, ranging from mild tingling sensations occurring 30 minutes to 48 hours before the eruption to shooting pains in the buttocks, legs, or hips occurring as long as 5 days before the eruption. Prodromal symptoms include itching, paresthesias, and pain around the lumbosacral dermatomes[11,12].

The duration of viral shedding is shorter in recurrences than in primary infection (4 days *vs*. 11 days). There are fewer lesions present (six lesions *vs*. 16 lesions), and lesions present more unilaterally[12].

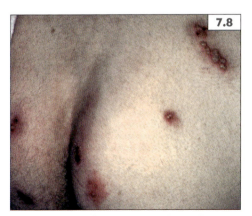

7.8 Herpes simplex virus on the buttocks.

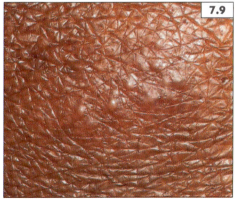

7.9 First stage of early recurrent infection with herpes simplex virus.

Subclinical shedding

This stage tends to appear within the first year of infection[9]. Despite the lack of any observable lesions, the virus can be transmitted to others[9]. Over time, the frequency of shedding tends to decrease[9].

LABORATORY STUDIES/ HISTOPATHOLOGY

A clinical diagnosis of genital herpes is confirmed by laboratory studies.

Viral culture is a widely available gold standard. This allows for definitive diagnosis and differentiation between HSV-1 and HSV-2 infections. The sensitivity depends on the stage of the episode. Viral culture is best used when lesions are still intact and nonulcerated. About 95% of vesicular lesions will grow HSV, as compared with 70% percent of ulcerative lesions and 30% of crusted lesions[12]. Viral culture results in the isolation of the virus within approximately 5 days. A negative culture does not negate HSV infection[9].

Polymerase chain reaction (PCR) is up to four times more sensitive than viral culture. PCR can be used to detect the DNA sequence of the HSV through molecular amplification[9,13]. DNA can be detected during periods of subclinical shedding, or from cerebrospinal fluid (CSF) (eliminating the need for brain biopsy in serious cases)[12]. PCR is more expensive and not routinely used, though it is emerging as a new gold standard.

Serologic testing can be used to detect HSV infection in the absence of lesions or with negative virus detection tests. It can also be used to screen patients with risk factors for HSV[12]. Type-specific immunoglobulin testing can distinguish HSV-1 from HSV-2 by detecting antibodies to glycoprotein 1 and 2 (G1 and G2) and is useful in differentiating past infections[12,13]. Two type specific antibody assays available include HerpeSelect HSV-1 and HSV-2 enzyme-linked immunosorbent assays and HSV-1 and HSV-2 immunoblot tests (FocusTechnologies)[12]. In patients with recurrent genital symptoms, atypical lesions, or healing lesions and negative HSV cultures, this testing can help confirm a clinical diagnosis[12].

Antigen detection direct fluorescence allows specific monoclonal antibodies to be used to detect and distinguish HSV antigens on a smear from the lesion[13].

Tzanck smear involves scraping of the base of the lesion to obtain vesicular fluid, which is then thinly smeared on a slide and stained with Giemsa or Wright stain (**7.10**). A positive result is marked by the presence of multinucleated giant acantholytic keratinocytes[13]. Although, on occasion, this test can be insensitive, when positive it is helpful as it immediately establishes the diagnosis.

Dermatopathology (**7.11–7.13**) examination reveals multinucleated giant keratinocytes, multilocular intraepidermal vesicles due to ballooning and reticular epidermal degeneration, acantholytic keratinocytes with steel-gray nuclei and margination of the peripheral nucleoplasm, and intranuclear inclusion bodies[13].

HSV enters the body through skin or mucosal surfaces and initiates cytolytic replication in local epithelial cells. These virions are seen histologically as intranuclear inclusions[10]. HSV also induces cells to fuse and form multinucleated giant cells[10]. Cell damage in the skin causes epithelial cells to detach (acantholysis) and form fluid-filled blisters containing cellular debris, inflammatory cells, (multinucleated) acantholytic keratinocytes, and progeny virions[10].

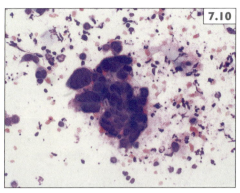

7.10 Positive Tzanck smear with a Giemsa stain (×400), showing an acantholytic multinucleated giant cell.

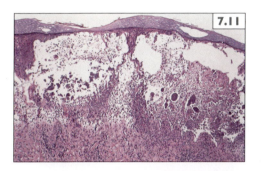

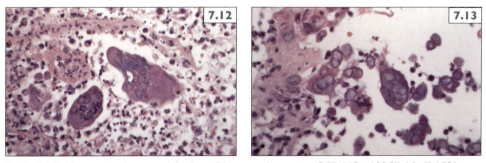

7.11–7.13 Herpes simplex virus histology. (Hematoxylin-eosin, ×5 [**7.11**]; ×100 [**7.12, 7.13**].)

COURSE, PROGNOSIS, AND COMPLICATIONS

After primary infection, the viral genome resides indefinitely in a latent state in neurons. Periodic reactivation follows, resulting in symptomatic or asymptomatic infection[12]. Most incidents are asymptomatic[8].

About 70–90% of people with symptomatic HSV-2, and 20–50% with symptomatic genital HSV-1 will have a recurrence within the first year[9]. As lesions progress, skin ulcers crust, whereas lesions in the mucous membranes heal without crusting[12] (**7.14**). Genital herpes tends to resolve and is rarely life-threatening, if the patient has a normal immune system[9]. The frequency of recurrent outbreaks is variable and tends to decline over time[9].

Initiating treatment following the first episode suppresses other sequelae of HSV infection. Episodic therapy is most effective when started immediately upon the earliest sign of outbreak[9].

Chronic antiviral medication utilization does not fully eliminate viral shedding, but does help with acute symptoms and speed of recovery. The daily use of treatment improves clinical outcome. Antiviral treatment is safe and well-tolerated[8,9].

Central nervous system (CNS) complications of genital herpes include aseptic meningitis (most frequent), sacral radiculopathy, transverse myelitis, and benign recurrent lymphocytic meningitis[12]. Meningeal signs occur more frequently in women. Approximately one-third of women and 1 in 10 men with primary infection have meningeal signs[12].

Other complications include extragenital lesions, and autonomic dysfunction including urinary retention that might require catheterization[11]. Although infre-quent, encephalitis and blindness can be complications of HSV-1 infection. Erythema multiforme may occur simultaneously or within 3–14 days following an outbreak[8] (**7.15**).

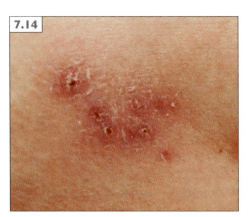

7.14 Crusted older lesions of herpes simplex virus.

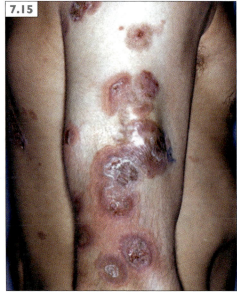

7.15 Erythema multiforme secondary to genital herpes.

Eczema herpeticum is a widely disseminated HSV eruption that is rare. It is most commonly seen in patients with atopic dermatitis, burns, pemphigus, ichthyosis vulgaris, Darier disease, and extensive mycosis fungoides or Sezary's syndrome (**7.16, 7.17**).

There is an increased risk of human immunodeficiency virus (HIV) associated with genital herpes, because lesions provide an avenue for transmission. Patients with HSV-2 have an increased risk of acquiring HIV by at least twofold[2,7]. Patients who are coinfected with HSV and HIV are noted to have more severe outbreaks of HSV.

Maternal–fetal transmission of genital herpes can occur during vaginal delivery and is associated with significant morbidity and mortality. Neonatal HSV can manifest as cutaneous, CNS, or disseminated multiple organ disease. The highest risk of transmission to a neonate is in women who develop primary infection during their third trimester. Cesarean delivery may be recommended[11].

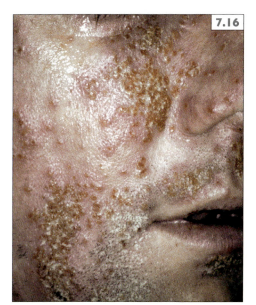
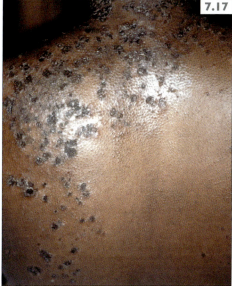

7.16, 7.17 Eczema herpeticum of the face (**7.16**) and back (**7.17**).

DIAGNOSIS

Approaches to the diagnosis of HSV are presented in *Table 7.2*.

The differential diagnosis is presented in *Table 7.3*.

TREATMENT

While HSV cannot be cured, antiviral medications can shorten the course, diminish symptoms associated with acute outbreaks, and reduce the risk of transmission to partners[7]. After antiviral drugs are discontinued, they no longer have

Table 7.2 Herpes simplex virus (HSV) diagnostic approaches

	Culture, PCR, or antigen detection for HSV-2	Type-specific HSV-2 IgG antibody	Type-specific HSV-1 IgG antibody	Interpretation
First assessment of lesion	(+)	(−)	(+)/(−)	Acute HSV-2
	(+)	(+)	(+)/(−)	Recurrent HSV-2
No lesions	n/a	(−)	(−)	At risk for HSV-1 or HSV-2 infection
	n/a	(−)	(+)	At risk for HSV-2
	n/a	(+)	(+)	HSV-1 and HSV-2 infection
Recurrent genital lesions	(+)	(+)	(+)/(−)	Recurrent HSV-2
	(−)	(+)	(−)	Recurrent HSV-2, consider alternative cause

Ig: immunoglobulin; PCR: polymerase chain reaction. (Adapted from Gupta *et al*., [2007]. *Lancet* **370**:2127–37[11].)

Table 7.3 Differential diagnosis of genital herpes

- Trauma
- Primary syphilis, chancre (*Treponema pallidum*)
- Chancroid (*Haemophilus ducreyi*)
- Lymphogranuloma venereum
- Donovanosis/granuloma inguinale *(Klebsiella granulomatis)*
- Gonococcal erosion
- Candidiasis
- Fixed-drug eruption
- Contact dermatitis
- Aphthous ulcers
- Lichen planus (bullous or erosive type)
- Crohn's disease

an effect on the risk, frequency, or severity of recurrences[14]. Resistance is rare in patients who are not immunocompromised. The concomitant use of topical therapy with antiviral drugs is discouraged and offers minimal clinical benefit[14].

During the first clinical episode, all patients should receive antiviral therapy (*Table 7.4*).

For recurrent episodes, suppressive therapy can be used to reduce the frequency of outbreaks by up to 80% (*Table 7.5*). For recurrent episodes, episodic therapy can

Table 7.4 Recommended regimens for the treatment of first clinical episode of herpes simplex virus infection

Acyclovir	400 mg orally	3 times a day	7–10 days
OR			
Acyclovir	200 mg orally	5 times a day	7–10 days
OR			
Famciclovir	250 mg orally	3 times a day	7–10 days
OR			
Valacyclovir	1 g orally	2 times a day	7–10 days

Treatment can be extended if healing is incomplete after 10 days therapy

(Adapted from CDC [2010]. *MMWR Recomm Rep* **59**(RR-12):1–110[14].)

Table 7.5 Recommended regimens for the treatment of recurrent episodes of herpes simplex infection

Acyclovir	400 mg orally	2 times a day
OR		
Famciclovir	250 mg orally	2 times a day
OR		
Valacyclovir	500 mg orally*	1 time a day
OR		
Valacyclovir	1 g orally	1 time a day

* Valacyclovir 500 mg once a day might be less effective than other valacyclovir or acyclovir dosing regimens in patients who have very frequent recurrences (i.e. ≥10 episodes per year)

(Adapted from CDC [2010]. *MMWR Recomm Rep* **59**(RR-12):1–110[14].)

be initiated within the first day of outbreak or during the prodrome that precedes some outbreaks. Patients should be given a supply or prescription for the medication with instructions to commence treatment when symptoms appear (*Table 7.6*).

For severe disease, intravenous (IV) acyclovir therapy should be given. The recommendation is acyclovir 5–10 mg/kg IV every 8 hours for 2–7 days or until clinical improvement is noted, followed by oral antiviral therapy to complete at least 10 days of total therapy. The dose can be adjusted in individuals with renal impairment[14].

In addition to antiviral medications, counseling can be provided to address the psychological impact of infection on the patient and/or partner. Patients should also be counseled with regard to the natural history of genital herpes and ways to minimize transmission. These include modification of sexual practices to reduce risk of transmission, disclosure of infection to partners, abstinence during outbreaks, and correct condom use.

Table 7.6 Recommended regimens for the episodic treatment of recurrent episodes of herpes simplex infection

Acyclovir	400 mg orally	3 times a day	5 days
OR			
Acyclovir	800 mg orally	2 times a day	5 days
OR			
Acyclovir	800 mg orally	3 times a day	2 days
OR			
Famciclovir	125 mg orally	2 times a day	5 days
OR			
Famciclovir	1 g orally	2 times a day	1 day
OR			
Famciclovir	500 mg orally	1 time a day	1 day
	Then:	2 times a day	2 days
	250 mg orally		
OR			
Valacyclovir	500 mg orally	2 times a day	3 days
OR			
Valacyclovir	1 g orally	1 time a day	5 days
OR			
Valacyclovir	2 g orally	2 times a day	1 day

(Adapted from CDC [2010]. *MMWR Recomm Rep* **59**(RR-12):1–110[14].)

CHAPTER 8

Genital Warts

Bobby Y. Reddy, MS, MD, and W. Clark Lambert, MD, PhD

DEFINITION

Genital warts is a disease of the skin and mucous membranes, caused by the human papillomavirus (HPV). The disease is mainly sexually transmitted; however, direct skin contact or autoinoculation can also be the cause of infection. It is highly contagious, occurring mainly among young sexually active individuals. The estimated incidence in the USA alone, is 1 million cases annually[1].

Synonyms for genital warts are: condylomata acuminata, venereal warts, and venereal vegetations.

ETIOLOGY AND EPIDEMIOLOGY

Genital warts are the most common observable manifestation of HPV infection[2]. They are present in approximately 1% of the sexually active population, with 90% of cases attributable to HPV types 6 and 11[2]. Infection with other types of HPV (16, 18, 33, 34, 42, 54, and 55) is also possible but is less common. The primary route of HPV infection is through sexual intercourse, either vaginal or anal, but sexual intercourse is not necessary for transmission, as infection only requires a period of skin to skin contact[3]. HPV remains one of the most common sexually transmitted infection, with approximately 5.5 million new infections worldwide, annually[4]. The infection often occurs within 2–10 years of initial sexual exposure, with a peak prevalence of infection between the ages of 20 and 24 years in women and between the ages of 25 and 29 in men[2,4]. Although the use of a male condom prevents HPV transmission, it does not confer full protection. A recent study indicated that regular and consistent condom use results in only a 70% reduction in HPV infection[5]. Factors enhancing the risk of transmission are predominantly related to sexual behavior, such as an early age for first coitus, the number of current sexual partners, and the total number of lifetime partners; however, other known risk factors include belonging to a non-Hispanic black race, having a lower socioeconomic status, and achieving only a lower education level[6,7].

NATURAL HISTORY

Genital warts result from HPV infection of basal keratinocytes. Studies demonstrate that infection is dependent upon microabrasion of the genital epithelium, in a manner which results in epithelial denudation but preservation of the epithelial basement membrane[3]. HPV initially binds to the exposed basement membrane before infiltrating keratinocytes, which most likely occurs as keratinocytes migrate to the basement membrane to re-epithelialize a wound[3]. Most HPV infections are subclinical; however, the virus can also replicate within actively dividing keratinocytes, ultimately

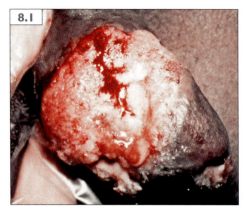

8.1 Condylomata acuminata on the glans penis.

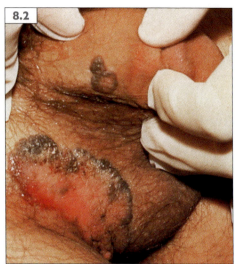

8.2 Condylomata acuminata.

manifesting as exophytic clinical lesions known as genital warts. The typical incubation period is 3 weeks to 8 months, with most warts appearing approximately 2–3 months after HPV infection[1]. Warts are highly contagious and an estimated 65% of noninfected individuals who engage in sexual intercourse with an infected partner will develop warts[1]. Approximately 20–30% of genital warts will spontaneously regress, but relapse of lesions is common[1].

CLINICAL PRESENTATION

Genital warts may present internally or externally. Large internal warts may produce severe obstructive symptoms, such as painful sexual intercourse, urinary retention, and rectal pain[2]. External warts can present on the penis, scrotum, and anus in men, and the vulva, vagina, anus, and the cervix in women. In both sexes, immunosuppression (medical or acquired immunodeficiency syndrome [AIDS] associated) results in widespread and more numerous lesions.

Penile warts

The most common type of penile wart is the condyloma acuminatum, an exophytic wart caused by HPV-6 and -11. The wart(s) usually occur(s) on the surfaces subject to trauma: the penile corona, the glans, the frenulum, and the inner aspect of the prepuce (**8.1, 8.2**). They may appear in the urethral meatus, on the scrotum, or in the groin (**8.3, 8.4**). The individual warts are usually soft, gray or pinkish in color. They can be elongated, filiform, or pedunculated, solitary or multiple. Initially small, they may grow and coalesce, forming 'cauliflower-like' lesions (**8.5, 8.6**). The other common type of wart found on the penis is small, discrete, flat warts, frequently present on the shaft of the penis. These could be either the only warts present or associated with typical condylomata on the glans. Subclinical HPV infection on the penis is not uncommon and it can be revealed by application of 5% acetic acid. It is of particular importance due to the possibility of unwitting infection of a sex partner.

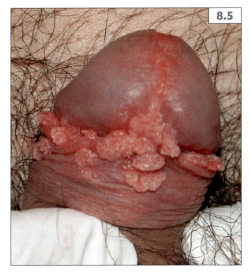

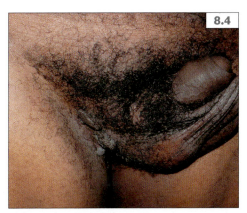

8.3 Confluent condylomata acuminata on the skin of the upper inner aspect of the thigh.

8.4 Warts in the groin.

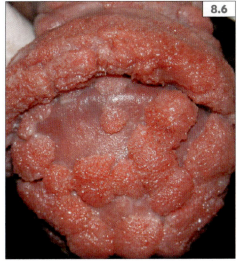

8.5, 8.6 Warts on the penis. (Courtesy of Dr. Tomasz F. Mroczkowski.)

Anal warts

Anal warts occur more often in men than in women. They are even more common in men who have sex with men (MSM) and engage in anal-receptive intercourse (**8.7**). Due to the warmth, moisture, and mechanical friction, these warts usually become large (**8.8**) and may be secondarily infected. Anal warts may extend into the anal canal, requiring anoscopy for their identification. Both anal and anorectal warts often assume a cauliflower-like appearance.

Vulval and vaginal warts

The predilection site of anogenital warts in women is the vulva and, in particular, the posterior commissure. They may also involve the skin of the labia and the perineum, as well as the vaginal, urethral, and anal mucosae, plus the cervix. Condylomata acuminata in women usually start as small soft verrucous papules which at times may coalesce to give an almost velvety appearance over large areas, forming a cock's comb-like excrescense (**8.9**). Between the labia majora and minora and the introitus, the warts may form small warty or fleshy streaks. In rare instances, the warts may develop into sessile, grape-like masses that completely mask the vulva. In pregnant women, genital warts may grow rapidly and become severe, with enlargement and maceration, prone to secondary infection. As in men, grossly inapparent warts may appear on the vulva or in the vaginal wall. They can be visualized by application of 5% acetic acid and are best seen by colposcopy.

Cervical warts

Condylomatous lesions on the cervix may present as typical exophytic papillary condylomata acuminata or flat warts. The latter are macroscopically invisible and can be visualized by application of 5% acetic acid and colposcopy. The flat warts on the cervix are frequently indistinguishable from cervical intraepithelial neoplasia and may escape detection by colposcopy, thus necessitating the use of biopsy and cytology in the diagnosis.

Fabry–Buschke–Lowenstein tumor

Fabry–Buschke–Lowenstein (FBL) tumors are rare giant condylomata. Based on their clinical appearance and histologic features, they have been called 'carcinoma-like condylomata' or 'condylomata-like carcinomas'. FBL tumors have a fungating or malignant gross appearance, and they differ from typical condylomata by their deep penetration and compression of adjacent tissues. Despite 'malignant' morphology, they are histologically benign[1] and never metastasize. FBL tumors may appear on the penis, vulva, scrotum, anus, and in the inguinal areas (**8.10**). They are generally associated with HPV-6 and HPV-11 infection.

All genital warts regardless of location may also be accompanied by pruritus, burning, tenderness, discharge, or even bleeding[4]. Although warts are benign and have no association with mortality, they may serve as a source of significant psychological distress, which can negatively influence sexual relations.

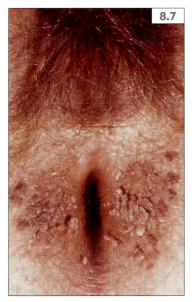

8.7 Anal warts.

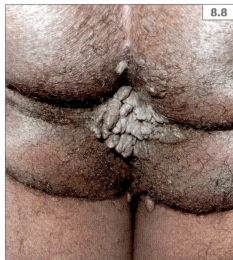

8.8 Large anal warts.

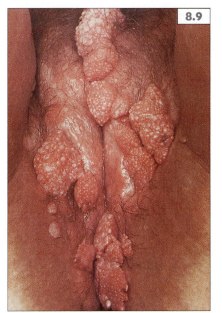

8.9 Cock's comb-like warts in a woman. (Courtesy of Dr. Tomasz F. Mroczkowski.)

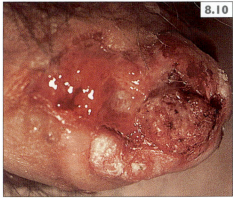

8.10 Fabry–Buschke–Lowenstein tumor on the penis. (Courtesy of Dr. Tomasz F. Mroczkowski.)

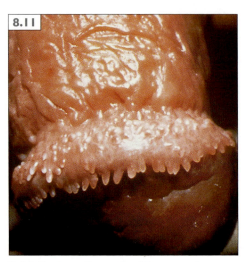

8.11 Pearly penile papules. (Courtesy of Dr. Tomasz F. Mroczkowski.)

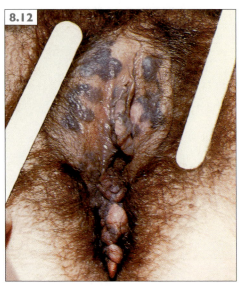

8.12 Bowenoid papulosis of the vulva. (Courtesy of Dr. Tomasz F. Mroczkowski.)

DIAGNOSIS AND DIFFERENTIAL DIAGNOSIS

There are no currently widely-accepted screening methods for detecting genital warts. The diagnosis of genital warts is established through a careful examination of the genitalia for characteristic clinical features. The use of a magnifying glass or colposcope may be helpful. All patients suspected of having anal warts should undergo anoscopy to determine the presence of warts in the anal canal[8]. The application of 5% acetic acid produces a whitish discoloration after several minutes; however, this test is nonspecific and may be positive in other skin diseases (e.g. candidiasis, lichen planus, microtrauma, and psoriasis)[8].

The differential diagnosis for genital warts includes, but is not limited to, condylomata lata (secondary syphilis), seborrheic keratoses, microglandular hyperplasia, nevi, pearly penile papules (**8.11**), skin tags, molluscum contagiosum, genital herpes, lichen planus, fibromas, and precancerous or cancerous lesions, such as bowenoid papulosis (**8.12**), malignant melanoma, and squamous cell carcinoma (**8.13**).

Anal warts should be distinguished from carcinoma and hemorrhoids, whereas cervical lesions should be separated from intraepithelial dysplasia.

LABORATORY STUDIES (HISTOPATHOLOGY)

A biopsy is warranted if the diagnosis remains uncertain or if lesions have an atypical appearance, in the form of pigmentation, ulceration, or induration[8]. Biopsies should also be obtained if the patient is immunocompromised, if there is a suspicion of neoplasia, or if lesions are resistant to treatment. The histopathology of typical condyloma acuminatum in the early stage shows disk-like thickening of the epithelium

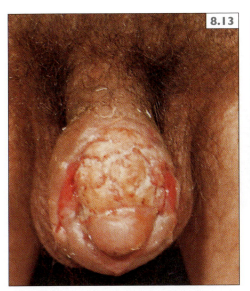

8.13 Squamous cell carcinoma of the penis. (Courtesy of Dr. Tomasz F. Mroczkowski.)

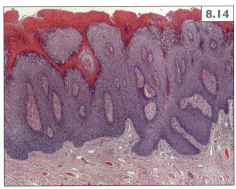

8.14 Condyloma acuminatum. The papillae are enlarged with rounded tops, with prominent koilicytic changes and halos surrounding hyperchromatic nuclei. This is in contrast with the sharply pointed papillae often seen in verrucae vulgares and the flat, ulcerated surfaces characteristic of 'condylomata lata' seen in syphilis (H&E, ×86).

above a flattened area of papillary dermis with dilated capillaries. The fully developed condyloma acuminatum reveals extreme acanthosis and papillomatosis. The most characteristic feature, however, is koilocytic atypia with enlarged cells, perinuclear vacuolization (halos), and hyperchromatic nuclei[4] (**8.14**).

TREATMENT
Treatment is not recommended for subclinical HPV infections. Also, treatment of warts does not cure HPV infection or decrease infectivity, because latent virus activation in adjacent areas of normal skin will result in recurrence[8]; hence, patient education is an important aspect of treatment. The primary objective of treatment is to remove visible and symptomatic genital warts. No conclusive evidence exists to suggest that any of the available treatment modalities are superior to any another. The 2010 USA Centers for Disease Control and Prevention (CDC) sexually transmitted disease guidelines recommend that treatment should be based on patient preference and factors such as size of lesion, morphology, anatomic site, treatment costs, and adverse effects of treatment[4].

The two main types of topically applied treatment are immunomodulators and cytotoxic agents. Immunomodulators include imiquimod and alpha interferon. Imiquimod possesses no direct antiviral activity; rather, its effectiveness lies in stimulation of immune response-modifying cytokines, such as alpha interferon, tumor necrosis factor, and interleukins 1, 6, and 8[8]. Imiquimod treatment results in a 50% clearance rate and is accompanied by a 10–20% recurrence rate[8]. Alpha interferon has direct antiviral activity and demonstrates a 20–60% clearance rate, with a 20–40% recurrence rate[8]. More recently, additional immunomodulators in

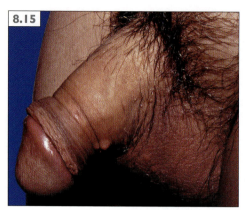

8.15 Warts on the skin of penis and in the groin (after treatment with trichloroacetic acid).

this category have been introduced but have not been evaluated for use in the genital area as of this writing.

Cytotoxic topical medications for genital warts include: podofilox, podophyllin, and 5-fluorouracil. Podophyllin, an antimitotic agent which requires physician application, is contraindicated during pregnancy and is not recommended for the treatment of warts in the vagina, urethra, perianal area, or cervix[9]. Keratolytic topical acids, such as trichloroacetic acid (**8.15**) and bichloroacetic acid, may also be used for the treatment of genital warts and are considered safe during pregnancy. Surgical options include cryotherapy, excision, curettage and electrodesiccation, and laser vaporization. Cryotherapy is often a first-line treatment for anal warts with excellent response rates and few adverse effects[8].

PREVENTION

Although there is currently no cure for genital warts, a USA Food and Drug Administration (FDA)-approved quadrivalent vaccine (Gardasil) has been shown to be a safe and effective method of preventing infection from HPV types 6, 11, 16, and 18, which would subsequently prevent most cases of genital warts[10]. This vaccine consists of noninfectious virus-like particles, which stimulate a potent immune response to the L1 capsid of HPV[10]. Currently, the vaccine is only approved in the USA for girls and women aged 9–26 and is given in three doses, with the second and third doses administered 2–6 months after the initial dose. In the UK, HPV vaccine against HPV types 16 and 18 (Cervarix) is given to girls at age 12–13. Because both men and women are carriers of HPV and have significant roles in its transmission, controversy remains on the issue of vaccinating boys and men. Preliminary data from Australia demonstrate that vaccination of girls and women leads to a reduction in the occurrence of genital warts in boys and men, suggesting that herd immunity occurs with vaccination[11]. Ongoing research is aimed at further determining the efficacy of vaccinating young men.

Molluscum Contagiosum

Freda Sansaricq, MD, and Vesna Petronic-Rosic, MD, MSc

DEFINITION

Molluscum contagiosum (MC) is a common viral infection that affects the skin and mucous membranes. Found to have higher incidences in tropical climates within developing countries, the disease is benign yet highly contagious[1]. It can be a source of significant cosmetic concern and social discomfort. The infection mostly targets the pediatric population, sexually active young adults, and those who are immunocompromised. It requires limited medical intervention and usually results in complete recovery within 6–12 months. In special populations, such as the immunocompromised or those suffering from underlying skin barrier disorders, recovery is more challenging and prolonged.

ETIOLOGY AND EPIDEMIOLOGY

The MC virus (MCV) is the responsible infectious agent. MCV, a member of the deoxyribonucleic acid (DNA) poxviruses, is one of the largest viruses known, thus far. It has a linear duplex DNA structure of 120–200 MDa mass. The four major subtypes, MCV-1, MCV-2, MCV-3, and MCV-4, are clinically indistinguishable[2]. Of the different subtypes, MCV-1 (genome of 180 kb) is responsible for most of the infections found in the pediatric population, and MCV-2 (genome of 195 kb) for those in immunosuppressed and sexually active patients.

MCV infects the epidermis, preferentially targeting keratinocytes. Replication within the cytoplasm stimulates the cell to undergo hypertrophy and hyperplasia. This results in the characteristic clinical lesions. Formerly thought to be a pediatric disease, MC infection is found in a worldwide geographic distribution and within a broad demographic range regardless of race. The disease is common in warm, humid climates and within living conditions that foster close quarters and poor hygiene. There is no appreciable difference in the level of incidence based on gender or seasonal variations. There is a bimodal age distribution with the first peak in early childhood and the second in early adulthood. Due to the mild and self-limited nature of the disease and the consequent lack of medical attention sought by infected individuals, the actual incidence may be grossly underestimated.

The virus is transmitted person to person through direct contact with an infected individual or with object surfaces that harbor the MCV, such as clothing, towels, bathing sponges, toys, or gymnastic equipment. Swimming pools, steam baths, saunas, and communal spray baths may also be potential sources of viral spread even though the mechanisms are still unclear[3]. Contact sports, such as wrestling, have been implicated in its transmission, and there has also been a case report published of a surgeon spreading the virus to patients.

Sexual contact is a major contributor to viral spread, especially among adolescents who present with the characteristic MC infection in the genital area. These individuals should be tested for other sexually transmitted diseases. Skin conditions such as atopic dermatitis (AD) may predispose to infection with MCV because of the associated skin barrier and immune cell dysfunction.

CLINICAL PRESENTATION

MC lesions present as pearly white, pink or flesh-colored 2–5 mm dome-shaped papules with central umbilication (**9.1**). The number of individual papules is usually between 10 and 20, but this can vary (**9.2–9.4**). Initially smooth, firm and painless, they may become itchy, red or swollen. Single and clustered lesions are commonly found on the trunk, arms, legs, axillae, and antecubital and popliteal fossae[4] but may also be widespread. When spread through sexual transmission, papules appear in the genital area including the upper thighs and lower abdomen (**9.4, 9.5**). Rarely, it can affect the palms, soles, oral and genital mucosa, or conjunctiva. MC infection on the eyelids can lead to keratoconjunctivitis or chronic conjunctivitis.

There may be focal redness and scaling due to inflammation or scratching, or a frank dermatitis around the lesions (molluscum dermatitis). The core of the papule has a central plug of white, waxy or cheesy material containing the virus. MC papules can emerge from hair follicles leading to subsequent comedo and secondary abscess formation.

Immunocompromised patients, including those infected with human immunodeficiency virus (HIV)/acquired immunodeficiency syndrome (AIDS) and organ transplant recipients, characteristically develop giant lesions that are ≥15 mm, more numerous and refractory to therapy[5–7]. An increase in facial molluscum has been linked to low CD4 cell counts and is used as a marker of HIV disease severity.

LABORATORY STUDIES

The MCV has not been successfully grown *in vitro*, and, therefore, laboratory studies are limited. However, human foreskin fragments have been effectively infected with patient-derived isolates of MCV and implanted into the renal capsule of athymic mice[8]. MCV infects humans almost exclusively with no known animal reservoirs, even though rare cases have been reported in animals[9].

COURSE, PROGNOSIS, AND COMPLICATIONS

The incubation period is estimated to be between 2 weeks and 6 months and is followed by an eruption of tiny papules. In an immunocompetent patient, infection with MC is self-limited and will spontaneously resolve in 6–12 months, requiring little to no medical intervention. In persistent cases complete resolution may take up to 5 years. There is no residual scarring unless the patient employs excessive scratching during the course of the infection. Scarring can also result from complications of medical intervention. The infection is more persistent in immunocompromised patients, following an aggressive course that results in giant lesions ≥15 mm in diameter and a larger number of papules[10].

Autoinoculation results from scratching or rubbing a lesion and then touching other areas of the body. Children are more prone to autoinoculation and should be instructed to avoid this action as this may prolong recovery. Possible complications include persistence, spread, or recurrence of lesions, secondary bacterial infections, and permanent scarring or skin discoloration. Generally, these can be avoided through proper medical management and limiting scratching or contact with the lesions.

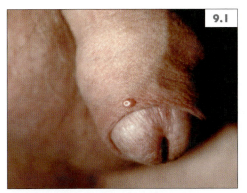

9.1 Typical dome-shaped papule with central umbilication. (Courtesy of Dr. Tomasz Mroczkowski.)

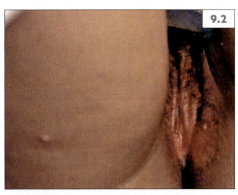

9.2 Molluscum contagiosum on the skin of the thigh and vulva. (Courtesy of Dr. Tomasz F. Mroczkowski.)

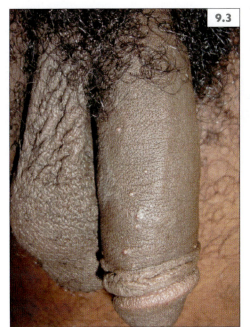

9.3 Molluscum contagiosum on the penis. (Courtesy of Dr. Tomasz F. Mroczkowski.)

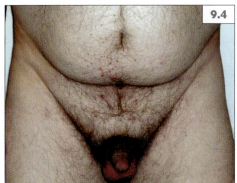

9.4 Numerous 1–2 mm erythematous, umbilicated papules on the abdomen and pubis.

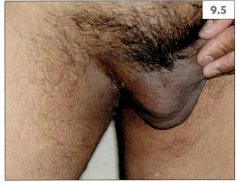

9.5 Confluent papules involving the inguinal crease, scrotum, and penile shaft.

DIAGNOSIS AND DIFFERENTIAL DIAGNOSIS

MC is most often a clinical diagnosis, based upon the typical appearance and any associated symptoms. In difficult situations, the diagnosis can be confirmed via histopathologic evaluation of a skin biopsy. There is epidermal hyperplasia with a central cavity (**9.6**) that contains 'molluscum bodies', also known as Henderson–Patterson bodies, eosinophilic inclusions that form above the stratum basale (**9.7**)[11]. The abundant granular eosinophilic cytoplasm of molluscum bodies contains virions and a small peripheral nucleus. Although easily visualized on routine hematoxylin–eosin stained sections (**9.6**), they are preferentially stained with Giemsa, Wright, Gram, and Papanicolaou stains. A Tzanck smear preparation of the thick white material expressed from the center of a papule will reveal molluscum bodies and is easily performed in the clinical setting. MC may present as an opportunistic infection in patients infected with HIV. Giant lesions, recurrent bouts of infection, and persistence, despite appropriate therapy, are characteristics of underlying immunodeficiency.

The differential diagnosis includes basal cell carcinoma, keratocanthoma, verruca vulgaris, warty dyskeratoma, and epidermal inclusion cyst. For lesions presenting in the genital area, condyloma acuminatum and vaginal syringoma are also a consideration. In immunocompromised patients, one might suspect fungal infections such as cryptococcosis, histoplasmosis, coccidioidomycosis, or penicilliosis. On the eyelid, MC may mimic a chalazion, lid abscess, or foreign body granuloma.

TREATMENT

In healthy, immunocompetent individuals, treatment is optional. The lesions typically undergo complete resolution within 6–24 months, although they may occasionally last up to 5 years. Autoinoculation prolongs disease duration. Treatment is warranted in the presence of itching, discomfort, complications from underlying disorders such as AD or secondary bacterial infections, and chronic keratoconjunctivitis. Also, intervention is indicated to prevent autoinoculation or spread to others. Social situations may require the patient to undergo immediate treatment due to cosmetic concerns, community isolation, or embarrassment.

Effective treatment options include cryotherapy, curettage, electrosurgery, pulsed dye laser therapy, or application of keratolytics[12]. More specifically, oral therapy with cimetidine has been shown safe and well tolerated; however, it tends to work better for lesions on the body than for those on the face[13]. Topical therapy with podophyllotoxin 0.5% cream is probably best restricted to men due to its teratogenicity[14]. Other topical therapies available for treatment of MC include iodine, salicylic acid, potassium hydroxide, tretinoin, benzoyl peroxide, cantharidin, and imiquimod[15]. In immunocompromised patients, intralesional interferon has been used[16].

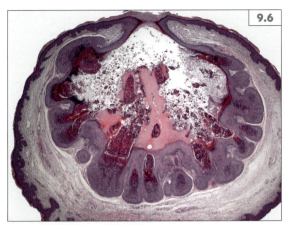

9.6 A characteristic histopathologic section demonstrating epidermal hyperplasia surrounding a central cavity (H & E, ×2).

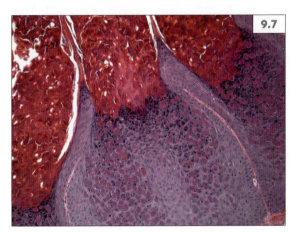

9.7 Microscopic examination revealing Henderson–Patterson bodies (molluscum bodies) that are eosinophilic inclusions which form above the basal layer (H & E, ×10).

CHAPTER 10

HIV Infection/AIDS

Laila M. Castellino, MD

DEFINITION

On June 5, 1981 the USA Centers for Disease Control and Prevention (CDC) published what became the first account of the acquired immunodeficiency syndrome (AIDS) in *Morbidity and Mortality Weekly Report*[1]. Two years later, a novel retrovirus, human immunodeficiency virus (HIV), was recognized as being the etiologic agent of the disease.

A surveillance case definition for AIDS was established early in the epidemic, which listed the opportunistic infections and malignancies associated with declining cell-mediated immunity. With advances in the understanding of the pathogenesis of AIDS, as well as serologic tests to detect HIV, the definition of AIDS was expanded to incorporate the CD4 cell count, in addition to other clinical diseases associated with HIV.

Currently, AIDS is defined as laboratory-confirmed evidence of HIV infection, in addition to a CD4+ T-lymphocyte count of <200 cells/μL, a CD4+ T-lymphocyte percentage of total lymphocytes of <14, or the diagnosis of an AIDS-defining condition (*Table 10.1*).

With advances in the treatment of HIV, the distinction between HIV and AIDS has become clinically less relevant, although this remains a useful tool in the public health realm.

ETIOLOGY AND EPIDEMIOLOGY

The disease is caused by HIV, capable of transcribing viral ribonucleic acid (RNA) into linear double-stranded DNA that is integrated into the host genome. The virus specifically targets CD4+ T cells, as well as macrophages and dendritic cells. The decline in CD4+ T cells leads to a loss of cell-mediated immunity, leaving the host increasingly susceptible to opportunistic infections.

Thirty years after its recognition, HIV remains a global epidemic. The World Health Organization (WHO) in its 2009 global report estimates that there are 33.3 million people living with HIV. In 2009 alone, 2.6 million people were newly infected with HIV, and 1.9 million people died of AIDS. The majority of cases are in sub-Saharan Africa (estimate 22.5 million), followed by south and south-east Asia (estimate 4.1 million). Two and a half million children (<15years) are estimated to be living with HIV. In the USA, the CDC estimates there are more than one million people living with HIV. Every year 56,300 Americans are estimated to be newly infected, and more than 18,000 people die of the disease.

Initially, HIV was primarily seen among men who had sex with men (MSM) and in injection drug users. Today, it is increasingly an epidemic of persons of color, women, heterosexuals, and injection drug users. While MSM still account for 53% of new infections,

Table 10.1 AIDS-defining conditions

- Bacterial infections, multiple or recurrent*
- Candidiasis of bronchi, trachea, or lungs
- Candidiasis of esophagus
- Cervical cancer, invasive
- Coccidioidomycosis, disseminated or extrapulmonary
- Cryptococcosis, extrapulmonary
- Cryptosporidiosis, chronic intestinal (>1 month's duration)
- Cytomegalovirus disease (other than liver, spleen, or nodes), onset at age >1 month
- Cytomegalovirus retinitis (with loss of vision)
- Encephalopathy, HIV related
- Herpes simplex: chronic ulcers (>1 month's duration) or bronchitis, pneumonitis, or esophagitis (onset at age >1 month)
- Histoplasmosis, disseminated or extrapulmonary
- Isosporiasis, chronic intestinal (>1 month's duration)
- Kaposi's sarcoma
- Lymphoid interstitial pneumonia or pulmonary lymphoid hyperplasia complex*
- Lymphoma, Burkitt (or equivalent term)
- Lymphoma, immunoblastic (or equivalent term)
- Lymphoma, primary, of brain
- *Mycobacterium avium* complex or *Mycobacterium kansasii*, disseminated or extrapulmonary
- *Mycobacterium tuberculosis* of any site, pulmonary, disseminated, or extrapulmonary
- *Mycobacterium*, other species or unidentified species, disseminated or extrapulmonary
- *Pneumocystis jirovecii* pneumonia
- Pneumonia, recurrent
- Progressive multifocal leukoencephalopathy
- *Salmonella* septicemia, recurrent
- Toxoplasmosis of brain, onset at age >1 month
- Wasting syndrome attributed to HIV

   *Only among children aged <13 years.

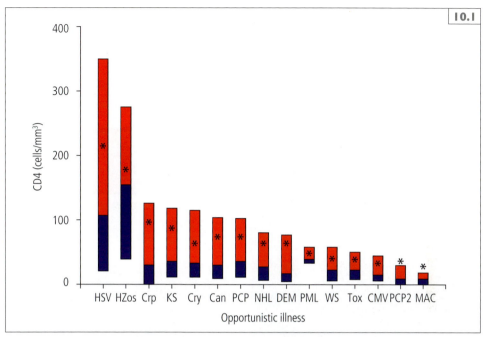

10.1 Boxplot of the median (line inside the box), first quartile (bottom of the box), third quartile (top of the box), and median (asterisk) CD4+ lymphocyte count at the time of the development of opportunistic disease. Can: *Candida* esophagitis; CMV: cytomegalovirus infection; Crp: cryptosporidiosis; Cry: cryptococcal meningitis; DEM: acquired immunodeficiency virus dementia complex; HSV: herpes simplex virus infection; HZos: herpes zoster; KS: Kaposi's sarcoma; MAC: *Mycobacterium avium* complex bacteremia; NHL: non-Hodgkin lymphoma; PCP: primary *Pneumocystis carinii* pneumonia; PCP2: secondary *Pneumocystis carinii*; PML: progressive multifocal leukoencephalopathy; Tox: *Toxoplasma gondii* encephalitis; WS: the wasting syndrome. (From: CDC (2008). Revised surveillance case definitions for HIV infection among adults, adolescents, and children aged <18 months and for HIV Infection and AIDS among children aged 18 Months to <13 years – United States, *MMWR Recomm Rep* **57**(RR10):1–8.)

heterosexual contact now accounts for 31% of new infections, injection drug use for 12%, and MSM who inject drugs for 4% [2]. It is estimated that in the USA, 21% of persons living with HIV remain undiagnosed[2].

CLINICAL PRESENTATION

In a study of 46 patients with primary HIV infection, 89% reported clinical manifestations consistent with an acute retroviral syndrome, of which the most commonly reported symptoms were fever, sore throat, fatigue, weight loss, and myalgia[3]. The most common findings on physical examination were lymphadenopathy, oral ulcerations, exudative pharyngitis, thrush, genital or rectal ulcerations, signs of neuropathy, orthostatic hypotension, and aseptic meningitis. Occasionally, a macular erythematous truncal eruption and thrombocytopenia have also been reported[4]. In untreated patients, the rate of progression from primary HIV infection to AIDS is estimated to be approximately 11 years[5]. As the CD4 count declines, the incidence of specific opportunistic infections varies (**10.1**)[6]. After seroconversion, while many patients will remain asymptomatic until diagnosed with a specific opportunistic

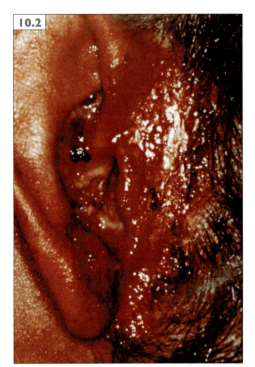

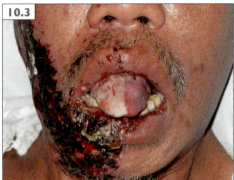

10.3 Herpes simplex infection accentuated in an AIDS patient.

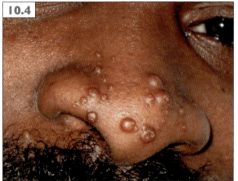

10.2 Herpes zoster, an exaggerated presentation in an AIDS patient.

10.4 Molluscum contagiosum, an exaggerated presentation in an AIDS patient.

infection, a large percentage of patients will go on to develop persistent generalized lymphadenopathy.

Specific cutaneous manifestations that are seen more often in HIV-infected individuals include those due to viral infections such as varicella zoster (**10.2**), herpes simplex (**10.3**), and molluscum contagiosum (**10.4**). Kaposi's sarcoma is a neoplastic disease that is associated with human herpes virus type 8 and

is seen predominantly in HIV-infected MSM (**10.5–10.8**). While the skin is the organ predominantly affected, the oral cavity, lungs, and gastrointestinal tract (including rectum) are also often involved. The characteristic purplish nodules and plaques are clinically indistinguishable from the lesions seen in bacillary angiomatosis, another disease that is seen more frequently in patients with HIV but is ascribed to the *Bartonella* organisms.

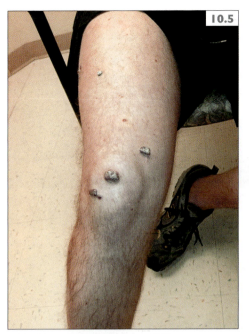

10.5 Kaposi's sarcoma in an AIDS patient.

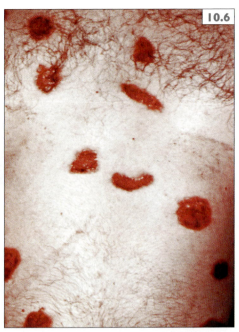

10.6 Kaposi's sarcoma in an AIDS patient.

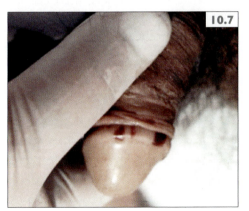

10.7 Kaposi's sarcoma on the penis in a patient with AIDS. (Courtesy of Dr. Tomasz F. Mroczkowski.)

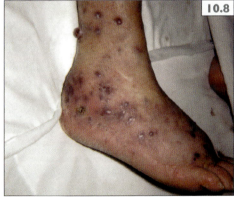

10.8 Kaposi's sarcoma on the leg in a patient with AIDS. (Courtesy of Dr. Tomasz F. Mroczkowski.)

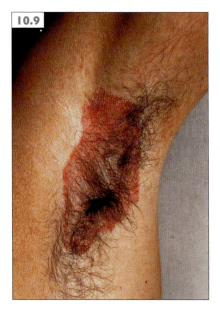

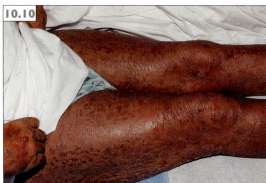

10.10 Psoriasis flare in an AIDS patient.

10.9 Seborrheic dermatitis in an AIDS patient.

Other cutaneous disorders that are well-described in patients with HIV include seborrheic dermatitis (**10.9**), psoriasis (**10.10**), prurigo nodularis, bacterial folliculitis, especially with methicillin-resistant *Staphylococcus aureus* (MRSA), scabies, including crusted scabies, and eosinophilic folliculitis. HIV-associated psoriasis is often severe, with frequent exacerbations. Rarely, cutaneous manifestations of endemic mycoses such as histoplasmosis, *Penicillium marneffei* infection, coccidioidomycosis, and paracoccidioidomycosis are also seen.

Given that HIV is a sexually transmitted disease (STD), it is not surprising that other sexually transmitted diseases are frequently diagnosed in persons with HIV[7]. Early in the HIV epidemic, the phrase 'gay bowel syndrome' was used loosely to describe a constellation of rectal and perianal diseases seen in MSM. Although the term did not connote a specific disease, it encompassed a wide range of etiologies that manifest as clinical proctitis, including that due to chlamydial, gonococcal, syphilitic, *Shigella*, or *Giardia* infection.

While specific genital and perianal diseases are covered in other chapters, special mention must be made of syphilis (**10.11, 10.12**) and lymphogranuloma venereum (LGV), which disproportionately affect the HIV-positive MSM population. Clinical manifestations of syphilis in the HIV-infected population are generally no different from those found in the non-HIV-infected population, although some reports suggest neurosyphilis may be more likely to develop[8]. Unusual serologic responses, such as higher than expected titers or higher rates of serologic treatment failure, are seen more commonly in HIV-infected patients, and close follow-up of these patients is warranted.

LGV in the developed world is an uncommon STD. Recently, there has been an increase in incidence, particularly in HIV-positive MSM in Europe and the USA[9]. Clinically, the disease is characterized by genital ulcerations, lymphadenopathy, and symptoms of proctocolitis.

LABORATORY STUDIES

Once the diagnosis of HIV is established, the CD4 T cell count and HIV viral load should be measured. In addition, HIV genotypic resistance testing should also be obtained at baseline, irrespective of the decision to start treatment. This has increasingly become a standard as an estimated 17% of patients with newly diagnosed HIV infection already have at least one drug resistant mutation[10].

Additionally, tests to screen for syphilis and other STDs should be obtained, as well as serologies for hepatitis A, B, and C viruses and cytomegalovirus (CMV). Tuberculin skin tests or interferon-γ release assay, as well as *Toxoplasma gondii* serology, should be obtained to determine the risk of disease, and hence, the need for prophylaxis. Women should also have a pap smear performed.

Complete blood count, chemistry profile, transaminase levels, blood urea nitrogen (BUN) and creatinine, fasting blood glucose, serum lipids, and urinalysis should also be obtained.

COURSE, PROGNOSIS, AND COMPLICATIONS

Untreated, most patients with HIV will go on to develop AIDS with its associated opportunistic infections. A small subset of patients are considered to be long-term nonprogressors, who remain asymptomatic and show no evidence of immunologic decline.

With the advent of effective therapy for HIV, the incidence of opportunistic infections has decreased dramatically in the USA, although esophageal candidiasis, *Pneumocystis jiroveci* pneumonia, disseminated *Mycobacterium avium* complex, and CMV disease remain the major incident opportunistic illnesses observed[11]. With advances in HIV therapy having led to a significant decline in morbidity and mortality in the USA, there has been a concomitant rise in the incidence of noninfectious complications, such as cancer, hyperlipidemia, and heart disease. An increasing number of deaths among HIV-infected persons are now ascribed to non-HIV-related causes, such as cardiovascular disease, non-AIDS-defining cancers, and substance abuse[12].

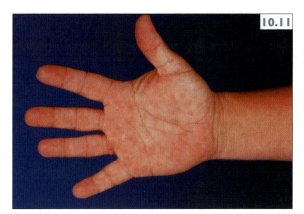

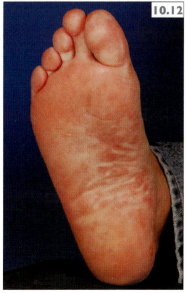

10.11 Secondary syphilis in an AIDS patient

10.12 Secondary syphilis in an AIDS patient.

DIAGNOSIS

Diagnosis of HIV infection is achieved most commonly by detection of HIV-specific antibodies in serum, and less commonly by demonstration of viremia by means of detection of HIV antigens or RNA. Initial testing for HIV most commonly is achieved by an enzyme immunoassay (EIA) that is quick and cost effective; however, while the EIA is highly sensitive, it does give false-positive results. A reactive test result must always be confirmed with a highly specific test such as a Western blot, or by detection of actual viral RNA. Most tests in use today can detect antibodies within a few weeks of initial infection. In situations where acute infection is suspected, tests to detect the presence of the virus (such as viral nucleic acid detection or p24 antigen) must be specifically requested. These are generally reactive within days of acquiring infection, at which time a serological test will likely be nonreactive.

Given that an estimated one in five individuals infected with HIV are not aware of their status[13], the CDC recommends routine screening for all individuals aged 13–64. More frequent screening is recommended for high-risk groups, such as injection drugs users and persons with multiple sexual partners. In addition, all persons who are being evaluated for STDs should be tested for HIV.

Sadly, in a high-risk population that reported symptoms and signs consistent with an acute retroviral syndrome and sought medical attention, only 25% received a correct medical diagnosis[2]. This reinforces the CDC recommendation that HIV testing be a part of routine medical screening. In patients presenting with acute retroviral syndrome, it is important to obtain both a serologic and a virologic test.

TREATMENT

Detailed discussion of the management of HIV infection is beyond the scope of this chapter. In general, individuals diagnosed with HIV should be referred to a specialist well versed in the treatment of HIV and its complications. In the USA, the Department of Health and Human Services regularly updates guidelines for the use of antiretroviral agents in HIV-1 infected individuals[14].

The decision to start antiretroviral therapy is based on several factors, including the patient's willingness and commitment to lifelong treatment. Specific indications include a history of an AIDS-defining illness, CD4 cell count of <350 cells/mm^3, pregnancy, presence of HIV-associated nephropathy, and patients with hepatitis B, when treatment of hepatitis B is indicated. In resource rich settings, initiation of therapy is recommended regardless of the CD4 cell count level, as there is increasing evidence that achieving viral suppression decreases mortality and HIV-related morbidity, while decreasing the risk of transmission to sexual partners.

At present, there are broadly six classes of antiretroviral medication, which include the nucleoside/nucleotide reverse transcriptase inhibitors, non-nucleoside reverse transcriptase inhibitors, protease inhibitors, fusion inhibitors, CCR5 antagonists, and integrase strand transfer inhibitors.

While HIV cannot be eradicated, the goal of treatment is to suppress viral replication in order to preserve the immune system and thus reduce the risk of opportunistic infection and other HIV-associated morbidity. In order to achieve this, all antiretroviral regimens currently in use contain at least two, preferably three, drugs from two or more classes of antiretrovirals.

With advances in therapy, HIV is increasingly considered to be a manageable chronic illness. Amazingly rapid progress has been made, moving from recognition of a syndrome to assignation of a causative agent, and to the development of specific molecularly designed effective therapies for HIV. Despite vast strides in the understanding of the pathogenesis and treatment, a vaccine to prevent HIV remains elusive. Clinicians and public health personnel must continue to reinforce the message of prevention.

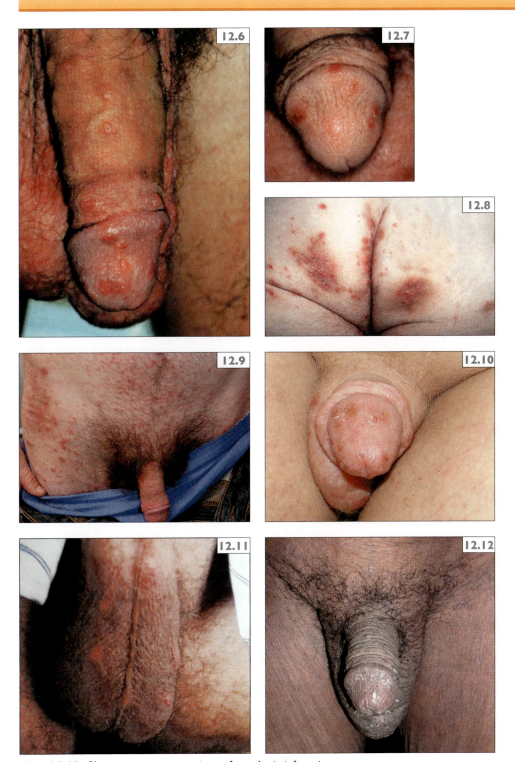

12.6–12.12 Characteristic presentations of a scabetic infestation.

In infants, the elderly and immuno-compromised hosts, all skin surfaces are susceptible, including the scalp and face, giving the picture of crusted scabies (**12.13**)[2].

Commonly, small erythematous papules are present, associated with variable numbers of excoriations. Vesicles, indurated nodules, eczematous dermatitis, and secondary bacterial infection are common. The pathognomonic sign is the burrow, representing the tunnel that a female mite excavates while laying eggs. Clinically, the burrow is wavy, thread-like, grayish-white and 1–10 mm in length (**12.14**)[1].

LABORATORY STUDIES

Polymerase chain reaction (PCR) of cutaneous scales can be used to confirm the existence of mites[6]. On histopathologic examination there is a patchy to diffuse infiltrate of eosinophils in the reticular dermis and a scabies mite may occasionally be seen within the epidermis. Pink 'pigtail'-like structures attached to the stratum corneum (which represent fragments of the adult mite exoskeleton) can serve as a clue to the diagnosis of scabies when mites, scybala, or eggs are not identified (**12.15**)[7].

COURSE, PROGNOSIS, AND COMPLICATIONS

Prognosis is excellent if the scabies are identified and treatment is initiated. Although *S. scabiei* var. *hominis* is not a known vector for any systemic disease, secondary bacterial infections with group A *Streptococcus pyogenes* or *Staphylococcus aureus* may occur if left untreated.

DIAGNOSIS

Clinical confirmation can be achieved with mineral oil examination in which skin scrapings from infested areas are inspected under light microscopy for adult mites, eggs, and/or scybala (**12.16**). In some patients, dermoscopy can be helpful for direct *in vivo* visualization of mites and eggs[8]. A skin biopsy can confirm the clinical diagnosis, but only if the specimen obtained happens to contain the mite or its eggs. Commonly, the diagnosis is based on clinical impression and response to treatment.

TREATMENT

The treatment regimen recommended by the CDC is permethrin 5% cream applied to all areas of the body from the neck down, and washed off after 8–14 hours; or ivermectin 200 µg/kg orally, repeated in 2 weeks; however, if a patient cannot tolerate or has failed with these therapies then lindane 1% lotion or cream applied in a thin layer to all areas of the body from the neck down and thoroughly washed off after 8 hours can be used. Lindane is not recommended as first-line therapy because of toxicity. For those with crusted scabies, a combined treatment is recommended with a topical scabicide and oral ivermectin or repeated treatments with ivermectin 200 µg/kg on days 1, 15, and 29[3].

Pruritus and lesions can persist for 2–4 weeks after successful treatment. Patients should realize that such reactions do not imply treatment failure, but rather represent the body's response to dead mites that are eventually sloughed off (within 2 weeks) along with natural epidermal exfoliation. Most patients, however, experience relief from pruritus, usually within 3 days[3].

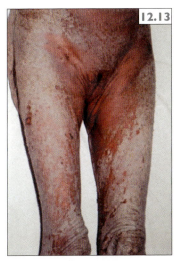

12.13 Crusted scabies.

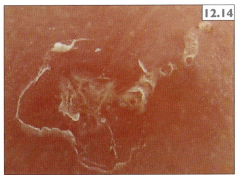

12.14 Scabetic burrow.

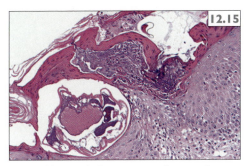

12.15 Histopathologic section showing the mite engulfed (H & E, ×200).

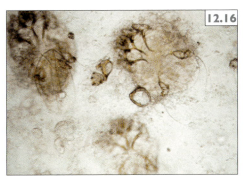

12.16 Skin scraping showing two mites and some eggs (×10).

CHAPTER 13

Sexual Abuse

Tunisia Finch, MD, and Vesna Petronic-Rosic, MD, MSc

DEFINITION

Sexual violence is defined by nonconsensual completed or attempted sexual activity and encompasses a range of behaviors that may not always include physical contact between the victim and the perpetrator. Forms of sexual violence include a completed or attempted sex act, abusive sexual contact, and noncontact sexual abuse, all of which are considered to be sexual abuse even when they are committed against a subject who is incapable of consent or refusal[1].

A sex act is defined by contact of the penis either with the vulva, anus, or mouth, in addition to anal or genital penetration of another person by hand, finger, or other object. Abusive sexual contact includes nonconsensual, intentional touching of the genitalia, anus, groin, breast, inner aspect of the thigh, or buttocks. Noncontact sexual abuse is limited to forms of sexual abuse that do not include physical contact, such as voyeurism, unwanted exposure to pornography, verbal or behavioral sexual harassment, or photographing another person without his or her consent[1].

For the purposes of this chapter, we will concentrate on the forms of sexual violence that are more likely to result in physical injuries to the victim, such as completed and attempted sex acts. Many victims of sexual abuse lack definitive medical findings and, ironically, the role of the medical provider has evolved into one in which the medical provider confirms that the victim is physically uninjured and initiates appropriate testing for the unwanted consequences of abuse[2].

ETIOLOGY AND EPIDEMIOLOGY

Sexual violence is a significant social and public health problem in the USA and other countries. Anyone can be a victim of sexual abuse and more often than not, the perpetrator is someone known to the victim. Approximately 11% of adult women and 2% of adult men reported experiencing forced sex over their lifetime, with 60.4% of female victims and 69.2% of male victims being raped by the age of 18; moreover, 25.5% of women and 41% of men were first raped before age 12. Among high school students nationwide, about 8% reported having been forced to have sex. Among students, 20–25% of women reported an attempted or completed rape experience while in college[3]. It is important to emphasize that these numbers often underestimate the problem of sexual violence, as many victims fear revealing their experiences.

Perpetrators are more likely to be men, have friends who are sexually aggressive, have witnessed or experienced violence as a child, have abused alcohol or drugs, or have been exposed to societal norms that support sexual violence and male superiority. Reports from female and male victims indicate that perpetrators were often intimate partners, family members, and friends[3].

CLINICAL PRESENTATION

A normal physical exam is seen in 80–95% of cases of sexual abuse; therefore, the examiner must use historical, physical, and laboratory data to confirm a diagnosis of sexual abuse[2,4]. Children often present with a variety of nonspecific complaints such as sleep disturbances, abdominal pain, enuresis, encopresis, or phobias. If the history is highly suggestive of abuse, a health care professional who is experienced in forensic examinations should perform a thorough physical examination within 72 hours of the event. In many cases, victims of sexual abuse do not disclose a history of sexual abuse until long after the event. The healing process in the anogenital region occurs quickly, and the greater the time interval to examination, the less likely it is that injuries will be appreciated[4,5]. The clinician must also have an understanding of the appropriate interview techniques, developmental milestones, normal sexual behaviors, and normal anatomic variations within the pediatric population. When possible, all genital findings should be photodocumented after obtaining consent[4].

Physical examination of prepubertal and pubertal children

The butterfly ('frog-leg') position and knee–chest position are the more commonly used examination positions used in child abuse cases. It is important to document the examination position and whether labial traction is used in girls, as these both may influence the findings[4,5]. A speculum is not typically used in prepubescent girls, because the genitalia can be visualized adequately with proper technique and positioning.

Colposcopy is now recommended for adequate sexual assault evaluation, because it aids in evaluation and documentation with digital imaging. Toluidine blue is an important tool to detect and document genital and perianal injuries after sexual assault. Application of toluidine blue dye and its subsequent removal from unstained areas by means of a destaining reagent (vinegar) has been shown to increase the detection rate of posterior fourchette lacerations from 16% to 40% in adult rape victims. The presence of lacerations, however, does not necessarily implicate the penis as the inflicting agent; fingers, tampons, foreign objects, and even improperly handled examining specula could be indicated. Therefore, the toluidine blue test should be performed before any digital or speculum examination and thus before the collection of forensic evidence[6,7]. Toluidine blue dye may cause some discomfort in children[7].

Clinicians should evaluate for the presence of erythema, ecchymoses, lesions, abrasions, lacerations, scarring, bite patterns, or discharge with regard to anatomic location in all children. Circumferential injuries to the shaft or glans penis are suggestive of abuse. Penile, vaginal, and anal secretions should be cultured for sexually transmitted diseases (STDs), and secretions should be examined for semen if penetration is suspected. Anal dilatation of any size is considered a normal reflex, if stool is present in the rectal vault or if dilatation occurs after the child has been in the prone knee–chest position for more than 30 seconds. Anal dilatation of 20 mm or greater, without stool in the rectal vault, is highly suspicious for abuse[5].

Physical examination of adult men and women

In cases of sexual abuse involving adult women, the clinician should perform an external examination and document findings of the external genitalia, perineum, vagina, and cervix specifically for injury, foreign materials, and other findings. When the vaginal examination is performed, the speculum should be lubricated with tap water because other lubricants may affect test results and decrease sperm motility.

In cases of sexual abuse involving adult men, the clinician should examine the external genitalia and perineum for injury, foreign materials, and other findings.

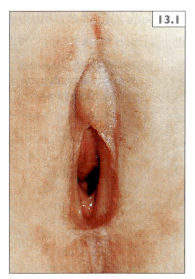

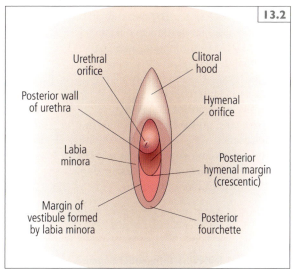

Urethral
orifice

Clitoral
hood

Posterior wall
of urethra

Hymenal
orifice

Labia
minora

Posterior
hymenal margin
(crescentic)

Margin of
vestibule formed
by labia minora

Posterior
fourchette

13.1, 13.2 Anatomy of genitalia in a 5-year-old girl. (From *The Great Ormond Street Colour Handbook: Paediatrics and Child Health*, CRC Press, with permission.)

Anoscopy may be performed if rectal injury is suspected. As in children, toluidine blue dye and colposcopy aid in identification and documentation of injuries[7].

Physical findings in children (13.1–13.3)
Categories of sexual abuse include signs that are suggestive of and those specific for abuse. Normal or nonspecific findings include hymenal tags, hymenal bumps, labial adhesions, anogenital erythema, perianal skin tags, anal fissures, and anal dilatation with stool in the ampulla[2,5]. Findings that are highly specific for sexual abuse are:
• Clear evidence of penetrating anogenital trauma, without alternative or accident-related explanation, namely acute hymenal laceration or ecchymoses, laceration, healed hymenal transection, absence of hymenal tissue in the posterior sector, perianal lacerations or scarring extending into the anal sphincter, or marked and immediate dilatation of the anus in a knee–chest position, with no constipation, stool in the vault, or neurologic disorder.

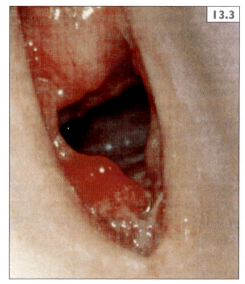

13.3 Laceration of the hymen and posterior fourchette following a rape one week earlier. (From *The Great Ormond Street Colour Handbook: Paediatrics and Child Health*, CRC Press, with permission.)

- The presence of semen/sperm/acid phosphatase/foreign deoxyribonucleic acid (DNA) in the vagina, anus, or external genitalia.
- Pregnancy without a history of consensual intercourse.
- Positive evidence of *Chlamydia trachomatis*, gonorrhea, or syphilis in the absence of perinatal transmission.
- Human immunodeficiency virus (HIV) infection not acquired perinatally or via transfusion of blood products.

Visible oral injuries or infections are infrequently found; bruising or petechiae of the hard or soft palate, and tears of the frenulum may indicate evidence of forced oral penetration. The differential diagnosis for sexual abuse is broad, as a variety of conditions can present with similar manifestations (*Table 13.1*)[2,5].

Table 13.1 Differential diagnosis of child sexual abuse

- Behçet's disease
- Bullous pemphigoid
- Congenital variations of perineum (periurethral bands, intravaginal ridges, midline perianal skin folds)
- Crohn's disease
- Dermatitis (seborrheic, atopic, or contact)
- Foreign bodies
- Hemangiomas
- Hemolytic uremic syndrome
- Kawasaki syndrome
- Labial adhesions
- Langerhans cell histiocytosis
- Lichen planus
- Lichen sclerosus et atrophicus*
- Masturbation
- Molluscum contagiosum
- Neurogenic anus
- Pinworm infestation
- Psoriasis
- Sarcoma botryoides
- Scabies
- Streptococcal infection
- Trauma (hair tourniquet, zipper entrapment injury, straddle injury)
- Urethral caruncle and prolapse
- Vulvovaginitis

*Most common condition mistaken for sexual abuse

Physical findings in adults

In adults, general body trauma occurs more often than genital trauma. Common findings in general body trauma include lacerations, abrasions, or contusions, with the extremities most commonly injured, followed by the head and neck[8,9]. In women, virginal and younger sexually experienced patients sustain genital injury more frequently; moreover, anogenital injuries are more frequent in patients who are examined within 24 hours after the assault, as well as in those who are victims of anal assault[9]. In one study of 1112 patients presenting after sexual assault, external genital, hymenal, vaginal, rectal, or cervical trauma was noted on examination in approximately 52% of female sexual assault victims, and external genital or rectal trauma was noted in 35.5% of male sexual assault victims[8].

LABORATORY STUDIES

Forensic evidence should be collected, typically within 72 hours of an acute event of sexual abuse[2,4,5,10]. Medical issues after sexual assault include acute injuries and evaluation of potential STD and pregnancy. The USA Centers for Disease Control and Prevention (CDC) have guidelines for sexually transmitted infection (STI) testing in cases of suspected sexual abuse. An initial examination should include the following procedures:

- Culture or FDA-cleared nucleic acid amplification tests for either *Neisseria gonorrhoeae* or *Chlamydia trachomatis*.
- Wet mount and culture of a vaginal swab specimen for *Trichomonas vaginalis* infection. If vaginal discharge, malodor, or itching is evident, the wet mount should also be examined for evidence of bacterial vaginosis (BV) and candidiasis.
- Collection of a serum sample for immediate evaluation for HIV, hepatitis B (HBV), and syphilis.

- Circumstances with a high risk for STDs and a strong indication for testing in children include the child has or has had symptoms or signs of an STD, or of an infection that can be sexually transmitted, even in the absence of suspicion of sexual abuse.
- A suspected assailant is known to have an STD or to be at high risk for STD.
- A sibling or another child or adult in the household or child's immediate environment has an STD.
- The patient or parent requests testing.
- Evidence of genital, oral, or anal penetration or ejaculation is present[10]. It has been shown that about 0.8% of prepubertal girls and 5% of adolescents will have a positive screening test, even though they do not report symptoms[5].

At the initial examination and at follow-up examinations, patients should be counseled regarding: (1) symptoms of STDs and the need for immediate examination if symptoms occur; and (2) abstinence from sexual intercourse until STD prophylactic treatment has been completed. Following an acute sexual assault, a serum or urine pregnancy test and emergency contraception should be offered. Examination for STDs should be repeated within 1–2 weeks of the assault. In situations where the transmission of syphilis, HIV, or HBV is a concern but initial tests are negative, an examination at 6 weeks, 3 months, and 6 months after the last suspected sexual exposure is recommended to allow time for antibodies to infectious agents to develop. Results of HBV surface antigen testing must be interpreted carefully, because HBV can be transmitted nonsexually. Decisions regarding which tests should be performed must be made on an individual basis[7,10].

COURSE, PROGNOSIS, AND COMPLICATIONS

After a detailed physical examination, the clinician is charged with the task of reassuring the child and his/her family that she is healthy and that her genital examination is normal. Assurance of a normal genital examination helps begin the process of healing[4,5]. The pain and physical scars may heal, but the emotional, psychological, and medical sequelae of sexual abuse may endure and be more devastating. Pregnancy and STD in all victims may result in lifelong effects that may be life threatening. Other long-term physical consequences include chronic pelvic pain, gastrointestinal disorders, migraines, and back pain. Adverse psychological and social consequences include shock, denial, depression, suicidality, post-traumatic stress disorder, and strained interpersonal relationships. Health behavior consequences include engaging in high-risk sexual behavior, substance abuse, and eating disorders[2,3]. Victims of sexual abuse should be referred for psychological counseling to discuss and treat psychological and health behavioral consequences[2].

DIAGNOSIS

Confirming sexual abuse requires a multidisciplinary approach. Due to the overlap in physical findings secondary to the naturally occurring variations and physical changes among individuals in a given population, physical examination cannot independently confirm or exclude nonacute sexual abuse as the cause of genital trauma[4,5]. Positive physical findings of sexual abuse are infrequently found; therefore, the history given by the child is often paramount in cases of sexual maltreatment. If a health care provider has reasonable cause to suspect abuse, he or she should report the abuse to the appropriate authorities to safeguard the child from further injury. Health care providers should contact their local child-protection service agency regarding child-abuse reporting requirements in their area[10].

TREATMENT

Presumptive treatment for gonorrhea and chlamydia is not recommended for prepubertal patients due to the low incidence, the low risk of ascending infection, and the frequent need for confirmatory testing. Exceptions to this recommendation are HIV and HBV prophylaxis, when indicated. It is important to highlight that the presence of an STI does not always mean a child was sexually abused; the clinician must carefully evaluate whether the child could have obtained these infections via a nonsexual mechanism such as acquisition at the time of birth or autoinoculation[5,10].

For postpubertal adolescents and adults, routine preventive therapy after a sexual assault is frequently recommended because follow-up of survivors of sexual assault can be difficult. A prophylactic regimen is suggested as preventive therapy in *Table 13.2*.

The frequency of HIV seroconversion in persons whose only known risk factor was sexual assault is probably low. Children may be at higher risk of transmission given the higher frequency of multiple episodes of assault. Factors impacting on the medical recommendation for postexposure prophylaxis (PEP) with zidovudine depend on several factors including:

- The likelihood of the assailant having HIV.
- Exposure characteristics that might increase the risk of HIV transmission.
- The time elapsed after the event.
- The potential benefits and risks associated with the PEP[10].

Table 13.2 Postexposure prophylaxis following sexual abuse in adults and postpubertal adolescents

- Postexposure HBV vaccination, without HBV immune globulin, should adequately protect against HBV infection. HBV vaccination should be administered to sexual assault victims at the time of the initial examination if they have not been previously vaccinated

- Follow-up doses of vaccine should be administered 1–2 and 4–6 months after the first dose

- An empiric antimicrobial regimen for chlamydia, gonorrhea, trichomonas, and BV:

  Ceftriaxone 250 mg IM in a single dose
  OR
  Cefixime 400 mg orally in a single dose
  PLUS
  Metronidazole 2 g orally in a single dose
  PLUS
  Azithromycin 1 g orally in a single dose
  OR
  Doxycycline 100 mg orally twice a day for 7 days

- Emergency contraception should be offered if the assault could result in pregnancy in the survivor

SECTION 2
CUTANEOUS DISEASES OF THE ANOGENITAL REGION

CHAPTER 14

Anatomic Abnormalities

Rim Ishak, MD and Abdul-Ghani Kibbi, MD

- **Congenital phimosis**
- **Hypospadias**
- **Epispadias**
- **Pearly penile papules**
- **Ectopic sebaceous glands of Fordyce**
- **Endometriosis**
- **Median raphe cyst**

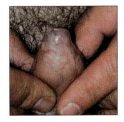
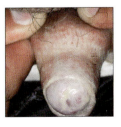
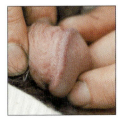
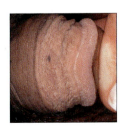

Congenital phimosis

DEFINITION

Phimosis, from the Greek word *phimos*, refers to the inability to retract the foreskin over the glans penis. Physiologic phimosis occurs in newborn boys up to 3 years of age, while pathologic phimosis develops usually secondary to distal scarring of the foreskin[1].

ETIOLOGY AND EPIDEMIOLOGY

Physiologic phimosis results from adhesions between the epithelial layers of the inner prepuce and glans. The majority of male newborns (96%) have physiological phimosis[2]. As the boy grows, these adhesions spontaneously resolve with repetitive foreskin retraction and erections. By the age of 3 years, only 8% of children will suffer from phimosis, and this further decreases to 1% by age 14[3].

Pathological phimosis in childhood is rare, and its causes are variable. Poor hygiene, recurrent episodes of balanitis, and forceful retraction of the foreskin with resultant tears at the preputial orifice may lead to scarring of the preputial orifice and phimosis[1]. Other causes include preputial stenosis and frenulum breve (short frenulum), which prevent retraction of the foreskin. Lichen sclerosus et atrophicus (LSA) has been recently considered as one of the main causes of pathological phimosis and has been reported in 40% of patients in a cohort of 1178 boys (mean age 8.7 years)[4].

CLINICAL PRESENTATION

Physiologic phimosis is usually asymptomatic; the parents of the affected child may note the inability to retract the foreskin during routine cleaning or bathing, or may report 'ballooning' of the prepuce during urination. With pathologic phimosis, patients may have hematuria, recurrent urinary tract infections, preputial pain, or a weakened urinary stream. On physical examination, erythema, edema, tenderness of the prepuce, purulent discharge, and even a constricted white fibrous ring may be observed; however, in physiologic phimosis, the preputial orifice is unscarred and healthy (**14.1, 14.2**).

COURSE, PROGNOSIS, AND COMPLICATIONS

Phimosis carries a good prognosis, if treated appropriately. In acute cases that are complicated, paraphimosis may develop in which the glans becomes swollen and painful, and the foreskin is trapped behind the glans in a partially retracted position. Chronic complications consist of discomfort or pain during urination or sexual intercourse, urinary dribbling, and rarely urinary obstruction. Other potential complications include penile carcinoma with a relative risk of 3.5 in patients with history of phimosis[5].

DIAGNOSIS AND TREATMENT

Phimosis is a clinical diagnosis, and laboratory and imaging studies are not indicated. Phimosis in physiologic states is best treated by proper hygiene, frequent massaging, and the liberal use of emollients. In symptomatic cases, initial therapeutic options include topical steroids for a period of 4 weeks. If this fails, then surgical manipulation in the form of circumcision, dorsal slitting of the prepuce, or preputioplasty may be suitable alternatives[3].

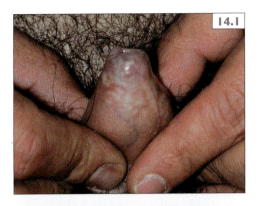

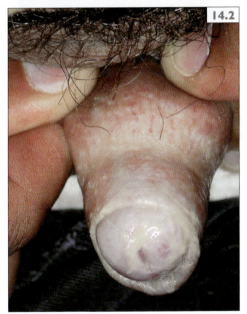

14.1, 14.2 Phimosis. (Courtesy of Dr. Shukrallah Zaynoun, Beirut, Lebanon.)

Hypospadias

DEFINITION

Hypospadias is a congenital anomaly in which the urethral opening is ectopically located on the ventrum of the penis proximal to the tip of the glans (**14.3**). The urethral opening may be located anywhere on the glans, and may even reach down to the scrotum or perineum.

ETIOLOGY AND EPIDEMIOLOGY

Hypospadias results when fusion of the urethral folds is faulty during organogenesis at between 8 and 15 weeks of gestation. Most cases of hypospadias are sporadic, and less than 7% of patients will have a positive family history. Many endocrine abnormalities have been implicated in its etiology; these include: deficient testosterone production by the testes, failure of conversion of testosterone to dihydrotestosterone (DHT), decreased numbers of androgen receptors in the penis, and reduced binding of DHT to the androgen receptors[6]. Estrogens and progestins given during pregnancy may increase the incidence of this anomaly.

Hypospadias is one of the most common congenital defects, occurring in approximately 1 in 250 live births[7]. In recent decades, its incidence has been increasing around the world partly owing to increased utilization of *in vitro* fertilization and maternal exposure to drugs such as progesterones, anti-inflammatory drugs, antihypertensives, diethylstilbestrol, and antipsychotics among others[8].

CLINICAL PRESENTATION

The position of the urethral meatus may be distal (glandular, coronal, or subcoronal), midpenile, or proximal (posterior penile, penoscrotal, scrotal, or perineal). The subcoronal position is the most common, accounting for 65% of cases. Proximal hypospadias is the most severe and is seen in 10–15% of cases[9]. A proximally displaced urethral meatus may typically have a stenotic appearance. With more proximal urethral defects, the penis develops an associated ventral shortening curvature or chordee. Approximately 8–10% of boys with hypospadias, especially of the more proximal types, may have cryptorchidism and 9–15% may have an associated inguinal hernia[10].

LABORATORY STUDIES

Laboratory studies are not indicated for either distal or middle hypospadias. Screening for a urinary tract anomaly by renal ultrasonography is in order in patients with proximal hypospadias and in those with additional clinical associations. Hormonal assays including 17-hydroxyprogesterone, testosterone, luteinizing hormone, and follicle stimulating hormone should be considered in more severe cases.

COURSE, PROGNOSIS, AND COMPLICATIONS

Children with hypospadias have normal onset of puberty and their fertility is not affected unless the patient has cryptorchidism, a chromosomal abnormality, or a varicocele. After corrective surgery, most patients are able to void in the standing position and are capable of completing normal sexual intercourse.

DIAGNOSIS AND TREATMENT

Hypospadias is essentially a clinical diagnosis. The only treatment of hypospadias is surgical repair with the objectives of reconstructing a straight penis (orthoplasty) with a slit-like meatus at the tip of the glans (urethroplasty), and allowing a forward-directed stream and normal coitus. The optimal timing for hypospadias surgery is at 6 months of age in an otherwise healthy newborn.

14.3 Hypospadias. (Courtesy of Dr. Tomasz F. Mroczkowski.)

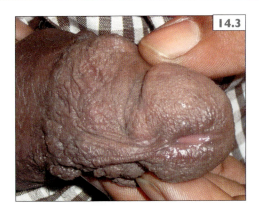

14.3

Epispadias

DEFINITION
Epispadias is a rare congenital anomaly in which the urethra opens on the dorsum of the penis, with deficient corpus spongiosum and loosely attached corpora cavernosa.

ETIOLOGY AND EPIDEMIOLOGY
Epispadias results from the faulty migration of the genital tubercle primordii to the cloacal membrane, resulting in a malformed genital tubercle, at around the 5th week of gestation. The incidence of complete epispadias is approximately 1 in 120,000 boys and 1 in 450,000 girls[11].

CLINICAL PRESENTATION
Depending upon the location of the opening, male epispadias may be classified as glandular, penile, or penopubic. The penopubic form is the most serious, and clinically these patients will have an associated dorsal groove extending through the glans, and an underlying separation of the pubic bones resulting in disruption of the bladder neck and incontinence. Epispadias may also be coupled with a dorsal chordee. Epispadias of the girl occurs when the urethra is displaced anteriorly, exiting in the clitoris or even more proximal. The clitoris is typically bifid, the mons is flattened, the labia are separated, and incontinence is the rule. Approximately 90% of cases of male epispadias are associated with bladder exstrophy, which occurs once in every 50,000 live births[12].

COURSE, PROGNOSIS, AND COMPLICATIONS
The prognosis for epispadias depends on the extent of the defect. Boys with minor epispadias will lead normal lives, and their fertility will not be affected. With more serious defects, patients may suffer complications such as incontinence, infertility, depression, and sexual dysfunction, even after successful surgery. Epispadias in girls can be surgically repaired, with minor residual deformities, and unaffected fertility.

DIAGNOSIS, LABORATORY STUDIES, AND TREATMENT
Epispadias is clinically identified at birth. With more proximal defects, or with associated bladder exstrophy, imaging studies are indicated. Voiding cystourethrography may uncover reflux, which if untreated can eventually lead to renal failure. Magnetic resonance imaging may be helpful in assessing the urethral defect and planning surgical correction.

Treatment consists of correction of penile curvature, reconstruction of the urethra, and fixing the bladder neck in incontinent patients. The surgery should be performed during the first 7 years of life.

Pearly penile papules

DEFINITION

Pearly penile papules (PPP), also known as Tyson's glands, hirsutoid papillomas, papilla in the corona glandis, hirsutis papillary corona of the penis, and corona capilliti[13], are angiofibromas of the glans and the corona of the penis.

ETIOLOGY AND EPIDEMIOLOGY

PPP are structurally related to acral angiofibromas[14], since their histology closely resembles adenoma sebaceum, fibrous papules of the nose, subungual and periungual fibromas. No agreement has been reached on the exact incidence and prevalence of PPP, and reports on prevalence vary between 8% and 48%. One group[15] found these lesions in 20% of men between the ages of 16 and 78 years, whereas a higher prevalence of 48% was documented in a genitourinary medicine clinic in Cambridge, UK[16]. They have been described in boys as young as 11 years[17] and in men as old as 52 years[16], but seem to be most frequently present in pubertal boys and young men. The incidence is generally higher among black people and uncircumcised men[13].

CLINICAL PRESENTATION

PPP are commonly seen in clinics for sexually transmitted diseases (STD) and are a reason for anxiety in adolescents and young men. The papules are typically smooth, measure 1–4 mm in diameter, and are asymptomatic. They may be pink, white, yellow, or translucent. They are typically seen in single or double rows on the corona of the glans, and may partially or completely encircle the glans (**14.4–14.7**). They tend to be most prominent on the dorsum of the glans and diminish as they approach the frenum. Two reports have described ectopic PPP on the penile shaft, one in an 11-year-old boy without having the typical lesions on the corona[17], and another on the ventral aspect of the penis simultaneously with typical coronal lesions[18].

COURSE, PROGNOSIS, AND COMPLICATIONS

PPP are benign and are considered a physiologic variant of the normal penis. They harbor no malignant potential. Once they appear, they tend to persist throughout life; however, they gradually become less noticeable with increasing age.

DIAGNOSIS

Diagnosis is typically made on clinical grounds. No laboratory tests or imaging studies are indicated for PPP, although dermoscopic findings can be useful. Characteristic dermoscopic features include whitish-pink cobblestone appearance in a few rows, with central vessel structures surrounded by crescent-shaped rims[19]. Confirmation of the diagnosis may be achieved by histopathologic analysis. Typically, one sees enlarged vascular spaces, stellate fibroblasts, and dermal fibrosis. No human papillomavirus deoxyribonucleic acid could be identified in PPP when tested by polymerase chain reaction[20].

TREATMENT

PPP are benign, asymptomatic, and require no treatment except reassurance. Some individuals, however, elect to remove them for cosmetic reasons. Many therapies have been tried including cryotherapy, electrodessication, and CO_2 laser. CO_2 laser appears to be the most effective, with excellent cosmetic results, with the continuous wave CO_2 laser giving better results than the pulsed CO_2 laser[21]. The 2940 nm Er:YAG laser may also be used. A report revealed that 45 patients with PPP were successfully treated and at 1 year there were no complications[22].

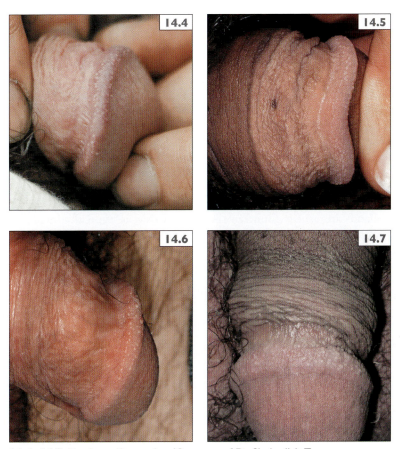

14.4–14.7 Pearly penile papules. (Courtesy of Dr. Shukrallah Zaynoun, Beirut, Lebanon.)

Ectopic sebaceous glands of Fordyce

DEFINITION

Ectopic sebaceous glands of Fordyce, also known as sebaceous gland prominence, Tyson's glands, and sebaceous hyperplasia, are normal variants of the skin of the scrotal sac and penile shaft. They are considered to be free sebaceous glands not connected to any hair follicles.

ETIOLOGY AND EPIDEMIOLOGY

Sebaceous glands are usually found in the skin in association with hair follicles as the pilosebaceous units. Ectopic sebaceous glands are considered to occur without hair follicles, typically in areas that are devoid of hair. They appear as tiny yellow papules on the vermillion border (Fordyce's spots), areola of the breast and labia (Montgomery tubercles), and prepuce and glans penis (Tyson's glands). Ectopic sebaceous glands of Fordyce are very common and are thought to occur in approximately one-third of men[23].

CLINICAL PRESENTATION

Ectopic sebaceous glands appear as asymptomatic, uniformly distributed 1–2 mm yellow papules on the penile shaft. The most common location in males is the inner aspect of the foreskin, followed by the frenulum. In women, they are classically located on the labia majora and the inner aspects of the labia minora. They may reach to numbers more than 100, and when inflamed, they may get larger and more prominent (**14.8**).

DIAGNOSIS AND TREATMENT

Diagnosis is typically made clinically; however, a biopsy can be performed for confirmation. Histology reveals sebaceous glands in the upper dermis with lobules of varying sizes that appear hyperplasic, yet are similar to those found with normal sebaceous glands. Because they are harmless, the patient only needs to be reassured.

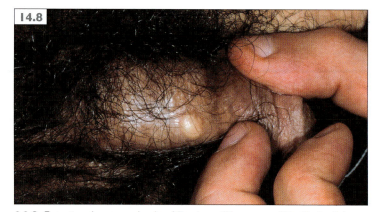

14.8 Ectopic sebaceous glands of Fordyce. (Courtesy of Dr. Shukrallah Zaynoun, Beirut, Lebanon.)

Endometriosis

DEFINITION, ETIOLOGY, AND EPIDEMIOLOGY

Endometriosis is the presence of ectopic endometrial glands and stroma outside the endometrial cavity. The most widely accepted assumption for the pathogenesis of endometriosis is the 'hypothesis of migration', whereby ectopic endometrial tissue migrates into the fallopian tubes and ovaries. Rarely, the same tissue can travel to the rest of the abdominal cavity and even appear in the umbilicus or vulvar regions as cutaneous nodules. There have been instances of vascular or lymphatic spread, and occasionally gynecologic surgery may trigger seeding into the abdominal cavity or cutaneous scars[24]. These ectopic endometrial foci respond to circulating hormones and may show secretory changes during the second half of the menstrual cycle. Endometriosis is a common gynecologic condition that affects up to 22% of all women[25]. Only 1.1% of all cases of endometriosis involve the skin, with scar endometriosis being the commonest form[26].

CLINICAL PRESENTATION AND LABORATORY STUDIES

The typical cutaneous finding is a blue tender nodule, often seen in the perineum, vagina, inguinal region, umbilical area, or within surgical scars. These lesions vary in size and tenderness with the menstrual cycle. Menstrual pain, dyspareunia, and infertility are the most common gynecologic complaints.

The possibility of simultaneous genital–pelvic endometriosis should be considered. Hormonal work-up is necessary when there is coexistent pelvic endometriosis.

COURSE, PROGNOSIS, AND COMPLICATIONS

The cutaneous lesions continue to wax and wane until identified. More widespread involvement leads to significant pain and distress. There have been case reports of malignant transformation in cutaneous endometriosis, especially in patients with long-standing and recurrent disease. Clear-cell carcinoma is the most common histological subtype, followed by endometrioid carcinoma[27].

DIAGNOSIS AND TREATMENT

Dermoscopy can be used to aid the diagnosis of endometriosis, and pathognomonic dermoscopic features include a homogenous reddish pigmentation that is regularly distributed, with small dark red globular structures within the pigmentation[28]. The mainstay of diagnosis is histology, where typical glandular and stromal tissue of the endometrium are seen lying within the dermis.

Excision is the mainstay of treatment of this condition, and local wide excision to ensure complete removal is curative. With more widespread disease, the choice lies between surgical excision and suppression of endometrial function. Danazol is the most commonly used drug, given at a dose of 400–800 mg daily for 6 months[29].

Median raphe cyst

DEFINITION

Median raphe cysts, also known as mucous cysts of the penis, genitoperineal cyst of the median raphe, parameatal cyst, hydrocystoma, and apocrine cystadenoma of the penile shaft[30], is an embryologic developmental abnormality of the male genitalia.

ETIOLOGY AND EPIDEMIOLOGY

Different histogenetic explanations have been implicated in the etiology of median raphe cysts, including an incomplete fusion of the urethral folds, or an abnormal formation of epithelial buds from the urethral epithelium that then became sequestrated and independent after closure of the median raphe[31].

CLINICAL PRESENTATION

The cysts most commonly develop on the ventral surface of the penis, typically near the glans, but they can occur anywhere from the urinary meatus to the anus. They most commonly present as asymptomatic, less than 1 cm dermal lesions in young men, and may appear suddenly after sexual intercourse-related trauma. The lesions are usually cystic, but sometimes they appear like an elongated structure called a raphe canal. Melanocytes may occasionally be present in the cyst wall, giving the cysts a pigmented appearance[32]. These congenital anomalies are rare, and are reported equally among pediatric and adult populations (**14.9**).

DIAGNOSIS

These lesions are typically diagnosed based upon clinical criteria. Excision reveals a well circumscribed cystic cavity with a well formed granular layer. The lining epithelium of these cysts differs according to the origin of the urethra in that segment, i.e. stratified in the distal part (ectodermal origin) and columnar pseudostratified in the remainder of the urethra (endodermal origin)[31]. The cysts never connect with the urethra.

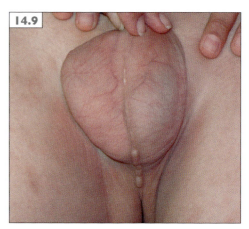

14.9 Median raphe cyst. (Courtesy of Dr. Shukrallah Zaynoun, Beirut, Lebanon.)

COURSE, PROGNOSIS, AND COMPLICATIONS

Median raphe cysts are benign lesions. The cysts tend to grow as the child grows, and, therefore, clinical symptoms are more likely to occur in adulthood. Although asymptomatic until adulthood, they may become traumatized and secondarily infected by *Neisseria gonorrhoeae* or *Staphylococcus aureus*, producing swelling, tenderness, and purulent discharge[33]. Spontaneous regression has been reported[34].

TREATMENT

The treatment of choice is simple excision followed by primary closure[35]. Some canals have been successfully treated by marsupialization or by surgical incision followed by electrosurgical destruction of the epithelial lining[36].

CHAPTER 15

Benign Tumors

Shaily Patel, MD, Arlene Ruiz de Luzuriaga, MD, and Vesna Petronic-Rosic, MD, MSc

- **Acrochordons (skin tags)**
- **Vestibular papillae of the vulva**
- **Seborrheic keratoses**
- **Lipoma**
- **Neurofibroma**
- **Epidermoid cyst (follicular cyst, infundibular type)**
- **Vaginal cysts of embryonic origin**
- **Steatocystoma**
- **Vulvar and penile melanocytic lesions**
- **Scrotal calcinosis**
- **Fox–Fordyce disease**
- **Hidradenoma papilliferum**
- **Syringoma**

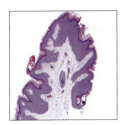
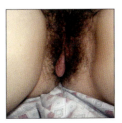
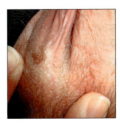
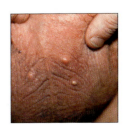

Acrochordons (skin tags)

DEFINITION, ETIOLOGY, AND EPIDEMIOLOGY

Acrochordons, or skin tags, are benign fleshy papules that commonly occur on the neck, axillae, and groin[1].

Acrochordons can be found in 25–60% of individuals. The incidence rises with age. Men and women are equally affected. Although the etiology is unknown, they occur with higher frequency in obesity, pregnancy, and diabetes. There may also be a familial tendency to the development of multiple skin tags[1].

CLINICAL PRESENTATION

Clinically, these lesions are small, flesh-colored or brown papules, 1–10 mm in size (**15.1**). Papules may be sessile or pedunculated[1].

COURSE, PROGNOSIS, AND COMPLICATIONS

Acrochordons are benign skin lesions that do not require treatment and may persist indefinitely. They can, however, become irritated by friction, jewelry, or clothing. If torsed, skin tags become painful and tender. Thrombosed skin tags can appear black and hemorrhagic and eventually will fall off on their own[1].

DIAGNOSIS

Diagnosis is based on clinical appearance and rarely requires a biopsy. The differential diagnosis may include nevi, seborrheic keratoses, and warts. Histopathologic evaluation will show a polypoid lesion with a flattened epidermis and loose to dense collagenous stroma with thin-walled dilated blood vessels in the center (**15.2**)[1].

TREATMENT

Asymptomatic acrochordons do not require treatment, although patients may request removal for aesthetic reasons. In such cases, scissor excision can be employed either with or without local anesthesia. Electrocautery and cryosurgery can also be used[1].

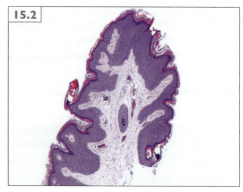

15.1 Acrochordons (skin tags) in the genital area. (Courtesy of Dr. Tomasz F. Mroczkowski.)

15.2 Acrochordon. Polypoid lesion with a loose collagenous stroma and dilated blood vessels (H&E, ×40).

Vestibular papillae of the vulva

DEFINITION, ETIOLOGY, AND EPIDEMIOLOGY

Vestibular papillae are small, smooth asymptomatic projections considered to be normal anatomical variants of the vulvar epithelium[2].

They are present in approximately 1% of women and are thought to be the female equivalent of pearly penile papules found on the corona of the glans penis[2,3].

CLINICAL PRESENTATION

Clinically, soft, flesh-colored, smooth, 1–5 mm papules are distributed in a symmetric, linear array, located on the inner surface of the labia minora[2] (**15.3**).

COURSE, PROGNOSIS, AND COMPLICATIONS

Since they are generally asymptomatic, no specific interventions are necessary. In rare cases, they may be accompanied by itching, pain, and burning that is managed with supportive care[2]. There are no complications associated with vestibular papillae[2-4].

DIAGNOSIS

Diagnosis is mainly based on clinical findings; however, vestibular papillae have often been confused with condylomata acuminata[3]. To clinically differentiate between vestibular papillae and condylomata acuminata, application of 5% acetic acid can be performed. The former should not whiten[4].

Dermatoscopy may also aid in the diagnosis and will demonstrate abundant irregular vascular channels within uniform cylindrical papillae with separate bases. This differs from condylomata acuminata, which have multiple irregular projections with tapering ends arising from a common base[4].

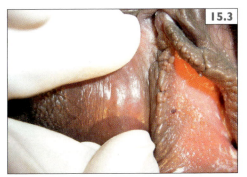

15.3 Vestibular papillae. Multiple smooth excrescences on the inner side of the labium minoris. (Courtesy of Dr. Tomasz F. Mroczkowski.)

Finally, if performed, a skin biopsy would reveal acanthosis and papillomatosis, without any viral cytopathic effects[2,4]. Polymerase chain reaction studies are negative for human papillomavirus[3].

TREATMENT

Given the benign course of these lesions, no treatment is required; however, establishing the correct diagnosis is essential to avoid unnecessary therapeutic interventions and to provide reassurance to patients[4].

Seborrheic keratoses

DEFINITION

Seborrheic keratoses are extremely common benign skin lesions that typically appear later in life and may occur at any site, invariably sparing the mucosal surfaces and the palms and soles[5].

ETIOLOGY AND EPIDEMIOLOGY

These lesions are the most common benign tumor in older individuals, affecting men and women equally. Incidence varies based on age, and can approach upwards of 80%. Although no specific etiologic factors have been identified, they occur more frequently in sunlight-exposed areas and may be hereditary[5].

CLINICAL PRESENTATION

There are many clinical and histological variants of seborrheic keratoses and a wide variety of clinical appearances. Classically, they present as oval, slightly raised, brown to black, sharply demarcated papules and plaques, 5–30 mm in size (**15.4**)[5]. The surface can be smooth, velvety, or verrucous, often with a 'stuck-on' appearance, keratotic plugging, and follicular prominence. In areas of friction, they tend to be smooth and pedunculated, resembling skin tags[6].

COURSE, PROGNOSIS, AND COMPLICATIONS

Seborrheic keratoses follow a benign course and tend to persist and grow slowly. If they become irritated or inflamed, lesions may be removed[5]. Typically, they do not result in complications, although development of malignant neoplasms within them or in a collision pattern has been described in 0.1–5% of cases[7].

DIAGNOSIS

Most seborrheic keratoses can be diagnosed clinically; however, they can resemble or harbor other proliferations including verrucae, squamous cell and basal cell carcinoma, solar lentigines, nevi, and melanoma[5-7]. Histopathologic evaluation reveals varying degrees of hyperkeratosis, acanthosis, and papillomatosis. Horn pseudocysts are characteristic (**15.5**)[5].

TREATMENT

No treatment is necessary for seborrheic keratoses, but they can be removed if they are symptomatic, become irritated and/or inflamed, or for cosmetic purposes. Removal techniques include shave excision, curettage, cryotherapy, laser ablation, and electrodessication[5].

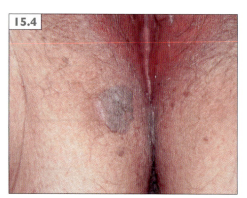

15.4 Seborrheic keratosis in the anogenital region. (Courtesy of Dr. Tomasz F. Mroczkowski.)

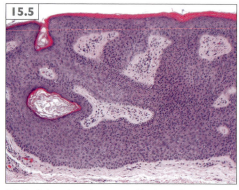

15.5 Seborrheic keratosis. Epidermal acanthosis with the presence of a horn pseudocyst (H&E, ×100).

Lipoma

DEFINITION
Lipomas are very common, benign subcutaneous tumors composed of fatty tissue. Most frequently, they are found on the trunk, but can also occur on the neck, extremities, axillae, scrotum, and vulva[8].

ETIOLOGY AND EPIDEMIOLOGY
Lipomas are the most common benign soft tissue neoplasm in adults, and may affect males slightly more than females[8,9]. The etiology is unknown; however, trauma has been suggested and alterations in chromosomes 12q13–15 and 13q12–22 may be detected[8]. Genital lipomas are rare, with only four reported cases of primary scrotal lipomas[9,10].

CLINICAL PRESENTATION
Lipomas present as asymptomatic, subcutaneous, mobile, rubbery soft, compressible nodules (**15.6**)[8]. In the groin, they are typically solitary[9]. Vulvar lipomas arise as subcutaneous masses and become pendulous and dependent. Similarly, primary scrotal lipomas can be pedunculated[9,10].

COURSE, PROGNOSIS, AND COMPLICATIONS
Lipomas are benign tumors that require no treatment[8]. They occasionally cause discomfort if they grow large enough to compress adjacent structures[9]. When multiple lipomas are present, there may be a familial component[8]. Complications are rare; still, any lipoma that continues to grow or becomes painful should be excised for further evaluation[9,10].

DIAGNOSIS AND TREATMENT
A majority of lipomas can be diagnosed clinically; however, for definitive diagnosis, biopsy should be performed. Histologically, a lipoma is an encapsulated, lobulated tumor containing normal adipocytes held together by fibrous strands of connective tissue (**15.7**)[8].

No treatment is required. Surgical excision or removal via liposuction may be performed if indicated and is usually curative[8].

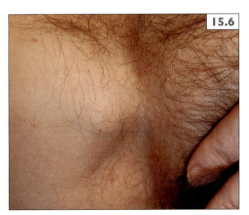

15.6 Lipoma. Subcutaneous soft compressible nodule.

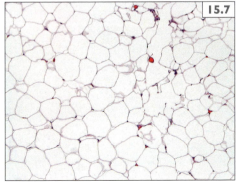

15.7 Lipoma. The lesion demonstrates mature adipose tissue with fibrous strands of connective tissue (H&E, ×200).

Neurofibroma

DEFINITION
Neurofibromas are benign tumors of neuromesenchymal origin that commonly occur on the trunk and head[11].

ETIOLOGY AND EPIDEMIOLOGY
Solitary neurofibromas are relatively common with no predilection for either gender. Patients with multiple neurofibromas or plexiform neurofibromas should undergo evaluation for neurofibromatosis[11]. Genital involvement is rare, but has been reported on the penis, scrotum, and vulva[12].

CLINICAL PRESENTATION
Neurofibromas are soft, skin-colored to pink-tan papules or nodules, usually 0.2–2.0 cm in size. They may become pedunculated and grow slowly, but are generally asymptomatic (**15.8**)[11]. Given their soft, compressible nature, they can be invaginated easily (the 'buttonhole sign'). Plexiform neurofibromas are considered pathognomonic of neurofibromatosis, and are typically large, baggy, pedunculated, or rope-like dermal and subcutaneous tumors[11,12].

COURSE, PROGNOSIS, AND COMPLICATIONS
Neurofibromas are benign. Occasionally, they may bleed or cause pain. A small percent of plexiform neurofibromas undergo malignant transformation, so regular clinical follow-up is recommended[11].

DIAGNOSIS AND TREATMENT
Diagnosis is based on clinical appearance in addition to histopathology, as the differential diagnosis includes nevi, soft fibromas, and dermatofibromas[11,12]. Histologically, neurofibromas are more or less well-circumscribed dermal and/or subcutaneous nodules composed of a fine fibrillary lattice of haphazardly organized spindle cells (**15.9**). The stroma can range from fibrotic to myxomatous. Mast cells, fibroblasts, Schwann cells, and perineural cells can all be present[11].

No treatment is necessary; simple excision is curative[11,12].

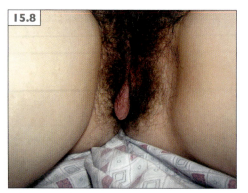

15.8 Neurofibroma. Soft, pink-tan pedunculated nodule.

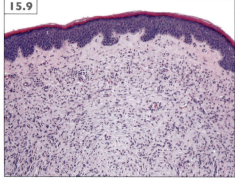

15.9 Neurofibroma. There is a proliferation of spindle cells in the dermis surrounded by an eosinophilic stroma containing mast cells (H&E, ×100).

Epidermoid cyst (follicular cyst, infundibular type)

DEFINITION
Epidermoid cysts are the most common cutaneous cyst and can occur anywhere on the body, most commonly on the face and upper trunk[13].

ETIOLOGY AND EPIDEMIOLOGY
Epidermoid cysts usually arise after puberty and affect men and women equally. They may be primary or arise from disrupted follicular structures or traumatically implanted epithelium[13]. Vaginal and scrotal cysts are common[14].

CLINICAL PRESENTATION
Epidermoid cysts present as firm, well-demarcated, mobile, dermal nodules that can range in size from a few millimeters to several centimeters. A punctum may be visible, which represents the hair follicle infundibulum from which the cyst is derived (**15.10, 15.11**)[13].

COURSE, PROGNOSIS, AND COMPLICATIONS
Epidermoid cysts are benign and most frequently asymptomatic. They can enlarge and become inflamed due to a foreign body reaction to keratin extruded into the dermis[13]. In such instances, removal is recommended.

DIAGNOSIS
Diagnosis is usually clinical. Histopathologic examination reveals a cystic cavity lined by stratified squamous epithelium with a granular layer. It is filled with laminated keratin (**15.12**). Occasionally, a foreign body granulomatous inflammatory cell infiltrate can be seen surrounding the cyst[13].

TREATMENT
No treatment is necessary for uncomplicated epidermoid cysts. Simple excision is curative if the entire cyst wall is removed. When inflamed, cysts may require incision and drainage, and occasionally antibiotic therapy. Intralesional triamcinolone may also aid in reducing inflammation[13].

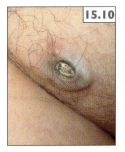 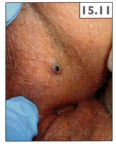

15.10, 15.11 Cyst. Firm, well-demarcated, mobile dermal nodule, with dilated punctum.

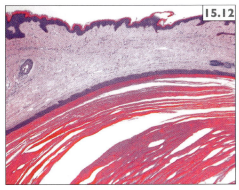

15.12 Epidermal cyst. Within the dermis is a cyst formed of squamous epithelium with a granular layer, and containing loosely-packed keratin fragments (H&E, ×40).

Vaginal cysts of embryonic origin

DEFINITION

Benign cystic lesions of the vagina and surrounding tissues originate from Müllerian or mesonephric remnants. The most common types are Müllerian cysts, Gartner's duct cysts, Bartholin's gland cysts, and Skene's duct cysts[14,15].

ETIOLOGY AND EPIDEMIOLOGY

The reported incidence of vaginal cysts is likely underestimated at 1 in 200 women, as many are not reported[14,16,17]. Müllerian cysts are formed from persistent Müllerian epithelial tissue in the vaginal wall[16]. Gartner's duct cysts arise from vestigial remnants of mesonephric ducts[14]. Bartholin's gland cysts are of urogenital sinus origin, and are homologous to the bulbourethral glands in males[14,18]. Skene's duct cysts are prostatic homologs that form after obstruction of the ducts, usually from infection[14].

CLINICAL PRESENTATION

Müllerian cysts are generally located in the anterolateral vaginal wall, and can range in size from 1 cm to 7 cm in diameter[14,16]. Gartner's duct cysts are often smaller, with an average size of 2 cm, but may enlarge[14]. Bartholin's gland cysts are unilateral, nontender cystic structures located medial to the labia minora and lateral to the introitus[14,18]. Skene's duct cysts rarely exceed 2 cm[14].

COURSE, PROGNOSIS, AND COMPLICATIONS

All these cysts are benign and can be followed clinically[14,15]. Occasionally, they may grow and become symptomatic causing dysuria and dyspareunia. They can also become infected and inflamed[14].

DIAGNOSIS

Histologic evaluation is necessary to establish the diagnosis. Müllerian cysts have a mucinous epithelium of endocervical, endometrial, or fallopian tube origin[16,17]. The lining is composed of simple columnar ciliated epithelium with abundant mucin within the cytoplasm. Small papillary infoldings can also be visualized[15]. In contrast, Gartner's cysts are lined by cuboidal, nonciliated, nonmucinous cells[14,17]. Bartholin's gland cysts may be lined by transitional, squamous, or mucinous columnar epithelium, depending on the site of origin[14,18]. Skene's duct cysts are lined by stratified squamous epithelium as they are derived from the urogenital sinus[14].

TREATMENT

No treatment is necessary; however, surgical excision is indicated for large or symptomatic cysts[15]. For a more conservative option, needle aspiration can also be performed[18].

Steatocystoma

DEFINITION

Steatocystoma is a rare benign cutaneous cyst of sebaceous origin. If solitary, it is referred to as steatocystoma simplex[19]. When multiple, it is referred to as steatocystoma multiplex, which may be sporadic or inherited as an autosomal dominant trait characterized by multiple cysts on the trunk and extremities[19,20]. Infrequently, they can involve the vulva, scrotum, and penis[19,21].

ETIOLOGY AND EPIDEMIOLOGY

Steatocystoma is rare, with an equal frequency in adult women and men[19]. It classically presents during adolescence and early adulthood[19-21]. Steatocystoma multiplex is due to mutations in *KRT17*, the gene that encodes for keratin 17; however, they are not found in spontaneous forms[19,20]. Given the fact that lesions tend to arise around puberty, a hormonal trigger has been implicated[21].

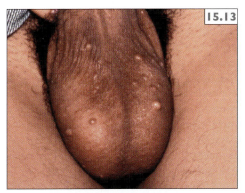

15.13 Steatocystoma multiplex. (Courtesy of Dr. Tomasz F. Mroczkowski.)

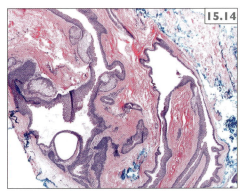

15.14 Steatocystoma (H&E, ×40). There is a cystic structure with a convoluted wall visible within the dermis.

CLINICAL PRESENTATION

Steatocystoma simplex is typically a 0.5–1.5 cm cyst. Rarely, they can be larger, with reports of solitary steatocystomas over 8 cm in size. The cyst contains an oily yellowish fluid that may house vellus hairs[19]. Steatocystoma multiplex classically presents with numerous uniform yellowish, cystic 2–6 mm papules (**15.13**). They tend to affect the trunk, upper extremities, and axillae more frequently but can be seen on the face, scalp, and genital area[19-21].

COURSE, PROGNOSIS, AND COMPLICATIONS

The course is chronic. A majority of these lesions are asymptomatic and do not lead to complications; however, they may become inflamed and infected requiring treatment[19]. In addition, steatocystoma multiplex can be part of pachyonychia congenita type 2[21]. These patients have numerous pilosebaceous cysts in addition to nail dystrophy, natal teeth, and hair abnormalities[19,21].

DIAGNOSIS

Diagnosis is based on clinical and pathological findings. Histological examination demonstrates a cystic structure lined by stratified squamous epithelium containing mature sebaceous glands (**15.14**).

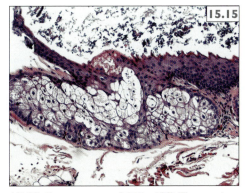

15.15 Steatocystoma (H&E, ×100). The cyst is lined by an eosinophilic cuticle. Sebaceous glands abut the cyst wall.

The luminal surface has a characteristic eosinophilic, corrugated cuticle (**15.15**)[19].

TREATMENT

Treatment is challenging, especially in extensive cases. Anti-inflammatory and antibiotic treatment, excision, needle aspiration, dermabrasion, cryotherapy, laser ablation, and incision and drainage with extraction have all been utilized with limited efficacy[19, 22,23]. Isotretinoin may be helpful in the suppurative variant[19].

Vulvar and penile melanocytic lesions

DEFINITION, ETIOLOGY, AND EPIDEMIOLOGY

Benign pigmented lesions of the genital region are melanotic macules, lentigines, and melanocytic nevi[24].

The overall prevalence of genital melanotic macules, lentigines, and melanocytic nevi is not well documented; however, pigmented lesions have been estimated to occur in about 10–20% of patients; the majority are lentigines[24-26].

CLINICAL PRESENTATION

Pigmented lesions of the genitalia present as brown to black macules/patches or papules/plaques, usually with a smooth surface and well-demarcated borders (**15.16–15.18**)[24-29]. They can range in size from several millimeters to many centimeters, and occur on both glabrous and nonglabrous skin[24-26]. Lentigines can be large and may have irregular, asymmetric borders (**15.19**)[24].

COURSE, PROGNOSIS, AND COMPLICATIONS

Typically, these lesions follow a benign clinical course. They tend to be asymptomatic and many patients are unaware of their presence. Occasionally, they will grow; this type of change often requires a biopsy to evaluate for malignancy[26,29]. If numerous, lentigines may indicate a multisystem disorder such as: Peutz–Jeghers syndrome, LEOPARD syndrome, Carney complex, Bannayan–Riley–Ruvalcaba syndrome, and Laugier–Hunziker syndrome, among others[24,28].

DIAGNOSIS

Genital melanotic macules, lentigines, and nevi require biopsy for diagnosis and to exclude malignant melanocytic proliferations. Melanotic macules demonstrate epithelial hyperplasia with basilar hyperpigmentation, predominantly of the rete tips[29]. If the melanocytes are present in a lentiginous pattern (single cells along the dermal–epidermal junction), they are referred to as lentigo[26].

Melanocytic nevi, in contrast, will contain nests of melanocytes, and resemble nevi at other locations (**15.20**)[24]. Of note, there is a special subset of nevi, referred to as atypical melanocytic nevi of the genital type, which can have features that overlap with melanoma[26]. These include dyscohesive and crowded nests of variable size, architectural disorder, cellular atypia, pagetoid spread, and dense fibrosis in the dermis[24,26,27]. It is exceedingly important to identify and distinguish these nevi on a special site from melanoma.

TREATMENT

Biopsy should be performed to evaluate for any atypical features. If benign, no treatment is necessary. Complete excision can be done for any atypical melanocytic proliferations that defy classification or clinically concerning lesions[24-26].

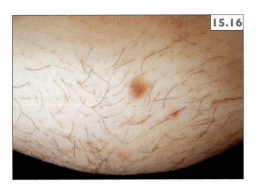

15.16 Nevus. Well-defined, tan, evenly pigmented macule.

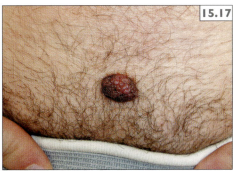

15.17 Nevus. Well-defined, pink-brown nodule with mamillated surface.

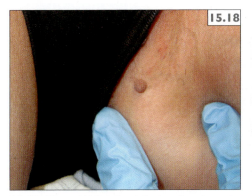

15.18 Nevus. Well defined, flesh-colored papule.

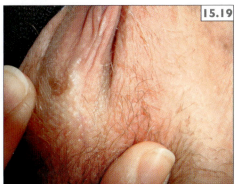

15.19 Lentigo. Light tan macule.

15.20 Nevus. There are nests of melanocytes both at the dermal–epidermal junction and in the dermis (H&E, ×40).

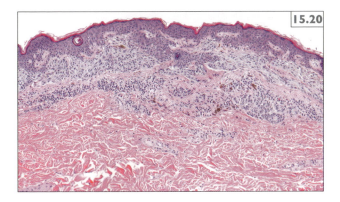

Scrotal calcinosis

DEFINITION
Scrotal calcinosis is a benign disorder in which calcified nodules occur on the scrotum[30]. It is the most common form of idiopathic calcinosis cutis[31].

ETIOLOGY AND EPIDEMIOLOGY
Some authors believe scrotal calcinosis results from calcification of scrotal epidermoid cysts, while others believe it is the result of dystrophic calcification[32]. Scrotal calcinosis is rare. It occurs any time from childhood to adulthood. Nodules tend to increase gradually in size and number over time[31,33].

CLINICAL PRESENTATION
Often multiple, these are firm, skin-colored to white, asymptomatic papules and nodules on the scrotum that range in size from several millimeters to 1 cm (**15.21, 15.22**)[31]. As they grow, lesions may become more yellowish and lobulated[30]. They are conspicuously hard on palpation[33].

COURSE, PROGNOSIS, AND COMPLICATIONS
Scrotal calcinosis is a benign condition that is mostly asymptomatic and uneventful. Occasionally, mild itching may be present. Some patients with numerous lesions report a sensation of heaviness[33]. Spontaneous breakdown can lead to discharge of white chalky material[30].

DIAGNOSIS AND TREATMENT
Scrotal calcinosis is usually a clinical diagnosis, although biopsy may be performed for histological confirmation. Examination of the biopsy specimen will reveal focal dermal collections of calcium that appear as deeply basophilic material when stained with hematoxylin and eosin (**15.23, 15.24**)[30,33]. A von Kossa stain will confirm the diagnosis. Occasionally, a foreign body reaction may develop around the deposits[33].

Clinical observation is recommended; however, surgical excision is curative for symptomatic or cosmetic purposes[31].

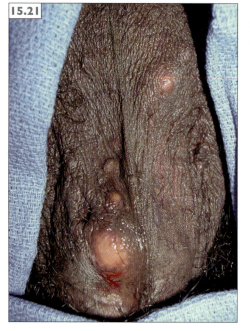

15.21 Scrotal calcinosis. Several firm, skin-colored to white, papules and nodules on the scrotum.

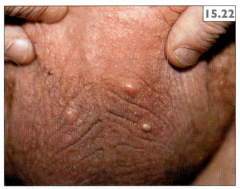

15.22 Scrotal calcinosis. Multiple small, firm, white and flesh-colored papules on the scrotum.

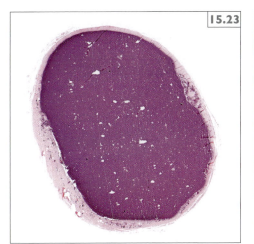

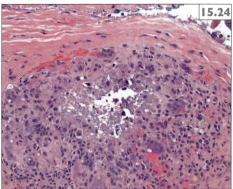

15.24 Scrotal calcinosis. Granulomatous inflammation in the dermis with some calcium deposits (H&E, ×200).

15.23 Scrotal calcinosis. The dermis contains an area of fibrosis with granulomatous inflammation and small collections of calcium (H&E, ×20).

Fox–Fordyce disease

DEFINITION, ETIOLOGY, AND EPIDEMIOLOGY

Fox–Fordyce disease, or apocrine miliaria, is characterized by multiple skin-colored papules that occur at sites with apocrine glands[34].

It is a rare condition that occurs in women at onset of adolescence or soon thereafter, with over 90% of cases occurring between the ages of 13 and 35 years. Rarely, it may occur in men or present postmenopausally[35]. No genetic defect or polymorphism has been identified[39]. It may be related to obstruction of the apocrine duct at its entrance to the follicular wall, which can lead to sweat retention, rupture, and inflammation[34,37].

CLINICAL PRESENTATION

Fox–Fordyce disease is characterized by uniform, flesh-colored to light brown, conical or dome-shaped 2–3 mm papules with a smooth surface[34–36]. They are folliculocentric and occur primarily in the axillae and areolae, but the umbilicus, pubis, labia majora, and perineum can also be involved[35]. Hairs are usually sparse in involved areas. They are extremely pruritic[37].

COURSE, PROGNOSIS, AND COMPLICATIONS

Fox–Fordyce disease is chronic and patients often present for treatment of pruritus, which can be severe[34]. Interestingly, pregnancy almost invariably leads to temporary improvement of the condition[35,36]. There are no known complications from the disease[34].

DIAGNOSIS

Diagnosis is based upon clinical and histopathologic features. As the differential is broad and includes various other conditions including lichen planus, lichen nitidus, eruptive syringomas, and folliculitis, biopsy should be performed to confirm the diagnosis[36,37]. The characteristic finding is obstruction of the follicular ostium by orthokeratotic cells. An inflammatory cell infiltrate composed primarily of lymphocytes surrounds the hair follicles and blood vessels. In addition, spongiosis of the infundibulum with vesiculation of the apocrine duct may be seen[35].

TREATMENT

Treatment can be challenging, and several methods have been employed. These include oral contraceptive pills, topical tretinoin, topical and intralesional steroids, topical clindamycin lotion, isotretinoin, and phototherapy[34,35]. In rare cases, surgical excision has been performed[37].

Hidradenoma papilliferum

DEFINITION, ETIOLOGY, AND EPIDEMIOLOGY

Hidradenoma papilliferum is a benign adnexal neoplasm of apocrine origin that almost exclusively arises on the vulva, perineum, or perianal region in women[19,38]. These lesions typically occur in postpubescent women, although there are exceedingly rare case reports of hidradenoma papilliferum occurring in men[19,39].

CLINICAL PRESENTATION

Clinically, the tumor is a firm, well circumscribed nodule, approximately 1 cm in diameter, covered by normal mucosa[19]. It tends to be solitary, flesh-colored, and cystic, commonly arising on the labia majora[40]. Occasionally, there can be multiple lesions[38].

COURSE, PROGNOSIS, AND COMPLICATIONS

Hidradenoma papilliferum is usually asymptomatic and follows a benign clinical course. Nevertheless, the lesion can ulcerate and bleed, which may require treatment. Some patients report pruritus[38,39].

DIAGNOSIS AND TREATMENT

Biopsy is typically necessary to confirm the diagnosis. Microscopic features include a pseudoencapsulated dermal nodule, with no epidermal connection (**15.25**). The nodule contains large cystic spaces with complex folds and papillary projections, lined by a single or double layer of columnar cells with eosinophilic cytoplasm. Decapitation secretion is usually present (**15.26**)[38].

Given the benign nature of this lesion, clinical observation is sufficient; however, for diagnostic confirmation or to treat symptomatic lesions, simple excision can be performed[19,38–40].

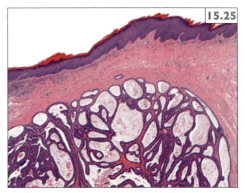

15.25 Hidradenoma papilliferum. There is a cystic lesion in the dermis forming a complex, papillary arrangement without apparent attachment to the dermis (H&E, ×40).

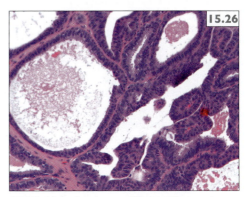

15.26 Hidradenoma papilliferum. The cystic lining is composed of columnar and cuboidal cells, some exhibiting decapitation secretion (H&E, ×200).

Syringoma

DEFINITION, ETIOLOGY, AND EPIDEMIOLOGY

Syringomas are benign eccrine neoplasms that most commonly occur around the eyes, but have been described on the neck, chest, axillae, hands, vulva, and penis[41–43].

Syringomas are fairly common. They tend to first appear around puberty and can increase in number with age[43]. Vulvar and penile lesions are far less common, with fewer than 100 cases reported in the literature; however, their prevalence is probably higher, as they often go unrecognized by both patients and physicians[41,43]. They are twice as common in women than in men[41].

CLINICAL PRESENTATION

Syringomas present as small, round to oval, yellow, brown, or pink papules[41]. Occasionally, they appear translucent or cystic. They are typically small, ranging from 1 mm to 3 mm in diameter, and are usually multiple. Their distribution can vary and may be linear, annular, or plaque-like, commonly symmetrical and/or bilateral[41,42]. In the eruptive variant, syringomas typically occur on the penis as well as the trunk[44].

COURSE, PROGNOSIS, AND COMPLICATIONS

Syringomas follow a benign but persistent course. Most are asymptomatic and as such are primarily a cosmetic concern to the patient; however, vulvar and penile syringomas can cause pain and pruritus[42,43]. Vulvar syringomas may also become more symptomatic and increase in size and number during pregnancy, premenstrually, or with oral contraceptives[41]. Patients with numerous syringomas or a familial predisposition should be examined carefully, as multiple lesions may occur in diabetes, Down, Brooke–Spiegler, Ehler–Danlos, Marfan, and Nicolau–Balus syndromes[41,42].

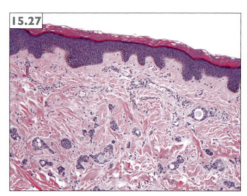

15.27 Syringoma. Within a fibrotic dermis are cords and strands of cuboidal cells, some featuring central lumina (H&E, ×100).

DIAGNOSIS

Although clinical appearance is typical, a biopsy may be performed for definitive diagnosis[45]. Dilated cystic spaces are lined by two layers of cuboidal cells and epithelial strands of similar cells (**15.27**)[41]. Some of the cysts have comma-like tails, resembling tadpoles or a paisley pattern[43]. In the clear cell variant, the cells have abundant clear cytoplasm[41].

TREATMENT

Treatment is largely for cosmesis and the goal is destruction of the lesion with minimal scarring. Various modalities have been utilized and include: surgical excision, electrocautery, electrodessication and curettage, laser ablation, cryotherapy, dermabrasion, and trichloroacetic acid; however, lesions often recur, and destructive treatments may lead to scarring. Reassurance and observation are recommended in most cases[41–44].

Skin Cancer of the Genitalia

Edward C. Monk, MD, and Anthony V. Benedetto, DO

- **Vulvar and penile intraepithelial neoplasia (squamous cell cancer *in situ*)**
- **Squamous cell cancer**
- **Basal cell cancer**
- **Melanoma**
- **Extramammary Paget's disease**
- **Kaposi's sarcoma**
- **Rare cancers of the genitalia**
- **So-called precancerous lesions**

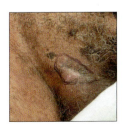
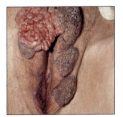
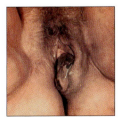
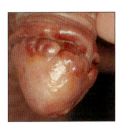

Skin cancer is not as common in the genital area as it is in the rest of the skin. This is likely due to the lack of ultraviolet light exposure as a carcinogen to this area; however, genital skin cancers are often more advanced and carry worse prognoses, when compared to their counterparts in other areas. This may be due to delays in diagnosis, differences in etiology, and differences in tumor environment; for example, a large portion of the genitalia is mucosa, which has high densities of blood and lymphatic vessels.

The most common malignancy of genital skin is squamous cell cancer (SCC). SCC accounts for approximately 90% of malignant tumors of the vulva and 5% of all gynecological cancers[1]. It represents 95% of penile cancers and 2% of all male genital cancers[2]. The sexually transmitted human papillomavirus (HPV) is mostly responsible for the high rate of SCC, as well as vulvar and penile intraepithelial neoplasias, essentially equivalents to SCC *in situ*. Although the other common skin cancers, basal cell cancer and melanoma, rarely present in the genitalia, they should be included in the differential diagnosis in certain clinical presentations and in at-risk patients. Extramammary Paget's disease is a rare skin cancer that has a proclivity toward the vulva when it occurs. Kaposi's sarcoma presents in certain at-risk populations and occasionally presents with a primary genital lesion. Finally, there are case reports of rare skin cancers presenting in the genitalia such as dermatofibrosarcoma protuberans and leiomyosarcoma.

Vulvar and penile intraepithelial neoplasia (squamous cell cancer *in situ*)

ETIOLOGY AND EPIDEMIOLOGY

Vulvar intraepithelial neoplasia (VIN) and its counterpart of the penis, PIN, are atypical neoplasias of keratinocytes confined to the epidermis, and considered to be precursors to invasive SCC[3,4] (**16.1**). VIN has undergone a recent change in classification, dropping the inclusion of low-grade lesions thought to have minimal potential for developing into invasive disease[4]. VIN can now be considered the equivalent of SCC *in situ* (SCCIS), encompassing Bowen's disease and bowenoid papulosis, which are clinical variants.

PIN has been graded based on dysplasia, with grades 2 and 3 considered to be the equivalent of SCCIS[3]. At this point there has not been a consensus in dropping low-grade (grade 1) PIN, which may carry minimal risk for developing into invasive disease.

VIN is classified, based on histological features into usual type, associated with HPV in 72–100% of cases and differentiated type, associated with chronic inflammation, most notably lichen sclerosus[4]. The usual type is more common and seen in younger patients. Some authors have recommended the same classification be adapted for PIN, which is associated with similar conditions to VIN, including HPV at a high rate similar to that of VIN[3]. The incidences of VIN and PIN have been increasing, likely related to the increase in all HPV infections[3,4].

CLINICAL PRESENTATION

Lesions of intraepithelial neoplasia (IN) may be red, white, or pigmented, with erosions or ulcers. Patients may experience pain or pruritus. In patients with a chronic inflammatory disease of the genitalia, such as lichen sclerosus or lichen planus, an eroded or irregular area may represent IN and should be biopsied. IN may be multicentric, and careful examinations of the cervix, vagina, and anus are warranted after diagnosis (**16.2**).

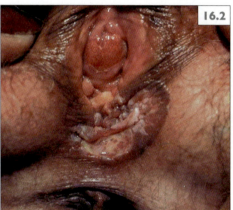

16.2 Discontiguous periurethral and perineal squamous cell cancer *in situ* demonstrating the field effect often seen in this region. Human papilloma virus testing was not available.

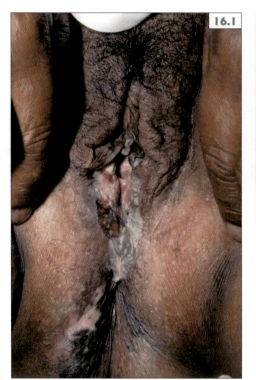

16.1 Squamous cell cancer *in situ* of the labia in a 60-year-old woman with surrounding lichen sclerosus.

IN has been given different names based on its clinical presentation. Bowen's disease is classically a well-demarcated plaque that may be scaly or ulcerated. It has been called erythroplasia of Queyrat, if located on the glans of the penis. Lesions of bowenoid papulosis are red to violaceous papules that may coalesce and resemble condyloma acuminata clinically (**16.3–16.5**).

DIFFERENTIAL DIAGNOSIS

The differential diagnosis includes condyloma acuminata, lichen sclerosus, lichen simplex chronicus, psoriasis, nummular eczema, tinea corporis, and extramammary Paget's disease.

LABORATORY STUDIES (HISTOPATHOLOGY)

The usual type, associated with HPV, may appear 'warty', with a papillomatous epidermal appearance along with cellular atypia; 'basaloid', with a thick yet flat epidermis containing undifferentiated cells and mitotic figures; or 'mixoid', a mix of the previous two. Differentiated type is associated with chronic inflammation, with atypia confined to the lower epidermis where cells are large and often form keratin pearls[4]. The differentiated type is subtler and may be confused with benign hyperplasia, despite its higher risk for invasive transformation versus usual type[4].

PIN has cellular atypia confined to the lower one-third and two-thirds of the skin in grades 1 and 2, respectively. There is full thickness atypia in grade 3 lesions[3].

PROGNOSIS

Measured rates of VIN progression to invasive disease vary greatly depending on the study and will likely be affected by the recent change in classification. There are cases of occult cancer when surgical specimens are analyzed that were preoperatively diagnosed as usual type of VIN, with rates of 3.8–18%[4]. The differentiated type of VIN consistently has shown a higher rate of progression than the usual type[4]. PIN has an overall rate of progression to invasive disease of 10–20% in higher-grade lesions. Bowenoid papulosis has a lower rate of invasive malignant transformation (1%)[3].

TREATMENT

Surgical and other destructive modalities, such as electrodessication and CO_2 laser ablation, have been employed to treat IN. These modalities carry high recurrence rates (20–40%)[3,4]. These high rates may be related to the associated HPV or chronic inflammation in tissue adjacent to IN, increasing the risk for dysplasias and eventual malignancy in this 'normal skin'. For this reason, a topical or more diffuse treatment regimen may benefit outcomes, or it may be employed in combination treatment with surgery. These treatments include antineoplastic methods, such as photodynamic therapy, topical 5-fluorouracil, and intralesional bleomycin. The antiviral agent, cidofovir, has been used for those lesions associated with HPV. Imiquimod, as an immune-modulator, also has efficacy in the treatment of IN[3,4]. While Mohs surgery is used for SCCIS in other locations with high success, data are limited to small case series for its use in the treatment of SCCIS in the genital area.

Vaccines exist designed to protect patients from the HPV types that are known to cause IN as well as SCC. There are case reports of clinical response to therapeutic administration of the vaccine to patients with IN[4].

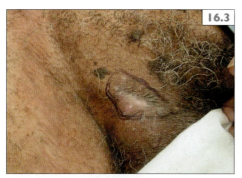

16.3 Squamous cell cancer *in situ* with discontinguous lesions of bowenoid papulosis in the surrounding area. While human papilloma virus testing was not available, there is a high likelihood for an association with the virus, and this demonstrates the way it can cause cancerous lesions by a field effect.

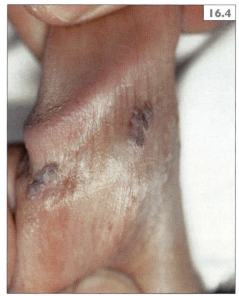

16.4 Bowenoid papulosis of the penile shaft.

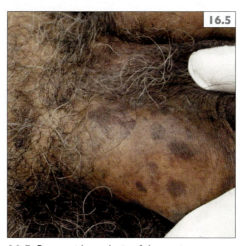

16.5 Bowenoid papulosis of the penis.

Squamous cell cancer

ETIOLOGY AND EPIDEMIOLOGY

SCC, similar to intraepithelial neoplasia (IN), is separated into HPV-independent and HPV-related disease. The associated HPV types are usually high risk, including 16, 18, 31, and 33[5].

Verrucous carcinoma, also known as giant condyloma of Buschke and Lowenstein (VC-GCBL) when located on the genitalia, is a less aggressive type of SCC, usually associated with HPV-6 and -11, low-risk types that are also associated with common condyloma acuminata[2]. Certain strains of HPV produce proteins that interact with host tumor suppressor function. For example, the gene products E6 and E7, coded for by high-risk HPV types associated with cancer, have been shown to lead to the dysfunction of the p53 and Rb tumor suppressor proteins, contributing to the development of cancer[1].

The second pathway is often associated with conditions of chronic inflammation, such as lichen sclerosus (**16.6, 16.7**). In women, this type of SCC is usually seen in the elderly, with risk factors including age and smoking[1]. In men, risk factors include age, smoking, chewing tobacco, lack of circumcision, balanitis, phimosis, poor penile hygiene, and lichen sclerosus[2].

CLINICAL PRESENTATION

Genital SCC may be white, brown, red, elevated, or ulcerated and may present with a cutaneous horn. Patients may be asymptomatic or experience itching, dyspareunia in women, soreness, or burning in association with genital SCC[1]. The most common location of vulvar SCC is the labia (80%), followed by the clitoris and the lower commissure[1]. The most common areas for penile SCC are the glans, prepuce, and shaft, in this order (**16.8, 16.9**). VC-GCBL presents clinically as a giant wart (**16.10**).

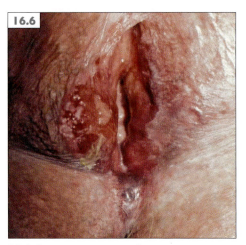

16.6 Invasive squamous cell cancer in surrounding lichen sclerosus.

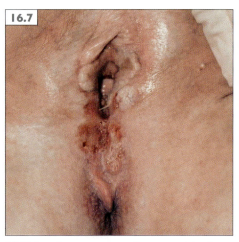

16.7 Invasive squamous cell cancer arising in lichen sclerosus in an elderly woman.

DIFFERENTIAL DIAGNOSIS

Differential diagnosis includes condyloma acuminata, lichen sclerosus, lichen simplex chronicus, psoriasis, extramammary Paget's disease, and chronic herpes virus infection in immunocompromised patients.

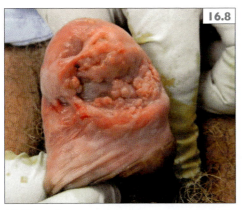

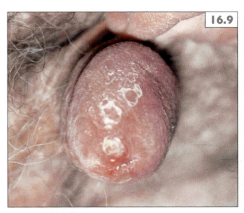

16.8 Invasive squamous cell cancer of the penis.

16.9 Invasive squamous cell cancer of the penis. Fibrinous tissue at the inferior edge represents the biopsy site.

LABORATORY STUDIES (HISTOPATHOLOGY)

SCC is a neoplasm of keratinocytes, in which cells are crowded, large, and pleomorphic. Individual keratinocytes mature and cornify abnormally, represented by parakeratosis, dyskeratosis, and the formation of keratin 'pearls'. Variations in level of atypia and pattern of invasion have led to numerous subclassifications of SCC.

VC-GCBL usually has squamous cancer cells in a well-differentiated, bulbous pattern histologically.

COURSE AND PROGNOSIS

Genital SCC has a high survival rate for localized disease. Lymph node involvement has the greatest prognostic value. The 5-year survival rate drops from over 90% to 50% when lymph nodes are involved[1,2,6].

In women, tumors >1 mm in depth or >2 cm in clinical width are associated with a high risk of lymph node disease, and are usually managed with lymph node evaluation or dissection[1].

In men poor prognosis and lymph node involvement are associated with lymphovascular invasion, corpus invasion, and poor histologic differentiation[2,6].

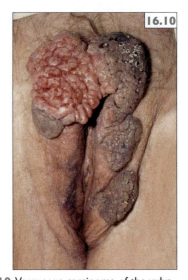

16.10 Verrucous carcinoma of the vulva.

DIAGNOSIS

Ultrasound and magnetic resonance imaging (MRI) are often used to evaluate local soft tissue invasion by the primary tumor[2]. Positron emission tomography-computed tomography (PET-CT) scans appear to be the most accurate modality for assessing subclinical lymph node and distant involvement[7].

TREATMENT

Traditionally, invasive SCC has been treated aggressively with penectomy or vulvectomy and lymph node dissection. Tissue-preserving procedures, including conservative local excision and laser surgery, have the benefit of limiting the psychological impact of treating SCC of the genitalia; however, they have a high overall recurrence rate (25–30%)[7]. Data for Mohs surgery for SCC of the genitalia are limited to case series. Recurrence rates appear to be higher than when Mohs is used for SCC in other locations[8,9]. Success with Mohs surgery decreases as lesions increase in width[8,9]. The high recurrence rates associated with these modalities are likely attributable to similar factors noted for VIN and PIN: locations in fields of tissue that are diffusely affected by contributing factors to malignancy such as HPV and chronic inflammation. Regardless of intervention, recurrence may develop years later. Patients with local recurrence maintain a high survival rate[7].

The use of sentinel lymph node biopsy for genital SCC is being investigated as an alternative to prophylactic dissection in patients with at-risk tumors with nonpalpable lymph nodes[1,6]. Lymph node involvement and more advanced disease may call for adjuvant radiation and/or chemotherapy.

Basal cell cancer

ETIOLOGY AND EPIDEMIOLOGY

Basal cell skin cancer (BCC) is the most common cutaneous malignancy, although genital BCC represents less than 1% of total BCCs. This is most likely due to the lack of exposure to UV radiation in this area. HPV is not believed to play a major role in the pathogenesis of BCC. On average, BCC of the genitalia presents in the eighth decade. Aside from age, the other major risk factors are previous radiation to the area, immunosuppression, and basal cell nevus syndrome[10].

CLINICAL PRESENTATION

BCC of the genitalia can mimic inflammatory dermatoses, although may also be nodular or ulcerated. Tumors are often larger due to delays in diagnosis[10] (**16.11**).

DIFFERENTIAL DIAGNOSIS

Differential diagnosis includes squamous cell cancer, psoriasis, nummular eczema, and extramammary Paget's disease.

LABORATORY STUDIES (HISTOPATHLOGY)

A biopsy should be performed and the histological subtype noted, because morpheaform, basosquamous, and metatypical types of BCC are assumed to have a higher likelihood of more invasive disease and metastatic potential, as they do in other locations. While there are some reports of metastatic BCC with primary lesions in the genital region, most lesions are localized[10] (**16.12**).

TREATMENT

Clinical borders are harder to delineate and recurrence rates are higher for BCC in the genital area[10]. This type of cancer is usually histologically conspicuous and generally contiguous, making Mohs surgery the ideal treatment. Nonsurgical methods have been used for BCC in other locations, and they may have a use in the genitalia.

16.11 Basal cell cancer of the scrotum in a 79-year-old man. Center of lesion with biopsy site.

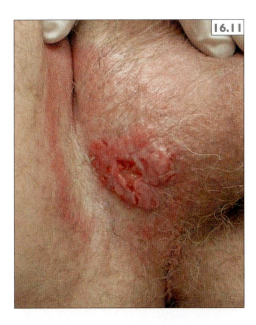

16.12 Basal cell cancer of the vulva.

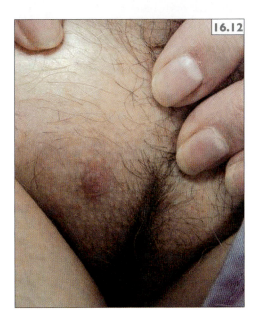

Melanoma

ETIOLOGY AND EPIDEMIOLOGY

Melanoma of the vulva represents 1–2% of all melanomas in women. It is the second most common malignancy of the vulva after squamous cell carcinoma. Case series have revealed that risk factors for melanoma of the genitalia include a family history of cutaneous melanoma and a personal history of atypical nevi[11]. The age of diagnosis for vulvar melanoma is notably older than that for cutaneous melanoma, with a median age of 66 years and a peak incidence ranging from the fifth to the eighth decade[12].

It is estimated that melanoma of the genitalia represents approximately 0.1% of all melanomas in men[13]. The reason for the low incidence in male versus female genitalia is not entirely clear, but it may have to do with melanocyte density being higher in the female genitalia[12].

The etiologic factors are less defined than those for genital SCC. Ultraviolet radiation is not usually a significant risk factor. Mucosal melanomas are associated with activating mutations in the KIT gene, which codes for a tyrosine kinase receptor[13]. They are less associated with the serine/threonine kinase BRAF mutations than cutaneous melanomas[13].

CLINICAL PRESENTATION

Melanoma of the genitalia is often asymptomatic and patients may be unaware of the lesions. Pain, pruritus, discharge, and bleeding are uncommon yet possible initial clinical manifestations. Lesions may present as being pigmented or amelanotic. They may be flat or nodular (**16.13**). Lesions may have subclinical areas or be multifocal (**16.14**).

DIFFERENTIAL DIAGNOSIS

Differential diagnosis includes labial lentigo, acquired nevus, angiokeratoma, pigmented seborrheic keratosis, pyogenic granuloma (differential diagnosis of amelanotic melanoma).

LABORATORY STUDIES (HISTOPATHOLOGY)

While an excisional biopsy is preferred for complete histologic analysis of a suspicious lesion, because of the sensitive area, one or more representative biopsies may be obtained from larger lesions, with a goal of obtaining sufficient depth for analysis.

Proportions of each melanoma histologic subtype in the genitalia vary in studies that usually have low sample sizes and often include both keratinized and mucosal sites together. A high proportion of mucosal melanomas have a mucosal lentiginous type of histology. Nodular and superficial spreading types may be seen in mucosal or keratinized sites[11].

PROGNOSIS

Melanoma of the genitalia has an overall worse prognosis than cutaneous melanoma. Cancers from mucosal and keratinized sites are often included in genital melanoma data, although they may vary in etiologic factors and prognosis. Studies that include only mucosal sites are small, though they support a poor prognosis[12]. Similar to cutaneous melanoma, depth of invasion, ulceration, and lymph node status are important prognostic factors[11] (**16.15**).

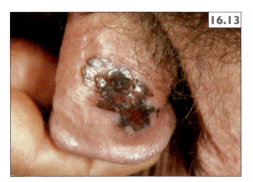

16.13 Melanoma. (Courtesy of Dr. Giuseppe Micali, Catania, Italy.)

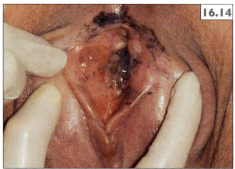

16.14 Melanoma. (Courtesy of Dr. Michael Mastrangelo, Philadelphia, PA.)

TREATMENT

Radical vulvectomy has not shown greater survival than limited vulvectomy in the treatment of vulvar melanoma. Current recommendations are similar to those for cutaneous melanoma with a 1 cm margin for lesions less than 1 mm in depth and a 2 cm margin for lesions >1 mm in depth. Prophylactic lymph node dissection is usually discouraged, and sentinel lymph node biopsies are usually performed for lesions >1 mm, though their prognostic value and role in the treatment of melanoma of the female genitalia are not yet known[11].

Melanoma of the penis has been treated with wide local excision, as well as partial or full penectomy, with variable lymph node management[12]. The significant association of mucosal melanoma with KIT mutations may lead to the utilization of tyrosine kinase inhibitors for advanced disease.

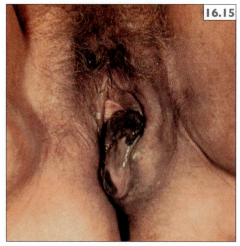

16.15 Advanced-stage melanoma in an elderly woman. (Courtesy of Dr. Marcia Ramos-e-Silva, PhD, Rio de Janeiro, Brazil.)

Extramammary Paget's disease

ETIOLOGY AND EPIDEMIOLOGY

Extramammary Paget's disease (EMPD) is a slow growing and rarely invasive cancer. Most cases of EMPD of the genitalia are primary epidermal neoplasms, though small proportions are associated with an underlying malignancy of an adnexal structure (4–17%) or distant organ (11–20%) such as the colon, cervix, or bladder[14]. The origin of cells in primary epidermal disease is unknown. They may represent malignant transformation of stem cells or ectopic cells that have spread to the epidermis from other structures, subsequently becoming malignant[14]. EMPD has a usual onset after age 50. It is more common in women, with 65% of all cases presenting on the vulva[14].

CLINICAL PRESENTATION

The vulva is the most common area of EMPD presentation (**16.16**). For men, the most common area of presentation is the perianal area, but it may also affect the peno-scrotal junction, the scrotum, or the inguinal folds[14] (**16.17**).

EMPD can present as an eczematous, erythematous, and/or ulcerated plaque, usually with asymmetric, though well-defined borders. Due to the similarity in appearance to inflammatory dermatoses, there may be a delay in diagnosis of years (**16.18**).

Patients with a diagnosis of EMPD must undergo a thorough work-up because there may be an association with underlying malignancy, especially if the cells stain with a pattern consistent with endodermal lineage (see below). Blood markers, such as carcinoembryonic antigen (CEA) may be elevated in advanced cases of EMPD[14].

DIFFERENTIAL DIAGNOSIS

The differential diagnosis includes squamous cell cancer *in situ*, eczematous dermatitis, and tinea corporis.

LABORATORY STUDIES (HISTOPATHOLOGY)

Microscopically, intraepithelial vacuolated cells with large nuclei are found that stain positively for mucin. Immunohistochemical (IHC) stains are positive for cytokeratin (CK)7 and negative for CK20 (ectodermal pattern) in primary epidermal EMPD or EMPD arising in an underlying adnexal structure. In contrast, IHC stains are positive for both CK7 and CK20 (endodermal pattern) in lesions associated with an underlying malignancy of another organ[14].

PROGNOSIS

Primary EMPD (with no underlying malignancy) progresses slowly and has a low mortality rate. The prognosis is worse if the tumor invades into the dermis. EMPD associated with an underlying adnexal or distant malignancy has a worse prognosis[14].

TREATMENT

The high prevalence of subclinical disease is reflected by the high rate of positive margins, despite wide excision, and high recurrence rates[15]. Mohs technique with IHC stain to guide margin analysis has been utilized[15]. There are case reports using topical treatments for primary EMPD. Imiquimod cream has been investigated with increasing frequency, with reports of success[16] and failure[17]. Lymph node analysis is usually recommended for any lesions that are beyond the epidermis, and while at least one group showed value in sentinel lymph node biopsy for invasive lesions, this technique has not been standardized for EMPD[18].

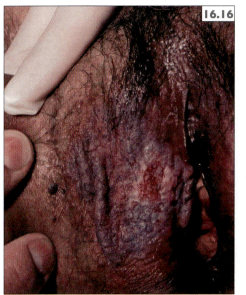

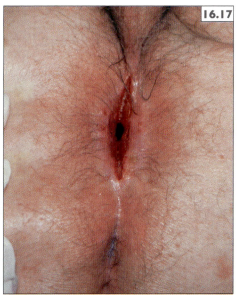

16.16 Extramammary Paget's disease of the vulva. Cytokeratin staining was unavailable.

16.17 Extramammary Paget's disease of the perianal area in a man. Cytokeratin staining was unavailable.

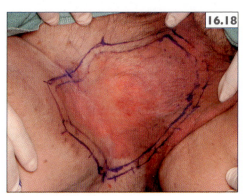

16.18 Primary extramammary Paget's disease of the inguinal fold and scrotum. (Courtesy of Dr. Curtis A. Pettaway, Houston, TX.)

Kaposi's sarcoma

ETIOLOGY AND EPIDEMIOLOGY

Kaposi's sarcoma (KS) is a lymphovascular malignancy. KS is clinically categorized into four groups: patients with human immunodeficiency virus/acquired immunodeficiency syndrome (HIV/AIDS) (epidemic), patients who are immunocompromised (iatrogenic), older patients from the Mediterranean or Eastern European regions (classic), or HIV-negative individuals, including children, from sub-Saharan Africa (endemic) (**16.19**).

Human herpes virus type 8 (HHV-8) is believed to be the major etiologic factor in KS, although secondary factors, such as immune suppression or genetic susceptibility, may be necessary since most people infected with HHV-8 do not get KS. This virus has been shown to up-regulate angiogenic and proliferation factors. Routes of transmission may be through saliva or sexual contact, which may explain why patients may present with genital lesions initially[19].

KS has mostly been seen in males; however, with HIV continuing to progress in some areas of Africa, the ratio of men to women with epidemic KS is becoming closer to 1:1 in certain regions of the continent[20]. Classic KS is consistently a male dominated disease.

Primary genital lesions are rare overall. Approximately 2–3% of HIV-associated KS patients present with primary lesions on the penis[19]. Most patients with classic KS present with lesions on the lower extremities, though there are a number of case reports of patients who presented with primary penile lesions.

The incidence and severity of KS in the USA have decreased through successful treatment of HIV with highly active antiretroviral therapy (HAART)[21].

CLINICAL PRESENTATION

Genital lesions may be the first presentation of KS. Lesions are typically red, brown, or purple patches, papules, or plaques. They may also present as nodules, wart-like lesions, pedunculated lesions, or regional swelling or pain or both[19] (**16.20**). Individual lesions typically progress from patches to plaques and nodules.

DIFFERENTIAL DIAGNOSIS

The differential diagnosis includes pyogenic granuloma, angiokeratoma, angioma, angiosarcoma, and condyloma acuminata.

LABORATORY STUDIES (HISTOPATHOLOGY)

Branched slit-like vascular spaces are seen in the dermis in patch-KS, while sheets of spindle cells are seen in nodular-KS. Stains for HHV-8 antigens are often used to confirm the diagnosis.

PROGNOSIS

KS associated with HIV can have an aggressive course affecting different organ systems. KS lesions will usually regress within a year of starting HAART therapy and this coincides with increasing CD4 counts and

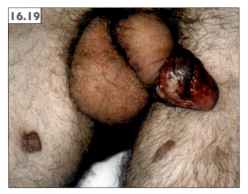

16.19 Kaposi's sarcoma of the penis in a human immunodeficiency virus-positive man. (Courtesy of Dr. Mariana Gusmão, Rio de Janeiro, Brazil.)

decreasing viral loads[21]; however, there are reported cases of persistent KS lesions despite treatment with HAART and improvement in lab values[22].

Classic KS tends to have an indolent course. In the limited number of cases of primary classic KS of the genitalia, there are reports of spontaneous regression, nonprogressive disease, and progression to involve the lower extremities over a course of months to years[22]. As lesions progress, there may be associated swelling, edema, and/or pain.

Endemic KS may present like classic KS with indolent disease; however, an aggressive course is possible and is usually seen in children with this type. Iatrogenic KS tends to be aggressive[21].

TREATMENT

In HIV-positive patients, HAART therapy has been shown to be the most important treatment for treating KS, and lesions have cleared in response to immune function recovery[21]. Surgical removal, destruction, and radiation have been employed for localized lesions of KS. Liposomal chemotherapy and biologics such as interferon-alpha to boost the immune system have been used to treat more widespread disease[21].

Rare cancers of the genitalia

There are case reports of rare malignancies presenting in the genitalia. Reported primary sarcomas include dermatofibrosarcoma protuberans, leiomyosarcoma, and angiosarcoma (**16.21**). Metastatic cancer of other genitourinary organs, including the prostate, cervix, kidney, or bladder, may present in the skin of the genitalia. Occasionally, these cancers will mimic benign processes, such as in the cases of leiomyosarcomas mimicking bartholin cysts of the vulva[23]. The presentation of any new lesion of the genitalia warrants close inspection and a possible biopsy to rule out malignancy. The lack of experience in dealing with these rare cancers would call for multidisciplinary involvement.

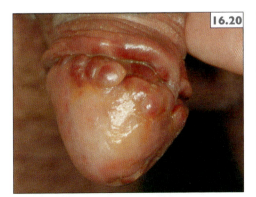

16.20 Kaposi's sarcoma. (Courtesy of Dr. Giuseppe Micali, Catania, Italy.)

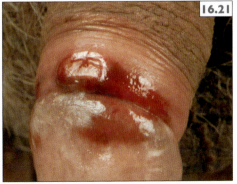

16.21 Angiosarcoma. (Courtesy of Dr. Giuseppe Micali, Catania, Italy.)

So-called precancerous lesions

Dermatologists are familiar with the term 'precancerous lesion', using it daily to describe actinic keratoses as possible precursors to SCCs. There is debate as to whether some or all actinic keratoses are actually very early SCCISs, or whether actinic keratoses represent a step in the evolution from normal skin to cancer, having accumulated some, but not all, the sun-induced genetic alterations of SCC. Obviously, actinic keratoses are very rare in the genital area due to the usual lack of sun exposure to this area; however, there are genital lesions that have significant risk to develop into skin cancers, specifically SCC.

VIN and PIN encompass skin lesions that have some level of dysplasia confined to the epidermis. Similar to actinic keratoses, their relationship to SCC has been debated. With recent changes in nomenclature, the authors consider these entities to be the equivalent of SCCIS (discussed in VIN/PIN/SCCIS section).

Some clinicians consider bowenoid papulosis to be a precancer, with its low rate of transformation into invasive disease. For this reason, we join those who consider it to be a low-grade SCCIS (discussed in VIN/PIN/SCCIS section). Both Bowen's disease and erythroplasia of Queyrat (Bowen's or SCCIS on the glans of the penis, **16.22**) are considered to be SCCIS, with a higher risk of invasive disease than bowenoid papulosis (discussed in VIN/PIN/SCCIS section).

Leukoplakia is more often described in the mouth, where it is a diagnosis of exclusion without consistent histopathologic findings. Oral leukoplakia is known to carry a risk for SCC. To confuse the issue, it is sometimes used to describe similar lesions on the genitalia, although the term is used less often in this region (**16.23**). Leukoplakia may have been used to describe lesions that actually represent other entities such as IN or lichen sclerosus et atrophicus[24]; however, there may be white plaques that develop on the genitalia that do not have diagnostic histological findings. In view of the natural history of oral leukoplakia, a risk for the development of SCC should be considered in such genital lesions.

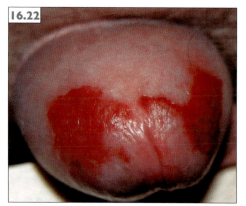

16.22 Erythroplasia of Queyrat. (Courtesy of Dr. Tomasz F. Mroczkowski.)

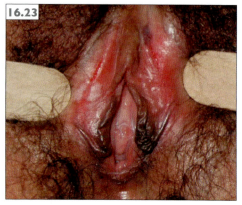

16.23 Leukoplakia of the inner side of the right labium. (Courtesy of Dr. Tomasz F. Mroczkowski.)

Anogenital Hemangiomas

Osamah J. Choudhry, BA, MD, Bobby Y. Reddy, MS, MD, and W. Clark Lambert, MD, PhD

DEFINITION

A hemangioma (infantile hemangioma) is a benign proliferative tumor of infancy, which usually resolves spontaneously by self-involution. Comprising about 1% of such tumors, hemangiomas of the anogenital region are a rare presentation[1].

ETIOLOGY AND EPIDEMIOLOGY

Although the exact pathogenesis is as yet unclear[2], studies have demonstrated that the endothelial cells of hemangiomas coexpress markers specific to the placental microvasculature (i.e. glucose transporter protein 1 [GLUT-1], Lewis Y antigen [CD 14], Fc y receptor II [CD 32], and merosin). This cannot be said of other vascular tumors, vascular malformations, or normal skin[3]. Gene activation patterns of the hemangioma endothelium also resemble those of the placental endothelial cell[4]. These findings collectively suggest that hemangiomas result from the embolization of placental stem cells to fetal tissues *in utero*[4]. This hypothesis of placental origin is supported by research demonstrating that infantile hemangiomas are more common in infants born to mothers with placental complications, such as placenta previa or abruptio placenta[3]. Furthermore, chorionic villus sampling is associated with a ten-fold increase in hemangioma incidence.

Hemangiomas are found in 9–13% of white non-Hispanics, 1.4% of black, and 0.8% of Asian infants, with a female to male ratio of 3:1[5]. The incidence increases significantly with preterm births weighing less than 1200 g (22–30%). In fact, it is estimated that hemangioma risk rises by about 40% per 500 g decrease in birth weight[5]. Maternal factors, such as advanced maternal age and pre-eclampsia, have also been found to increase the incidence of infantile hemangiomas[5].

CLINICAL PRESENTATION

Hemangiomas are clinically diverse. Appearance on presentation is dependent on the depth, location, and evolutionary stage[2]. Approximately 55% are present at birth, while the rest develop over the first weeks of life[2]. The initial presentation is generally a pale macule with thread-like telengiectasias. With proliferation, the more characteristic appearance of the tumor develops: a bright red, elevated and noncompressible plaque. Hemangiomas which lie deeper in the dermis may present with a slightly bluish tone.

Anogenital hemangiomas are predominantly found in the perineum, labia, and scrotum[1] (**17.1**). Infants can present with secondary complications such as ulceration, bleeding, or infection. The most frequent and worrisome of the complications is ulceration, which occurs in 5–13% of all hemangiomas[6]. Associated with the proliferatory phase within 4–5 months of birth, ulceration is much more commonly seen in anogenital hemangiomas because of the macerating influence of urine and stool[6]. The macerating effect also complicates wound healing, which predisposes the area to further ulceration and increases the risk of developing a secondary bacterial infection[1].

LABORATORY STUDIES (HISTOPATHOLOGY)

A biopsy is not indicated in the diagnosis or management of anogenital hemangiomas. Classically, hemangiomas appear as solid masses of plump, proliferating, endothelial cells with increased mitotic activity and narrow vascular channels.

COURSE

Hemangiomas are biphasic, with early proliferation followed by slow involution. Maximal growth is typically seen by about 6–8 months of age[7]. The involutionary phase is difficult to predict, but is usually noted by a change in color from bright red to gray or purple[7]. Complete resolution can be seen in approximately 60% of cases.

DIAGNOSIS

A thorough history and physical examination are essential to the diagnosis of anogenital hemangioma, with recognition of its characteristic appearance and rapid growth. While clinical assessment is sufficient to diagnose the more common intracutaneous anogenital hemangiomas, duplex sonography is necessary to confirm the subcutaneous location and exclude the presence of soft-tissue neoplasms[1].

The differential diagnoses for anogenital hemangioma are vast, with angiokeratoma (**17.2**), nevus flammeus, cherry hemangioma, capillary malformation, lipoma, pyogenic granuloma, Cobb syndrome (port-wine stain or angioma extending to the spinal cord), congenital syphilis, and Dabska tumor the more notable considerations[6]. In addition, syndromic associations are not to be overlooked, as in structural abnormalities of the gastrointestinal and urogenital systems such as PELVIS, SACRAL, and LUMBAR syndromes[8,9].

TREATMENT

The primary management goal in anogenital hemangioma is the prevention of ulceration[1]. This is accomplished by minimizing area contact with urine, stool, and excess moisture with frequent diaper changes and application of a topical barrier cream (e.g. zinc oxide paste)[1]. If ulceration does occur, topical antibiotics (e.g. mupirocin, neomycin, and silver sulfadiazine) are indicated to prevent secondary infection[6]. To hasten wound healing, the area should also be covered with a hydrocolloid dressing which can be changed twice weekly with gentle saline washes[6]. Pulsed dye laser may be used to alleviate pain and stimulate repair[10,11]. If bacteremia is suspected by the presence of signs such as fever and leukocytosis, systemic antibacterial therapy may be necessary.

There is rarely a need for surgical intervention or laser ablation for anogenital hemangiomas because aesthetic concerns are uncommon[12]. Aggressive intervention

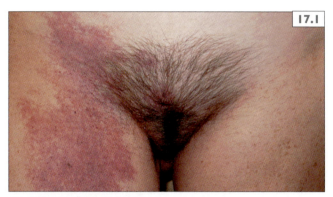

17.1 Anogenital hemangioma.

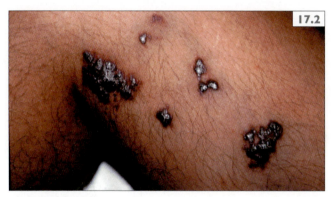

17.2 Angiokeratoma.

may also worsen the situation by causing ulceration. In particular, treatment with dye- and Nd-YAG laser can initiate ulceration of vulnerable skin[12]. Therefore, the 'wait- and-see' policy remains the best choice of management for nonulcerating anogenital hemangiomas.

CHAPTER 18

Allergic Dermatitis, Irritant Dermatitis, and Drug Reactions

Roman J. Nowicki, MD

- **Contact dermatitis (syn. contact eczema)**
- **Allergic contact dermatitis**
- **Irritant contact dermatitis**
- **Erythema multiforme, Stevens–Johnson syndrome, toxic epidermal necrolysis**
- **Fixed drug eruption**
- **Diaper dermatitis in adults**

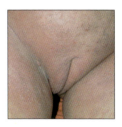
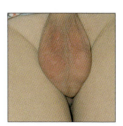
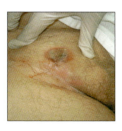
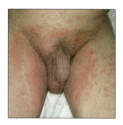

Genital allergy or irritant reaction should be considered as a possible diagnosis in all patients with genital soreness or irritation for which no infection or dermatosis can be identified, and in whom clinical manifestations remain unchanged or worsen with treatment.

Contact dermatitis (syn. contact eczema)

The term 'contact dermatitis' denotes an acute or chronic inflammatory skin disorder caused by allergens (allergic contact dermatitis, ACD) or chemical/physical irritants (irritant contact dermatitis, ICD). Despite their different mechanisms, they can be difficult to distinguish from one another at the clinical, histologic, and even molecular levels.

Allergic contact dermatitis

ETIOLOGY AND EPIDEMIOLOGY
ACD is a delayed type of induced allergy resulting from cutaneous contact with a specific allergen to which the patient has developed a specific sensitivity. Filaggrin barrier defects might predispose to ACD by allowing greater penetration of chemical haptens. Formaldehyde is a major cause of ACD. Certain preservative chemicals widely used in shampoos, lotions, other moisturizers, and cosmetics are termed formaldehyde releasers (i.e. quaternium-15 [Dowicil 200], imidazolidinyl urea [Germall 115]). Individuals may develop allergy to fragrances. Fragrances are found not only in perfumes, colognes, aftershaves, deodorants, and soaps, but also in numerous other products, often as a mask to camouflage an unpleasant odor. ACD is frequent in the perianal area as a result of the use of sensitizing medications and remedies (e.g. topical benzocaine). Individuals with pruritus ani and pruritus vulvae may become sensitized to benzocaine

and other medications applied to chronic pruritic processes. Women with lichen sclerosus et atrophicus frequently develop ACD, complicating the severe chronic vulvar dermatosis. Possible causes include contraceptives, deodorants and feminine hygiene sprays, antiseptic agents, antibiotics (often used by a partner), and condoms (latex, **18.1**), other rubber products, lubricants, or preservatives).

ACD is most common during adulthood, but it can affect all ages. A frequent cause of ACD in elderly patients is topical medication.

CLINICAL PRESENTATION
ICD is usually confined to the area where the trigger actually touched the skin, whereas ACD may be more widespread on the skin. Signs of both forms include the following:

Red eruption. This is the usual reaction. The eruption appears immediately in ICD; in ACD, the dermatitis sometimes does not appear until 24–72 hours after exposure to the allergen.

Blisters or wheals. Blisters, wheals, and urticaria often form in a pattern where skin was directly exposed to the allergen or irritant.

Itchy, burning skin. ICD tends to be more painful than itchy, while ACD often itches.

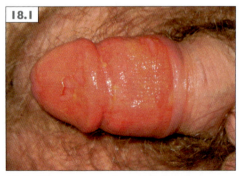

18.1 Allergic contact dermatitis (latex).

In women, the appearance is that of a dermatitis: erythema, edema, and vesicles with varying degrees of lichenification seen on the cutaneous side of the labia majora pudendi or the skin of the area.

In men, there may also be an eczematous process, but recurrent balanitis can also develop, probably due to an allergy to a product used by his partner (propane-1, 2-diol of lubricating gel) or for his partner (the nonoxynol-9 of condoms). ACD of the penis is usually associated with marked edema, because the skin covering the genitalia is thin and elastic. Most often, the glans and foreskin are involved, but the inflammation can spread to the shaft.

LABORATORY STUDIES

Patch testing can help to differentiate ICD from ACD. This diagnostic procedure may provide important information that can help in the management of recalcitrant and difficult-to-manage dermatosis.

Skin biopsy may help exclude other disorders, particularly tinea, psoriasis, and cutaneous lymphoma.

COURSE, PROGNOSIS, AND COMPLICATIONS

To develop ACD, two phases are necessary: sensitization and elicitation. Individuals with ACD typically develop dermatitis (within a few days of exposure) in areas that were exposed directly to the allergen. Certain allergens penetrate intact skin poorly, and the onset of dermatitis may be delayed for up to a week following exposure. A minimum of 10 days is required for individuals to develop specific sensitivity to a new contactant.

DIAGNOSIS

A detailed history and clinical examination are crucial to the diagnosis of ACD and ICD. Clinically, genital ACD is characterized by erythema and marked edema and, in time, with microvesiculation and exudation. When ACD is suspected, the medical history of the patient is important to enable appropriate patch testing and a correct diagnosis.

The differential diagnosis includes ICD, erythema multiforme, asteatotis, atopic dermatitis, tinea cruris, psoriasis, cutaneous lymphoma, and prurigo nodularis.

TREATMENT

The primary goal in preventing ACD is the prevention of further damage by removing/ avoiding the offending allergen. Toilet paper (tissue) and commercial wipes may need to be avoided as their use might contribute to irritation, especially when used to rub or scratch the area. Both may contain allergens such as formaldehyde, bezalkonium chloride, and fragrances. Urine, stool, and excessive vaginal secretions are known to contribute to local irritation. Cotton washcloths may be used to clean the area. Cool water compresses or sitz-baths are recommended to clean the area. Soap, an irritant itself, should be avoided.

All topical agents should be used with caution, as they can be irritants or allergens. An emollient applied twice a day after cleansing with clean water will both lubricate and protect the area.

Topical corticosteroids (TCS) are frequently the first-line pharmacologic therapy for those with ACD, where the allergen cannot be avoided or where etiology is mixed. Ointment-based formulations are preferred because they are less likely to contain allergens or irritants. Oral antihistamines may help to diminish the pruritus caused by ACD.

Irritant contact dermatitis

ETIOLOGY AND EPIDEMIOLOGY

Clinical manifestations of irritant contact dermatitis (ICD) may be associated with irritants. They have the potential to disrupt membranes or interfere with metabolic processes in the epidermis or dermis.

Chemical ICD (CICD) is either acute or chronic, and is usually associated with strong and weak irritants, respectively. Highly alkaline soaps, detergents, and cleaning products all have the common effect of directly affecting the barrier properties of the epidermis. These effects include removing fat emulsion, inflicting cellular damage on the epithelium, and increasing the transepidermal water loss (TEWL) by damaging the horny layer water-binding mechanisms and damaging the deoxyribonucleic acid (DNA), which causes the layer to thin. The cosmetic products responsible for irritation are mainly liquid foam hygiene products, used too frequently and/or for too long and/or badly rinsed. In women, depilatory products can also be to blame. Some patients complain of irritation due to the perfume of scented toilet papers.

Physical ICD (PICD) is a less researched form of ICD due to its various mechanisms of action and a lack of tests for its diagnosis. A complete patient history combined with negative allergic patch testing is usually necessary to reach a correct diagnosis. The simplest form of PICD results from prolonged rubbing, although the diversity of implicated irritants is far wider. Examples include paper friction and scratchy clothing.

The anogenital region is often the site of ICD: in men, promoted by sweat and rubbing, and in women, by aggressive hygiene. ICD affects very young and very old patients more severely. The greatest single risk for ICD is a history of atopic dermatitis.

CLINICAL PRESENTATION

ICD (**18.2**) consists of a spectrum of disease that ranges from a mild dryness (**18.3**), erythema (**18.4**, **18.5**), or chapping, to various types of eczematous dermatitis (**18.6**), widespread edema, or an acute caustic burn. The severity of dermatitis produced by an irritant depends upon the type of exposure, vehicle, and individual propensity. The lesions can be dry, lichenified (**18.7**), and sometimes fissured at the base of the folds. The dominant symptom is intense itching.

COURSE, PROGNOSIS, AND COMPLICATIONS

Itching, burning, and erythema occur, often followed by edema, papules, vesicles, and bullae in exposed areas of contact with an offending chemical irritant or allergen. Later, weeping, crusting, scaling, fissuring, excoriations, and secondary infections occur.

DIAGNOSIS

To diagnose ICD, clinically relevant contact allergies have to be excluded. Patients should be asked specifically about sexual practices, plus the use of condoms or spermicidal agents.

TREATMENT

As with ACD, the primary treatment for ICD is avoidance of the irritant. A new generation of cleansers (synthetic detergents or syndets) has emerged. Syndets with a pH of approximately 5.5 seem to be especially relevant, because they do not modify skin pH. Emollients and topical glucocorticosteroids are the mainstay of therapy. When choosing a steroid, it is helpful to match the vehicle to the morphology (ointment for dry scaling lesions, lotion or cream for weeping areas of dermatitis). Topical steroids are sometimes combined with antifungals and antimicrobials. Topical calcineurin inhibitors are an alternative[1-4].

18.2 Irritant contact dermatitis (K-Y jelly). (Courtesy of Dr. Tomasz F. Mroczkowski.)

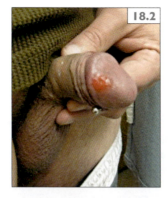

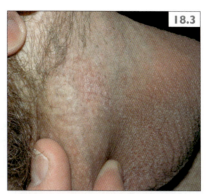

18.3 Irritant contact dermatitis (soap) – a mild dryness.

18.4 Irritant contact dermatitis (soap) – erythema.

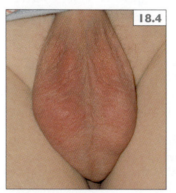

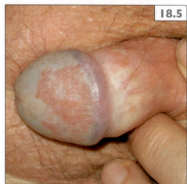

18.5 Irritant contact dermatitis (soap) – balanitis.

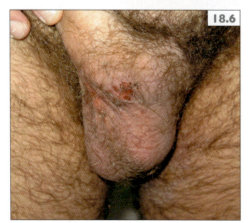

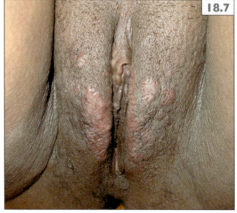

18.6 Irritant contact dermatitis (soap) – impetiginization.

18.7 Irritant contact dermatitis (soap) – lichenification.

Erythema multiforme, Stevens–Johnson syndrome, toxic epidermal necrolysis

DEFINITION

Erythema multiforme (EM) is an acute, and sometimes recurring skin condition considered to be a type IV hypersensitivity reaction associated with certain infections, medications, and various other triggers. EM may be present with a wide spectrum of severity. EM minor represents a localized eruption of the skin with minimal or no mucosal involvement. EM major is a term that may be used to refer to two conditions that constitute a spectrum of the same disease process: Stevens–Johnson syndrome (SJS) and toxic epidermal necrolysis (TEN) (also known as Lyell's syndrome). SJS and TEN are more severe, potentially life-threatening disorders.

In SJS, a person has blistering of mucous membranes, typically in the mouth, eyes, and vagina, and patchy areas of dermatitis. In TEN, there is a similar blistering of mucous membranes, but in addition the epidermis peels off in sheets from large areas of the body.

ETIOLOGY AND EPIDEMIOLOGY

Approximately 50% of cases of EM are idiopathic, with no precipitating factor identified. Many potential triggers have been implicated as possible causes of EM, SJS, and TEN. Most notable causes are infectious agents (herpes simplex virus [HSV], human cytomegalovirus [HCMV], Epstein–Barr virus, *Mycoplasma* spp. and histoplasmosis) and drugs. Nearly all cases of SJS and TEN are caused by a reaction to a drug, most often antibiotics, barbiturates, anticonvulsants (**18.8**), nonsteroidal anti-inflammatory drugs (NSAIDs), or allopurinol. A slow acetylator genotype is a risk factor for sulfonamide-induced SJS. Additionally, the antidepressant mirtazapine and tumor necrosis factor (TNF)-alpha antagonists infliximab, etanercept, and adalimumab have been reported as causes.

In up to one-half of cases, no specific etiology has been identified.

EM typically affects young individuals including children. One-half of the children with EM have a history of herpes labialis or progenitalis. SJS and TEN occur in all age groups but are more common among older people, probably because older people tend to use more drugs. SJS is also more likely to occur in people with acquired immunodeficiency syndrome (AIDS). In SJS, the male-to-female ratio is 2:1.

CLINICAL PRESENTATION

In EM, 50% of patients have prodromes, including a moderate fever, general discomfort, cough, sore throat, vomiting, chest pain, and diarrhea. These symptoms are usually present for 1–14 days before the cutaneous eruption occurs. The lesions usually begin on the acral areas and spread centripetally. Prominent mucosal involvement may occur. The genital areas may have painful, hemorrhagic bullae, and erosions. Mucosal lesions usually heal without sequelae. Generalized lymphadenopathy often accompanies EM.

In SJS, less than 10% of the body surface is affected (**18.9**). The mucosal involvement in SJS is more severe and more extensive. Genital lesions may result in urinary retention.

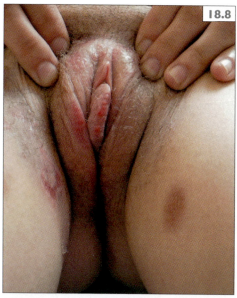

18.8 Stevens–Johnson syndrome (carbamazepine) – genital changes.

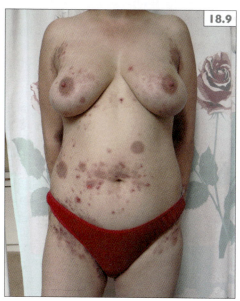

18.9 Stevens–Johnson syndrome (carbamazepine).

In TEN, large areas of skin peel off, often with just a gentle touch or pull: 30% or more of the body surface peels away. The affected areas of skin are painful, and the person feels very ill with chills and fever. In some people, the hair and nails fall out. The skin loss in TEN is similar to a severe burn and is equally life threatening. Huge amounts of fluids and salts can seep from the large, raw, damaged areas. A person who has this disorder is very susceptible to organ failure and infection at the sites of damaged, exposed tissues. Such infections are the most common cause of death in people with this disorder. The active stage of dermatitis and skin loss can last between 1 day and 14 days.

LABORATORY STUDIES

In severe cases, elevated erythrocyte sedimentation rate (ESR), moderate leukocytosis, and mildly elevated liver transaminase levels may be found. Specific HSV antigens have been detected within keratinocytes by immunofluorescence study. The HSV DNA has been identified primarily within the keratinocytes by polymerase chain reaction (PCR) amplification.

Histopathologic examination of a cutaneous punch biopsy may be used to confirm the diagnosis and to rule out the differential diagnoses. Initially, vacuolar change occurs at the dermal–epidermal junction and shows sparse lymphocytic and macrophage infiltration. This vacuolar change represents individual or small groups of necrotic (apoptotic) keratinocytes. Vacuolization then becomes confluent, which is clinically observed as blistering. The overlying epidermis shows full-thickness necrosis and sloughs off at the dermal–epidermal junction, exposing a relatively normal-appearing dermis. The upper dermis displays mild inflammation with perivascular lymphohistiocytic infiltrates.

Immunohistopathologic analysis shows a predominance of CD8 T cells and macrophages in the epidermis, whereas CD4 T cells form the perivascular infiltrates in the papillary dermis.

EM has a high density of cell infiltrate rich in T-lymphocytes. SJS/TEN is characterized by a cell-poor infiltrate of macrophages and dendrocytes, with strong TNF-alpha immunoreactivity. Immune complex deposition is variable and nonspecific.

COURSE, PROGNOSIS, AND COMPLICATIONS

Although most patients have an uncomplicated course, this cannot be predicted, especially among immunocompromised patients and those with secondary bacterial infections of the skin or the mucosa. Vaginal and urethral lesions are infrequent. The erosions may cause urinary retention and phimosis. Hematocolpos is the result of genital lesions in teenage women. It is often caused by the combination of menstruation with an imperforate hymen. Severe scarring of the genitourinary tract may cause vaginal and urethral stenosis.

EM has a mortality rate of less than 5%. Clearing may require 3–6 weeks. Skin lesions sometimes heal with hyperpigmentation and/or hypopigmentation. Scarring is usually absent, except after secondary infection.

DIAGNOSIS

The diagnosis is based mainly on the appearance of the skin lesion, especially when there is a history of risk factors or related diseases. Tests may include: Nikolsky's sign (a skin finding in which the top layers of the skin slip away from the lower layers when slightly rubbed) and skin lesion biopsy and microscopic examination of the tissue. Complete blood count usually reveals moderate leukocytosis with atypical lymphocytes. Eosinophil counts greater than $1000/mm^3$ may also be seen. Severely elevated total white blood cell counts indicate infection.

The skin lesions should not be confused with other conditions if rather rigid criteria of diagnosis are accepted. The distribution, symmetry, tendency to iris formation and bulla formation are characteristic. Drug eruptions, lupus erythematosus, bullous pemphigoid, fixed drug eruption, Behçet disease, staphylococcal scalded skin syndrome (SSSS), and toxic erythemas of unknown cause must be excluded.

TREATMENT

The cause of EM should be identified, when possible. If a drug is suspected, it should be immediately withdrawn. Infections should be appropriately treated after cultures and/or serologic tests have been performed. Suppression of HSV can prevent herpes-associated erythema multiforme (HAEM).

Mild cases of EM require only symptomatic treatment, which may include oral antihistamines, analgesics, local skin care; cold compresses with saline or Burow's solution; topical steroids; and soothing oral treatments such as saline gargles, viscous lidocaine, and diphenhydramine elixir. SJS and TEN can be life threatening and should be treated in a manner similar to thermal burns. The most severe cases should be managed in intensive care or burn units. Aggressive monitoring and replacement of fluids and electrolytes are of paramount importance. Topical treatment, including that for genital involvement, may be performed with a gauze dressing or a hydrocolloid. The use of liquid antiseptics (0.05% chlorhexidine) during bathing helps prevent superinfection. Oral antacids may be helpful for discrete oral ulcers. IV antibiotics may be necessary to treat secondary infections. Second-line treatment is intravenous immunoglobulin (IVIG). Third-line treatment is cyclosporine, cyclophosphamide, plasmapheresis, pentoxifylline, N-acetylcysteine, ulinastatin, infliximab, and/or granulocyte colony-stimulating factors (if TEN associated-leukopenia exists). Systemic steroids are unlikely to offer any benefits[5–8].

Fixed drug eruption

DEFINITION

The term fixed drug eruption (FDE) describes the development of one or more annular or oval skin erythematous patches as a result of systemic exposure to a drug. FDE normally resolves with hyperpigmentation and may recur at the same site with re-exposure to the drug.

ETIOLOGY AND EPIDEMIOLOGY

The exact mechanism of FDE is unknown. Recent research suggests a cell-mediated process that initiates both the active and quiescent lesions. The process may involve an antibody-dependent, cell-mediated, cytotoxic response. CD8+ effector/memory T cells play an important role in reactivation of lesions with re-exposure to the offending drug. FDE has been reported in association with several drugs, the most frequently implicated being barbiturates, sulfonamides, salicylates, phenazone derivatives, and tetracyclines. The most common cause is trimethoprim–sulfamethoxazole. Rarely, FDE can occur when the sexual partner has taken the drug, and it is assumed the toxic component of the drug is passed through vaginal fluid. The offending drug is thought to function as a hapten that preferentially binds to basal keratinocytes, leading to an inflammatory response.

FDE is the second or third most common skin manifestation of adverse drug events.

CLINICAL PRESENTATION

The initial eruption is often solitary and frequently located on the lip or genitalia (**18.10–18.12**). The penis is one of the more commonly affected areas of the body for FDE. Genital mucous membranes may be involved in association with skin lesions or alone. The lesions are usually round or oval, well demarcated and erythematous, but can be bullous with subsequent ulceration, usually developing within a few days of drug administration. Initially, FDE presents as a solitary lesion. Pruritus is rare, but burning and discomfort are possible.

LABORATORY STUDIES

Patch testing and oral provocation have been used to identify the suspected agent and check for cross-sensitivities to medications. Oral provocation is thought to be the only reliable way to diagnose FDE. Skin biopsy is the diagnostic procedure of choice. Histologic examination of inflammatory/acute lesions shows an interface dermatitis with vacuolar change and Civatte bodies. Dyskeratosis and individual necrotic keratinocytes within the epidermis may be prominent features. Spongiosis, dermal edema, eosinophils, and occasional neutrophils may be present. Pigmentary incontinence within the papillary dermis is a characteristic feature and may be the only feature seen in older, noninflamed lesions.

COURSE, PROGNOSIS, AND COMPLICATIONS

FDE generally appear within 2 days of initiation of drug therapy. With these eruptions, few lesions occur, sometimes limited to a single eruption, appearing as well-demarcated lesions with significant edema, usually associated with itching and burning at the site. Lesions may persist for from days to weeks and then fade slowly to residual oval hyperpigmented patches. Repeated exposure to the offending drug may cause new lesions to develop in addition to 'lighting up' the older hyperpigmented lesions. Subsequent re-exposure to the medication results in a reactivation of the site, with inflammation occurring within 30 minutes.

DIAGNOSIS

The most common clinical manifestation is a round or oval, sharply-demarcated erythematous/edematous area. The differential diagnosis includes melasma, bullous pemphigoid, cellulitis, drug-induced bullous disorders, lichen planus, insect bites, discoid lupus erythematosus, erythema annulare centrifugum, pityriasis rosea, erythema multiforme, erythema dyschromicum perstans, contact dermatitis, herpes simplex, pemphigus vulgaris, postinflammatory hyperpigmentation, and psoriasis.

TREATMENT

The main goal of treatment is the identification of the causative agent, in order to avoid it. TCS may be all that are required. In cases in which infection is suspected, antimicrobials and proper wound care are advised[9–12].

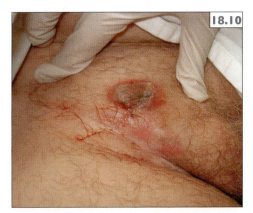

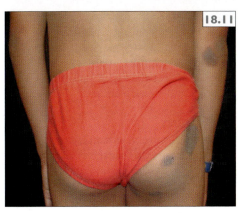

18.10, 18.11 Fixed drug eruption. (Courtesy of Dr. Oliverio Welch, Monterrey, Mexico.)

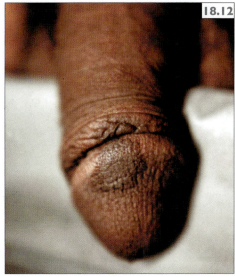

18.12 Fixed drug eruption on the head of penis caused by tetracycline. (Courtesy of Dr. Tomasz F. Mroczkowski.)

Diaper dermatitis in adults

syn. napkin dermatitis, diaper rash, nappy rash

DEFINITION, ETIOLOGY, AND EPIDEMIOLOGY

Diaper dermatitis (DD) is a term applied to skin eruptions in the diaper area that are caused by various skin disorders and/or irritants. Eruptions are directly or indirectly caused by the wearing of diapers. DD is caused by overhydration of the skin, plus maceration, prolonged contact with urine and feces, retained diaper soaps, and topical preparations. Mycoses and irritant dermatitis are the main causes of DD in the elderly. Increased wetness in the diaper area makes the skin more susceptible to damage by physical, chemical, and enzymatic mechanisms. Wet skin increases the penetration of irritant substances. Superhydration urease enzyme, found in the stratum corneum, liberates ammonia from cutaneous bacteria. Urease has a mild irritant effect upon nonintact skin. Lipases and proteases in feces mix with urine on nonintact skin and cause an alkaline surface pH, adding to the irritation.

Physical factors such as obesity, sweating, friction, incontinence, and soiling by excreta may cause erythema or fissuring and render the skin vulnerable to the effects of other agents. Initially, it is marked by soreness or slight itching and a superficial mild erythema of the opposed surfaces.

DD is a common skin disorder of the elderly and a frequent cause of dermatological consultation for bedridden patients.

CLINICAL PRESENTATION

Irritant diaper dermatitis (IDD) is characterized by confluent patches of erythema and scaling, often with papulovesicular or bullous lesions, fissures, and erosions, with the skin folds spared. The eruption may be patchy or confluent, affecting the abdomen from the umbilicus down to the thighs and encompassing the genitalia, perineum, and buttocks. Genitocrural folds are often spared in irritant dermatitis, but may be involved in primary candidal dermatitis (**18.13–18.15**).

LABORATORY STUDIES

In most cases, laboratory investigations are not necessary, except for mycological cultures of cutaneous swabs.

COURSE, PROGNOSIS, AND COMPLICATIONS

Factors that influence diaper skin condition are overhydration, skin irritants, mechanical friction, skin pH, diet, age, gestational age, antibiotic therapy, diarrhea, and medical conditions. DD with secondary bacterial or fungal involvement tends to spread to concave surfaces (i.e. skin folds), as well as convex surfaces, and often exhibits a central erythema with satellite pustules around the border. Secondary infection occurs rapidly, and DD may be perpetuated as an infectious dermatitis. In atopic dermatitis patients, there will be increased eczematization; in others, the dermatitis may progress to crusting, along with pustular or vegetating lesions.

For older patients, diaper skin breakdown may be associated with irritant dermatitis, skin tears, and pressure ulcers.

DIAGNOSIS

Signs and symptoms are restricted in most patients to the area covered by diapers. The differential diagnosis includes candidiasis, seborrhoic dermatitis, atopic dermatitis, psoriasis, and lichen planus.

TREATMENT

The most effective treatment is to increase the number of times the diapers are changed. The treatment goal is to minimize chemical and mechanical irritants from urine and feces. The skin should be cleansed as soon as possible after soiling to minimize fecal exposure time. Optimum cleansing systems maximize

18.13–18.15 Diaper dermatitis with secondary fungal involvement.

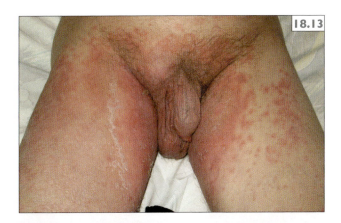

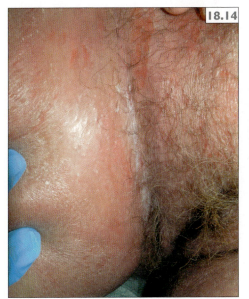

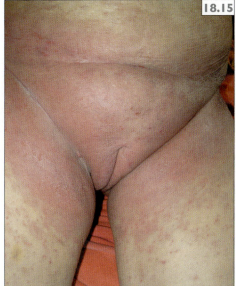

removal of skin contaminants, contain ingredients of low/no irritancy, minimize irritating residuals left on the skin, and require minimal rubbing. Excessive rubbing and over-cleaning can lead to mechanical stripping and skin barrier damage.

Thorough drying of the skin before diapering is a good preventive measure. The excess moisture, either from urine and feces or from sweating, creates the conditions for the development of DD. Various moisture-absorbing powders also help prevention. Another approach is to block moisture from reaching the skin, and commonly recommended remedies using this approach include oil-based protectants or barrier cream, petroleum jelly, and zinc oxide-based ointments. Not infrequently, topical steroids and/or antifungals are indicated[13–15].

Bullous Diseases

Juliana L. Basko-Plluska, MD, Jie Song, MD, and Vesna
Petronic-Rosic, MD, MSc

- **Pemphigus vulgaris**
- **Pemphigus vegetans**
- **Paraneoplastic pemphigus**
- **Bullous pemphigoid**
- **Pemphigoid gestationis**
- **Cicatricial pemphigoid**
- **Linear IgA bullous dermatosis**
- **Epidermolysis bullosa acquisita**
- **Hailey–Hailey disease**

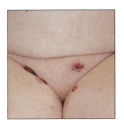
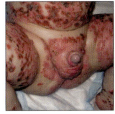
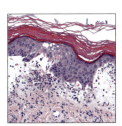
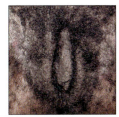

Pemphigus vulgaris

DEFINITION, ETIOLOGY, AND EPIDEMIOLOGY

Pemphigus vulgaris (PV) is a chronic autoimmune blistering disease of the skin and mucous membranes which may be fatal unless treated aggressively. PV is caused by circulating immunoglobulin (Ig)G autoantibodies directed against the keratinocyte desmosomal proteins, desmoglein 1 (Dsg1) and desmoglein 3 (Dsg3). Dsg1 and 3 play an important role in cell–cell adhesion. Binding of the autoantibodies to Dsg1 and 3 induces the loss of normal cell adhesion in the epidermis, and subsequent blister formation. In the mucosal variant, autoantibodies exclusively react with Dsg3, whereas patients with the mucocutaneous variant have antibodies against both Dsg1 and 3.

PV affects all races but is more common in individuals of Jewish and Mediterranean descent. Genetic predisposition is suspected, because PV occurs more frequently with certain major histocompatibility complex (MHC) class II molecules, such as DR4 and DRw6. Men and women are equally affected.

CLINICAL PRESENTATION

Typical lesions of PV are flaccid bullae which rupture easily and leave denuded, painful superficial erosions that heal slowly without scarring. Intact bullae are infrequently seen. Commonly, the disease begins in the oral mucosa with ill-defined, irregular, gingival (desquamative gingivitis), buccal, and palatal erosions. Other mucosal surfaces may be affected, including the conjunctiva, esophagus, vagina, cervix, urethra, and anus. Most patients develop cutaneous lesions several months later. Sites of predilection include the scalp, face, chest, axillae, groin, and umbilicus. The Nikolsky sign describes the clinical finding that physical trauma can shear the epidermis from normal-appearing skin, resulting in clinical lesions. It is a moderately sensitive but highly specific bedside tool for the diagnosis of intraepidermal blistering disorders, particularly pemphigus.

PV involves the female genital tract in up to 50% of patients[1,2]. Rarely, PV may be localized exclusively to the genital tract. Labia minora are the most frequently involved site, followed by the vaginal mucosa, labia majora, and cervix. Genital lesions usually persist even when otherwise successful control of generalized pemphigus is achieved. The resistance to treatment may be explained by the constant exposure of the genital tract to local trauma and friction from body movements, contraceptive devices, tampons, and coitus. Patients with genital disease complain of burning on micturition, discomfort during intercourse, adherence of undergarments to lesions, and foul odor. Interestingly, a case of PV localized exclusively to the vaginal mucosa presenting as chronic vaginal discharge has been reported[3].

PV of the male genital tract has also been described, with the glans penis being the most common site of involvement[4]. The urethral mucosa, with the exception of the distal portion, is spared because it is derived from endoderm and lacks Dsg1 and 3. Anal and perianal disease is uncommon, but may be encountered in patients with severe PV[5].

LABORATORY STUDIES

Histopathologic examination demonstrates suprabasal acantholysis and 'tombstoning' of the basal keratinocytes (**19.1**). The blister cavity contains acantholytic keratinocytes along with a few inflammatory cells, notably eosinophils, lymphocytes, and neutrophils. A mild-to-moderate perivascular mononuclear cell infiltrate may be present in the papillary dermis.

Direct immunofluorescence (DIF) of perilesional skin demonstrates intercellular IgG and complement C3 deposition throughout the epidermis. Indirect immunofluorescence (IIF) demonstrates the presence of circulating IgG autoantibodies that bind to the epidermis in 80–90% of patients. The titer of the antibody correlates with the activity of the disease process.

A Tzanck test, which is easily performed in the office, demonstrates acantholytic cells.

COURSE, PROGNOSIS, AND COMPLICATIONS

Before the advent of systemic corticosteroids, PV was associated with a high mortality rate, largely due to significant water loss and secondary bacterial infections of extensive denuded areas. With the use of systemic corticosteroids and immunosuppressive agents, the mortality rate is less than 10%. Therapy-related complications constitute the main cause of death.

DIAGNOSIS

Clinical, histopathologic, and immunopathologic findings can help differentiate PV from other bullous disorders. The differential diagnosis for cutaneous lesions includes bullous pemphigoid (BP), pemphigus foliaceus (PF), paraneoplastic pemphigus (PNP), and Hailey–Hailey disease. Mucosal lesions may resemble those seen in herpetic gingivostomatitis, erythema multiforme, Stevens–Johnson syndrome, lichen planus, and cicatricial pemphigoid (CP).

TREATMENT

Standard treatment consists of high-dose corticosteroids, preferably in combination with a steroid-sparing immunosuppressive agent such as azathioprine, mycophenolate mofetil, or cyclophosphamide. These drugs are usually started simultaneously, followed by a gradual tapering of the corticosteroid and continuation of the steroid-sparing agent until clinical remission is obtained. Plasmapheresis is useful for quickly reducing the titers of circulating antibodies and should be considered for severe pemphigus that is unresponsive to a combination of systemic corticosteroids and immunosuppressives[6]. Rituximab and high-dose intravenous immunoglobulin (IVIG) are additional effective treatment options for resistant disease[7,8]. Patients should minimize activities that may cause the blisters to rupture, including contact sports and consumption of foods that may irritate the oral mucosa. Patients with genital lesions should avoid sexual activity because trauma can induce new lesions and prevent existing lesions from healing. Daily topical care is important for anogenital disease. Patients are encouraged to soak in a bath tub with lukewarm water to which aluminum acetate powder and chlorhexidine gluconate have been added. These additives dry the weeping lesions and prevent infection[2,5].

19.1 Pemphigus vulgaris. Suprabasal acantholysis and 'tombstoning' of the basal keratinocytes (H & E, ×20).

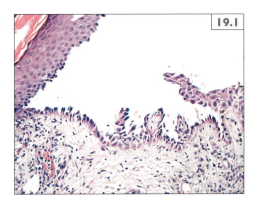

Pemphigus vegetans

DEFINITION, ETIOLOGY, AND EPIDEMIOLOGY

Pemphigus vegetans is an uncommon variant of PV with a predilection for intertriginous sites. The exact pathophysiology of pemphigus vegetans remains unknown. One hypothesis is that vegetative lesions on the skin folds develop as a result of the relative occlusion and maceration with subsequent bacterial infection. Another hypothesis suggests that pemphigus vegetans represents a reactive pattern of the skin to the autoimmune insult of PV. A role of TH_2-mediated immune reaction with involvement of IgG4–IgG2 autoantibody isotypes and cytokines that induce epithelial proliferation and eosinophilic chemotaxis has been proposed; however, this remains to be proven. The majority of patients with pemphigus vegetans have IgG autoantibodies against Dsg3 antigen, which leads to loss of cellular cohesion in the epidermis. Autoantibodies against Dsg1 are present only in a minority of patients.

Pemphigus vegetans has been reported in association with human immunodeficiency virus (HIV) infection, organ transplantation, drug intake, most notably captopril, and malignant neoplasms. It comprises only 1–20% of all pemphigus cases and is most common in North Africa. It predominantly affects middle-aged women, with a mean age of onset of 40–50 years.

CLINICAL PRESENTATION

Pemphigus vegetans presents with flaccid blisters and erosions that form papillomatous or vegetative plaques (**19.2**)[9]. The groin, axillae, and inframammary folds are most frequently involved. Oral lesions presenting as vegetative plaques on the vermilion border of the lips occur in most patients.

Erosive stomatitis and a cerebriform tongue, characterized by a pattern of sulci and gyri on the dorsal surface, are also features of pemphigus vegetans. Two different clinical variants have been recognized: the Neumann type and the Hallopeau type. The Neumann type is characterized by extensive flaccid bullae that erode and secondarily heal with papillomatous, vegetating plaques and a course similar to that of PV. The Hallopeau type, which has a relatively milder course, begins with grouped or annular pustules which evolve gradually to verrucous and papillomatous vegetations. Vegetative lesions may grow to a few centimeters in size, with new pustules developing at the periphery.

LABORATORY STUDIES

The histopathologic findings are similar in both types of pemphigus vegetans[9]. Epidermal hyperplasia, intraepidermal vesicles, eosinophilic abscesses, and suprabasal acantholysis are the most prominent features. A dense inflammatory infiltrate consisting of plasma cells and eosinophils may be present in the dermis.

Findings on DIF and IIF are identical to those seen in PV. There is intercellular IgG and C3 deposition in the epidermis.

COURSE, PROGNOSIS, AND COMPLICATIONS

Patients with the Hallopeau type often have a relatively benign disease, require lower doses of systemic corticosteroids, and usually have a prolonged remission. Patients with the Neumann type have a course similar to that of PV, need higher doses of systemic corticosteroids, and have relapses and remissions. Cutaneous lesions may be complicated by bacterial or fungal superinfection. Other complications include those due to systemic immunosuppression and corticosteroid use.

DIAGNOSIS

The most important differential diagnosis to pemphigus vegetans is pyodermatitis-pyostomatitis vegetans, which has the same clinical and histopathologic manifestations as pemphigus vegetans but can be differentiated on the basis of negative DIF. Condylomata lata, especially in the vulva or groin area, vegetating pyoderma, linear IgA pemphigus, BP, and Hailey–Hailey disease are also in the differential.

TREATMENT

Immunosuppressive drugs, in particular topical or intralesional corticosteroids for localized disease, and systemic corticosteroids for extensive disease, are the mainstay of treatment. However, systemic corticosteroids often are not sufficient to induce remission, especially in patients with the Neumann type. Combination therapy with azathioprine, dapsone, cyclosporine, or cyclophosphamide may be more effective. Combination of corticosteroids with etretinate has been recently reported as an effective treatment modality for lesions resistant to conventional therapy[10]. Extracorporal photophoresis and CO_2 laser have been effective in some case reports. Topical and oral antimicrobials are added when signs of secondary infection are present.

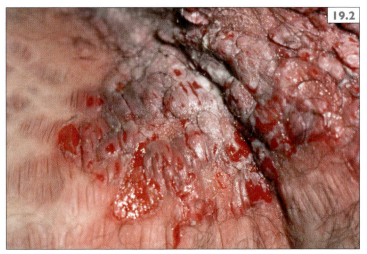

19.2 Pemphigus vegetans. Healing lesion in the genital area. (Courtesy of Dr. Larry E. Millikan.)

Paraneoplastic pemphigus

DEFINITION

Paraneoplastic pemphigus (PNP), also known as paraneoplastic autoimmune multiorgan syndrome, is an autoimmune blistering disorder that most often occurs in association with an underlying malignancy.

ETIOLOGY AND EPIDEMIOLOGY

Both humoral and cell-mediated immunity play a role in the development of PNP[11]. IgG autoantibodies to Dsg1 and 3 are thought to initiate loss of cellular adhesion of keratinocytes and intraepidermal blister formation. Autoantibodies to plakins, particularly envoplakin, periplakin, desmoplakin, plectin, and BP antigen type I (BPAg1) are very specific; however, their exact role in the pathogenesis of PNP remains unclear. The intracellular location of plakin proteins makes it unlikely that antiplakin autoantibodies initiate the pathologic process in PNP. Cell-mediated immunity may be responsible for the variable clinical manifestations of PNP.

PNP occurs in association with lymphoproliferative neoplasms, Castleman's disease, thymoma, and retroperitoneal sarcomas. Among the lymphoproliferative disorders, non-Hodgkin's lymphoma and chronic lymphocytic leukemia are the most common. PNP affects all age groups, including children, and has no gender predilection. In children, Castleman's disease is the most commonly associated tumor. Diagnosis of the underlying neoplasm usually precedes the development of PNP; however, in approximately one-third of patients the underlying neoplasm is undiagnosed at the time that PNP develops.

CLINICAL PRESENTATION

The most characteristic clinical feature of PNP is the presence of severe intractable stomatitis that extends onto the vermilion of the lip. Painful oral blisters, erosions, and ulcerations are frequently the presenting sign, and are most resistant to therapy. Ocular, esophageal, nasopharyngeal, vaginal, labial, and penile mucosal surfaces may also be affected. Cutaneous lesions are polymorphic and mimic other skin conditions, such as erythema multiforme, Stevens–Johnson syndrome, and toxic epidermal necrolysis. Patients may present with targetoid lesions, flaccid or tense bullae, erosions, and hemorrhagic crusts.

LABORATORY STUDIES

The histopathologic findings of cutaneous lesions show considerable variability, reflecting the polymorphism seen clinically. Suprabasal acantholysis similar to PV, necrosis of the epidermal keratinocytes (**19.3**), as well as vacuolar degeneration of basal cells similar to that seen in erythema multiforme are characteristic.

DIF of perilesional skin reveals intercellular deposition of IgG and C3, and variable staining along the basement membrane zone. IIF is preferentially done on murine bladder to detect IgG antibodies against plakin proteins and desmogleins. Because DIF is occasionally negative and antidesmoglein antibodies are not always present, the most reliable diagnostic tool is the detection of serum antiplakin antibodies.

Immunoblotting and immunoprecipitation are additional diagnostic tools that are used to demonstrate the presence of different antiplakin antibodies.

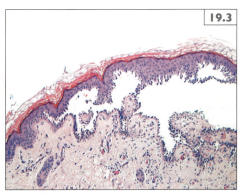

19.3 Paraneoplastic pemphigus. Suprabasal acantholysis and rare necrotic keratinocytes (H&E, ×10).

COURSE, PROGNOSIS, AND COMPLICATIONS

For the majority of patients with benign tumors, their condition improves substantially and/or clears completely following surgical excision of the tumor. Alternatively, mortality rate is higher than 90% when PNP occurs in the setting of a malignant neoplasm, in spite of treatment. Death results from complications of immunosuppressive therapy, such as sepsis, progression of malignancy, bronchiolitis obliterans, or gastrointestinal bleeding.

DIAGNOSIS

The diagnosis of PNP is made on the basis of clinical and histopathologic observations, immunofluorescence, and immunoprecipitation tests. No generally accepted diagnostic criteria have been defined thus far. The differential diagnosis includes erythema multiforme, PV, CP, Stevens–Johnson disease, toxic epidermal necrolysis, and graft-versus-host disease.

TREATMENT

The management of PNP includes treatment of the underlying neoplasm as well as suppression of the immune system to prevent production of pathogenic autoantibodies. Rituximab, an anti-CD20 antibody, has been used in patients with underlying non-Hodgkin's lymphoma; however, remission rates remain dismal. Immunosuppressive therapy consists of oral prednisone in combination with cyclosporine or cyclophosphamide. Further treatment options include azathioprine, mycophenolate mofetil, and high-dose IVIG, which may be used alone or in conjunction with corticosteroids. Cutaneous lesions respond more quickly to therapy than the stomatitis. Overall, PNP is recalcitrant to treatment.

Bullous pemphigoid

DEFINITION, ETIOLOGY, AND EPIDEMIOLOGY

Bullous pemphigoid (BP) is a chronic, autoimmune blistering skin disorder that predominantly affects the elderly and results in significant morbidity.

BP results from autoantibodies against two hemidesmosomal proteins, BPAg1 (also known as BP230), and BP antigen type II (BPAg2 or BP180 or type XVII collagen). BPAg1, a cytoplasmic protein belonging to the plakin family, plays an important role in promoting adhesion of the intermediate filaments to the hemidesmosomes in the plasma membrane. BPAg2 is a transmembrane protein with a large collagenous extracellular domain that is associated with the hemidesmosome-anchoring filament complexes in the basal keratinocytes. Binding of the autoantibodies to their target antigens leads to complement activation and recruitment of inflammatory cells, ultimately resulting in blister formation.

BP predominantly occurs in the elderly after the age of 60. Men and women are equally affected, and there are no known racial or ethnic predilections. Common triggers in patients with an underlying genetic predisposition include malignancy, trauma, UV irradiation, and drugs, most notably diuretics, analgesics, antibiotics, and captopril.

CLINICAL PRESENTATION

Clinically, two phases of BP are recognized. The nonbullous phase is characterized by nonspecific, eczematous, and urticarial papules and plaques which may persist for several weeks to months (**19.4**). These lesions may remain the only sign of the disease. Alternatively, they may progress to the bullous phase, during which tense bullae with serous or hemorrhagic fluid, erosions, and crusts develop on normal or erythematous skin (**19.5**, **19.6**). Pruritus and tenderness at the site of lesions are common. The skin

eruption may be localized to a particular body site, but is more often widespread, favoring skin folds. Axillae, medial thighs, groin (**19.6**), abdomen, flexor aspects of the forearms, and the lower aspects of the legs are the main sites of predilection. Mucosal involvement is rare.

Genital involvement is more common in children than adults with BP. Vulvar disease has been reported in 9% of adults and 40% of children with BP[12]. Rarely, BP in the vulva may be complicated by periclitoral adhesions. Localized vulvar pemphigoid is a rare variant of BP, which has been reported in children between the ages of 6 and 13. In this variant, blistering, erosions, and crusting remain localized to the vulva and are associated with a good prognosis. These patients have circulating autoantibodies directed against the same 230-kDa antigen as the antibodies in patients with generalized BP[13].

LABORATORY STUDIES

Histopathologic examination of a blister reveals a subepidermal split with superficial dermal inflammation consisting of eosinophils, histiocytes, and lymphocytes (**19.7**).

DIF of perilesional skin shows linear deposition of IgG and C3 along the dermal–epidermal junction (DEJ) in up to 100% of cases. IIF using the patient's serum reveals linear deposition of IgG and C3 at the DEJ of normal human skin in approximately 70% of patients. Antibody titers do not correlate with the disease course. When 1 mol/L sodium chloride (salt)-split skin is used as the substrate, circulating antibodies from the patient's serum deposit on the roof of the artificial blister at the DEJ.

COURSE, PROGNOSIS, AND COMPLICATIONS

BP is a chronic disease, with spontaneous exacerbations and remissions. The majority of patients experience clinical remission within 5 years. Patients with localized disease have the best prognosis and respond

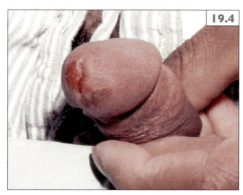

19.4 Bullous pemphigoid. Eczematous plaque on the head of the penis. (Courtesy of Dr. Larry E. Millikan.)

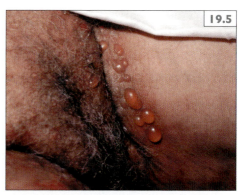

19.5 Bullous pemphigoid. Bullae in the groin. (Courtesy of Dr. Tomasz F. Mroczkowski.)

well to therapy. Patients with progressive or severe, widespread disease, those requiring high doses of corticosteroids and immunosuppressive agents, and those with underlying medical problems have an increased risk of death. Death most often occurs within the first 12 weeks of therapy mainly from infection complicated by sepsis and treatment-related adverse events.

DIAGNOSIS

The diagnosis of BP is made on the basis of clinical appearance, histology, and immunofluorescence studies. Nevertheless, the distinction of BP from other autoimmune blistering disorders can sometimes prove challenging. The differential diagnosis includes CP, epidermolysis bullosa acquisita (EBA) and linear IgA bullous dermatosis (LABD). Vulvar BP can present with clinical findings similar to those of lichen sclerosus et atrophicus or herpes simplex infection. In children, vulvar BP can raise false concerns about sexual abuse[14].

TREATMENT

The general goal of treatment is to decrease or stop blister formation, promote healing of existing blisters and erosions, and to control the associated pruritus. Localized disease may be successfully treated with

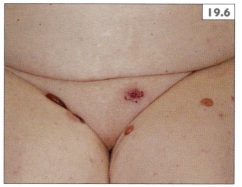

19.6 Bullous pemphigoid. Intact hemorrhagic bullae and healing erosion in the groin area.

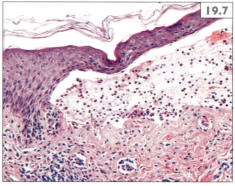

19.7 Bullous pemphigoid. Subepidermal blister with a dense eosinophilic infiltrate in the blister cavity and dermis (H & E, ×20).

topical corticosteroids or topical calcineurin inhibitors in the case of localized vulvar BP[15]. Patients with widespread skin disease should be started on systemic corticosteroids unless contraindicated. Addition of tetracycline plus niacinamide may allow for a quicker steroid taper. Patients with contraindications to corticosteroids are treated with dapsone, a combination of tetracycline and niacinamide, or immunosuppressive drugs, such as azathioprine, cyclophosphamide, mycophenolate mofetil, cyclosporine, or methotrexate. IVIG and plasmapheresis are recommended if all other treatments fail[6,8].

Pemphigoid gestationis

DEFINITION, ETIOLOGY, AND EPIDEMIOLOGY

Pemphigoid gestationis (PG) is a rare autoimmune blistering disease of pregnancy, which develops during the second or third trimester. PG, also known as herpes gestationis, is an autoimmune blistering condition that results from the recognition of placental proteins as foreign and the subsequent production of antiplacental antibodies that cross-react with the same proteins in the skin[16]. The main antigen is collagen XVII or BPAg2, which is present in both skin and placenta. It is now believed that an abnormal expression of major histocompatibility complex (MHC) class II molecules in the placenta leads to the presentation of this self-antigen to the maternal immune system. Subsequently, autoantibodies are formed, mainly of the IgG1 and IgG3 subclasses, which cross-react with collagen XVII in the skin. The major antigenic epitopes are restricted within the noncollagenous 16A (NC-16A) region of collagen XVII. Once the antibodies bind to collagen XVII, they activate complement C3 and recruit inflammatory cells, resulting in the formation of a subepidermal blister.

PG is a rare disorder, with an incidence of 1 in 50,000 pregnancies[16]. No racial differences have been reported. An increased incidence of HLA-DR3 and HLA-DR4, as well as autoimmune diseases, particularly Grave's disease, may exist amongst patients with PG. PG has also been reported in association with trophoblastic tumors, choriocarcinoma, and hydatidiform moles. Exacerbating factors include oral contraceptives and menses in cases that continue postpartum.

CLINICAL PRESENTATION

PG typically develops during the second or third trimester of pregnancy, but it may occur any time from the first trimester to the immediate postpartum period. It usually presents with intense pruritus, which precedes the onset of lesions by days to weeks. Typically, lesions begin as urticarial papules and plaques in and around the umbilicus and spread centrifugally to involve the trunk, extremities, palms, and soles (**19.8**). Subsequently, tense vesicles and bullae appear superimposed on the urticarial plaques and on normal skin. The face and mucous membranes are usually spared. Infants born to mothers with PG may also have cutaneous findings due to transplacental transfer of maternal immunoglobulins; however, this occurs rarely.

LABORATORY STUDIES

Histopathologic examination shows eosinophilic spongiosis of the epidermis, a subepidermal blister with eosinophils in the cavity, as well as a mixed dermal infiltrate of eosinophils and lymphocytes. Vacuolization and necrosis of the basal layer may be seen.

DIF of perilesional skin shows linear deposition of C3 along the basement membrane in 100% of cases, and linear deposition of IgG in 25–50% of cases. Similar findings are observed in the skin of neonates born to affected mothers, regardless of whether skin findings are present. IIF detects C3 in the sera of patients with PG in more than 90% of cases, but IgG is positive in less than 25%. A three-step complement-binding-IIF technique enhances the sensitivity and reveals the presence of IgG autoantibodies in virtually all patients' sera.

COURSE, PROGNOSIS, AND COMPLICATIONS
In the majority of cases, PG improves during the last weeks of pregnancy, only to flare again postpartum, within 24–48 hours of delivery. The eruption usually resolves within 3 months postpartum; however, in rare cases it may persist for years. The diagnosis of chronic PG versus conversion to BP has been considered in these cases[17]. PG often recurs with subsequent pregnancies, in which case it may have an earlier onset and a more severe course. Skip pregnancies have been reported in a few patients.

Infants born to mothers with PG rarely have cutaneous findings due to passive transplacental transfer of maternal immunoglobulins. However, they are usually born prematurely and are small for gestational age. In addition, infants born to mothers who were treated with oral corticosteroids during pregnancy are at risk of developing adrenal insufficiency, albeit very rarely.

DIAGNOSIS
The major differential diagnosis of PG is pruritic urticarial papules and plaques of pregnancy (PUPPP), which is the most common dermatosis of pregnancy and affects women in the third trimester of their first pregnancy. PUPPP presents with urticarial papules and plaques within the striae distensae, sparing the periumbilical area. When clinical distinction is not possible, DIF can be used, as it is invariably negative in PUPPP. Other differential diagnoses include BP, CP, and PV.

TREATMENT
Treatment of PG may present a challenge during pregnancy. Systemic therapy should not be initiated unless the severity of symptoms outweighs the potential risks for the fetus. The goals of therapy are to control the intense pruritus and suppress the formation of new lesions. Topical corticosteroids with or without antihistamines may be used for limited disease; however, they are usually insufficient to control the symptoms. Systemic corticosteroids are the mainstay of therapy as they are highly effective and relatively safe to use during pregnancy. Generally, low doses may suffice; however, the dose may be increased during the postpartum period to suppress any anticipated flare. Addition of immunosuppressive agents to oral corticosteroids is contraindicated during pregnancy and breast feeding[16]. Skin lesions in infants are transient and require no specific treatment.

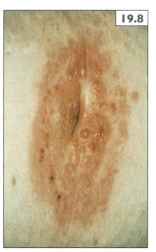

19.8 Pemphigoid gestationis. (Courtesy of St John's Institute of Dermatology (King's College), Guy's Hospital, London, with permission.)

Cicatricial pemphigoid

DEFINITION, ETIOLOGY, AND EPIDEMIOLOGY

Cicatricial pemphigoid (CP) is a rare, scarring autoimmune blistering disease that favors the mucosal surfaces more than the skin. CP, also known as mucous membrane pemphigoid, results from binding of IgG and less commonly IgA autoantibodies to the basement membrane of stratified squamous epithelia of mucosae and skin. These autoantibodies bind to specific extracellular components of the hemidesmosomes, namely the distal C-terminus of BPAg2 and epilegrin (also known as laminin 5). Patients with predominant ocular CP have IgG autoantibodies against the β_4 subunit of $\alpha_6\beta_4$ integrin. Binding of the autoantibodies to their antigenic substrates results in a subepidermal split.

CP is a rare condition that typically occurs in the elderly, with a mean age of onset of 66 years. There is a slight female predominance, with a female to male ratio of 1.5:1. There is no apparent racial or ethnic predilection although some studies have shown an association with specific HLA phenotypes, primarily HLA-DQw7, in both oral and ocular forms of the disease. Patients with antiepilegrin CP may be at a higher risk of developing adenocarcinoma[18].

CLINICAL PRESENTATION

The two most frequently involved sites are the oral and conjunctival mucosae. Oral mucosa is affected in ~85% of patients, and is frequently the only site of involvement. Clinically, patients present with painful erosive gingivitis, bleeding, and chronic erosions on the palate, tongue, and floor of the mouth. Intact blisters are rarely observed. Lesions invariably progress to scarring, which results in delicate, white, reticulated patches. Ocular lesions manifest as conjunctivitis or a foreign-body sensation. Chronic inflammation may result in progressive scarring and blindness. Other mucosal surfaces with a squamous epithelial lining, including the external genitalia and anus, may be affected.

Genital mucosa is affected in up to 50% of patients with CP (**19.9**). In women, painful erosions and fissures may affect the vulva and perineum. Examination of the vaginal mucosa may reveal erythematous, friable mucosa. Scarring and loss of vulvar architecture may occur due to chronic disease[19]. Agglutination or resorption of the labia minora, stenosis of the introitus and the urethral meatus, as well as phimosis of the clitoris may be seen. In men, adhesions can form between the prepuce and the glans penis. Involvement of the anorectal area is associated with pain on defecation, intermittent bleeding, and narrowing of the anal canal.

Skin involvement, which occurs in only 25–30% of patients, is variable. The scalp, face, neck, and upper trunk are most frequently involved. Tense, serous or hemorrhagic bullae, which heal with scarring and milia, are the typical presentation. Cutaneous CP involving the head and neck without mucosal involvement is known as the Brunsting–Perry variant of localized BP.

LABORATORY STUDIES

Histopathologic examination of an intact vesicle reveals a subepidermal blister with a variable degree of inflammation in the dermis, composed primarily of mononuclear cells (**19.10**). Older lesions tend to demonstrate fibrosis in the upper dermis. Biopsy from a mucosal lesion may contain plasma cells.

DIF of perilesional skin demonstrates linear IgG and/or C3 deposits, and less commonly IgA or IgM, along the DEJ. IIF is positive for circulating IgG or IgA/IgM autoantibody against the basement membrane in 20–30% of patients. Using salt-split skin, the majority of patients have autoantibodies that bind to the epidermal side of the split skin. Patients with antiepilegrin CP have antibodies that bind to the dermal side.

COURSE, PROGNOSIS, AND COMPLICATIONS

CP is a chronic, potentially devastating, but rarely fatal disease. The most important long-term complication is visual loss due to ocular involvement. Life-threatening complications due to laryngeal, esophageal, and tracheal disease are rare. Dyspareunia and narrowing of the introitus can result from CP of the vulva.

DIAGNOSIS

CP is differentiated from other blistering disorders on the basis of clinical, histopathologic, and immunopathologic findings. Differential diagnosis includes BP, LABD, and EBA. Genital lesions may mimic the findings of other inflammatory skin disorders, including erosive lichen planus and lichen sclerosus et atrophicus. Differentiating between the various conditions is important because they affect different organ systems and have different prognoses.

TREATMENT

The treatment of patients with CP depends upon the extent and severity of the disease. A multidisciplinary team should be involved in the care of patients with CP of various organ systems. Localized disease may be successfully treated with potent topical or intralesional corticosteroids. Systemic therapy is implemented for more extensive disease. Dapsone is a first-line therapy for oral and cutaneous disease. Ocular involvement is best treated with cyclophosphamide, either alone or in combination with systemic corticosteroids. Systemic corticosteroids alone are generally not sufficient. They are used in combination with other immunosuppressive medications, such as azathioprine and mycophenolate mofetil. High-dose IVIG and rituximab may be effective in treatment-resistant cases. Recently, it was proposed that patients with vulvar disease be treated with prednisone in combination with cyclophosphamide or azathioprine to prevent devastating complications from scarring[20]. Surgery is reserved for severe esophageal, laryngotracheal, and ocular disease.

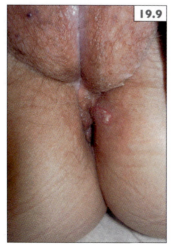

19.9 Cicatricial pemphigoid. Painful, macerated erosion with erythematous borders on the perineum.

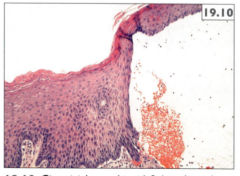

19.10 Cicatricial pemphigoid. Subepidermal blister with a mixed inflammatory infiltrate and red blood cells within the blister cavity as well as early fibrosis of the superficial dermis (H & E, ×20).

Linear IgA bullous dermatosis

DEFINITION, ETIOLOGY, AND EPIDEMIOLOGY

Linear IgA bullous dermatosis (LABD) is a rare autoimmune blistering disorder in children and adults, which may be triggered by drugs, infections, and malignant processes.

LABD, also known as chronic bullous disease of childhood in children, is defined by the presence of homogenous linear deposits of IgA along the DEJ. The autoantibodies target fragments of the extracellular domain of BPAg2, namely proteins with a molecular weight of 285 kDa, as well as 97-kDa and 120-kDa antigens. The 120-kDa soluble ectodomain of BPAg2 is the major target antigen. Binding of the autoantibody to the antigen leads to complement activation and neutrophil chemotaxis. These events result in loss of adhesion at the DEJ and blister formation.

LABD occurs in association with drugs, most notably vancomycin, infections, and lymphoproliferative disorders. An association with HLA-B8, CW7, and DR3 haplotypes has been reported. LABD has a bimodal age distribution, peaking in the first and sixth decades of life.

CLINICAL PRESENTATION

LABD consists of pruritic, annular papules, vesicles, and bullae on erythematous or normal-appearing skin. Targetoid, erythema multiforme-like lesions may also be present. The distribution of lesions differs between children and adults. In children, lesions are most frequently found on or near the genitalia, perioral region, and the lower trunk (**19.11**). The genital region is involved in more than 80% of children. In adults, there is a predilection for the extensor surfaces and the trunk, with a symmetric distribution. Involvement of the perineum and perioral region is not common. Oral and ocular disease ranges in severity from mild oral ulcers to severe oral or conjunctival disease.

Ocular involvement is associated with photosensitivity, blurred vision, scarring, and rarely blindness.

LABORATORY STUDIES

Histopathologic examination reveals a subepidermal blister with collections of neutrophils aligned along the basement membrane, occasionally forming microabscesses in the dermal papillae (**19.12**).

DIF of perilesional skin demonstrates linear IgA deposits along the DEJ. IIF demonstrates circulating IgA autoantibodies in the majority of patients.

COURSE, PROGNOSIS, AND COMPLICATIONS

The course of LABD is variable and unpredictable. Most cases spontaneously resolve within 5 years of onset. In drug-induced cases, immediate cessation of the suspected drug will lead to remission.

DIAGNOSIS

LABD is differentiated from the other bullous disorders based on the clinical, histopathologic, and immunofluorescence findings. Differential diagnosis includes dermatitis herpetiformis (DH), CP, BP, and EBA. Differentiation of LABD from DH is the most challenging. By definition, LABD is differentiated from DH on the basis of DIF. Whereas LABD is characterized by linear IgA deposits along the basement membrane, DH has granular depositions of IgA in the dermal papillae or in a continuous pattern along the basement membrane[21].

TREATMENT

The majority of patients with LABD respond well to dapsone or sulfapyridine therapy. Glucose-6-phosphate dehydrogenase (G6PD) levels should be measured prior to the initiation of therapy, because dapsone may cause hemolytic anemia or methemoglobinemia in the absence of G6PD. The treatment should be started with a low dose of dapsone, which can be

19.11 Linear IgA bullous dermatosis. Annular and herpetiform hemorrhagic bullae admixed with crusted erosions on erythematous skin involving the genitalia and the lower trunk of a child.

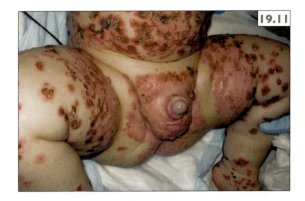

19.12 Linear IgA bullous dermatosis. Subepidermal blister with a predominantly neutrophilic infiltrate in the underlying dermis (H & E, ×10).

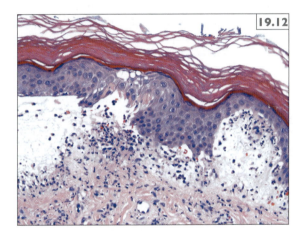

slowly increased to as high as 300 mg daily. Some patients with widespread disease may require addition of systemic corticosteroids along with dapsone in order to induce remission. Other reported effective therapies include oral antibiotics and colchicine. Mycophenolate mofetil, azathioprine, IVIG, and cyclosporine can be used as steroid-sparing agents in patients who do not respond to a combination of prednisone and dapsone, or in patients with severe disease.

Epidermolysis bullosa acquisita

DEFINITION, ETIOLOGY, AND EPIDEMIOLOGY

Epidermolysis bullosa acquisita (EBA) is a chronic autoimmune blistering disorder of the skin and mucous membranes associated with autoimmunity to type VII collagen. EBA results from IgG autoantibodies binding to the noncollagenous N-terminal domain (NC1) of type VII collagen, a major component of the anchoring fibrils, which attaches the basement membrane to the underlying dermis. A small group of patients may have IgG autoantibodies against the central collagenous domain or the NC2 domain. Upon binding, the autoantibodies interfere with the assembly of type VII collagen and its interactions with other matrix proteins. This results in a subepidermal blister at the level of the sublamina densa.

EBA affects middle-aged individuals and the elderly. It does not have any racial or gender predilection. An association with HLA-DR2 has been reported, implying the possibility of a genetic component. A number of systemic diseases have been reported in association with EBA, including Crohn's disease, systemic lupus erythematosus, rheumatoid arthritis, thyroiditis, and diabetes mellitus.

CLINICAL PRESENTATION

EBA presents with skin fragility and trauma-induced bullous lesions, which heal with milia, atrophic scars, and dyspigmentation (**19.13**). The oral, ocular, vaginal, and other mucous membranes may be involved. Three distinctive clinical variants of EBA are recognized: the noninflammatory variant, the generalized inflammatory variant, and the mucous membrane variant. The noninflammatory variant presents with noninflammatory, tense vesicles and bullae on extensor acral surfaces. The vesicles on mucous membranes rupture easily; therefore, erosions are most frequently encountered on the mucosal surfaces. The generalized inflammatory variant is characterized by widespread, tense vesicles and bullae, as well as generalized erythema, urticarial plaques and pruritus. The bullae form in areas that are not exposed to trauma and heal with little scarring. Mucous membranes may be involved. The mucous membrane variant affects predominantly the mucous membranes, including the vaginal and rectal mucosa, and is associated with significant scarring. Patients present with erosions on one or more mucosal surfaces, similar to CP.

LABORATORY STUDIES

Histopathology of a blister reveals a subepidermal split with a variable degree of mixed inflammatory infiltrate in the dermis, composed of neutrophils, eosinophils, or lymphocytes (**19.14**). In the noninflammatory lesions, there is minimal-to-absent cellular infiltrate.

DIF of perilesional skin demonstrates linear deposition of IgG and/or C3, and rarely IgA or IgM, along the DEJ in approximately 100% of cases. IIF using the patient's serum on normal human skin substrate demonstrates the presence of circulating IgG antibodies that recognize type VII collagen. These antibodies bind to the dermal side of salt-split skin.

Other tests may be performed to establish the diagnosis of EBA, including immunoelectron microscopy, immunoblotting, immunoprecipitation, and enzyme-linked immunosorbent assay; however, these tests are expensive and not readily available in most clinical practices.

COURSE, PROGNOSIS, AND COMPLICATIONS

EBA is a chronic disease that waxes and wanes with periods of partial remission and exacerbation. EBA can cause significant morbidity. Atrophic scarring may result in limited joint mobility. Acral involvement may be mutilating and cause 'mitten' deformities that hinder the daily activities of patients. Involvement of the aerodigestive tract may lead to dysphagia, laryngeal stenosis, and airway compromise. Ocular disease may be complicated by conjunctival scarring and blindness. Vaginal or rectal involvement may lead to strictures, dyspareunia, and difficulty with defecation.

DIAGNOSIS

The diagnosis of EBA is established on the basis of clinical, histopathologic and immunopathologic findings. The differential diagnosis includes BP, LABD, CP, and bullous systemic lupus erythematosus. The findings on DIF, IIF, and salt-split skin are especially useful in differentiating EBA from BP.

TREATMENT

EBA is generally refractory to treatment. Because of the rarity of this disorder, treatment is largely based on anecdotal reports. Topical steroids are used for localized disease. Systemic therapy is reserved for generalized disease. Options include prednisone, azathioprine, methotrexate, mycophenolate mofetil, dapsone, colchicine, and IVIG, alone or in combination with plasmapheresis[22].

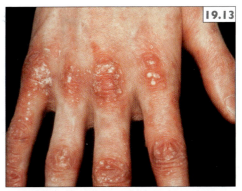

19.13 Epidermolysis bullosa acquisita. (Courtesy of St John's Institute of Dermatology [King's College], Guy's Hospital, London, with permission.)

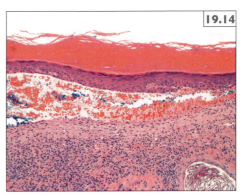

19.14 Epidermolysis bullosa acquisita. Subepidermal blister with red blood cells in the blister cavity and a dense, mixed inflammatory infiltrate in the underlying dermis (H & E, ×10).

Hailey–Hailey disease

DEFINITION, ETIOLOGY, AND EPIDEMIOLOGY

Hailey–Hailey disease (benign familial pemphigus) is an uncommon, autosomal dominant disorder, characterized by flaccid blisters and erosions that favor intertriginous areas.

Hailey–Hailey disease is caused by mutations in the *ATP2C1* gene, which encodes a Golgi-associated Ca^{2+} ATPase pump, resulting in depletion of intraluminal Golgi Ca^{2+} stores. Ca^{2+} depletion in the Golgi apparatus impairs complete processing of intercellular proteins, leading to acantholysis. The exact prevalence of Hailey–Hailey disease remains unknown. The mode of inheritance is autosomal dominant with variable penetrance; however, sporadic cases with a negative family history have been reported in about 15% of patients. The age of onset is usually the third to fourth decade.

CLINICAL PRESENTATION

The most common presentation is with recurrent macerated or crusted erosions, which tend to spread peripherally, producing a circinate border with small, flaccid, easily-ruptured vesicles and crusts. Chronic, moist, malodorous vegetations and painful fissures are common. Symptoms are exacerbated by heat, friction, and sweating. Healing occurs without scarring, leaving postinflammatory hyperpigmentation. The axillary folds, inguinum, perianal region, and lateral aspects of the neck are major sites of predilection (**19.15**). Asymptomatic leukonychia is present in about 70% of cases.

Solitary anogenital involvement is rare in Hailey–Hailey disease. Vulvar disease is characterized by a pruritic, painful, and persistent eruption that may resemble candidiasis, whereas vaginal disease may present with dyspareunia as the sole clinical manifestation. Verrucous papules resembling condylomata acuminata are an unusual presentation of perineal and perianal disease[23].

LABORATORY STUDIES

Histopathologic examination reveals extensive acantholysis resembling a 'dilapidated brick wall' and few dyskeratotic cells (**19.16**). In chronic lesions, epidermal hyperplasia, parakeratosis and focal scale-crust are found. DIF is negative.

COURSE, PROGNOSIS, AND COMPLICATIONS

The disease waxes and wanes with periods of remission and exacerbation. The clinical course is complicated by colonization and secondary bacterial, fungal, and viral infections. Kaposi's varicelliform eruption due to dissemination of herpes simplex virus is a rare and serious complication, characterized by fever and a rapidly spreading vesicular eruption, which should be treated promptly. Rare cases of squamous cell carcinoma arising *de novo* in skin lesions of Hailey–Hailey disease have been reported[24].

DIAGNOSIS

The diagnosis of Hailey–Hailey disease is made on the basis of clinical and histopathologic findings. Genital Hailey–Hailey disease may clinically resemble PV, erosive lichen planus, herpes simplex infection, inverse psoriasis, candidiasis, atopic dermatitis, and erythrasma. Extramammary Paget's disease must be ruled out.

TREATMENT

Topical steroids combined with topical antimicrobials and cleansers are the treatment of choice. Patients should be advised to wear light-weight clothing and avoid activities that result in sweating or friction to the skin. Intralesional steroids are used if lesions are refractory to topical steroids. Anecdotal reports have described a therapeutic benefit from topical cyclosporine, tacrolimus, and 5-fluorouracil. There is no strong evidence to support systemic therapy for Hailey–Hailey disease; however, oral cyclosporine, methotrexate, and acitretin have been shown to be effective in some case reports[25,26].

Surgical excision is reserved for refractory cases. Superficial ablative techniques, including dermabrasion, 5-aminolevulinic acid, photodynamic therapy, and erbium-YAG laser have been used with limited success.

Other cutaneous diseases with a bullous presentation in the anogenital region include bullous lupus erythematosus, bullous lichen planus, and bullous lichen sclerosus et atrophicus. These disorders are discussed in detail in other chapters.

19.15 Hailey–Hailey disease. Hyperpigmented and slightly erythematous plaque with peripheral erosions and fissures involving the inguinal folds.

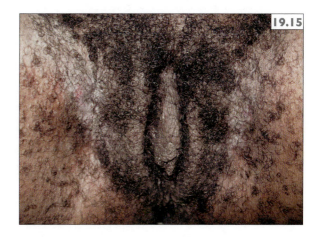

19.16 Hailey–Hailey disease. Extensive intraepidermal acantholysis resembling a 'dilapidated brick wall' and rare dyskeratotic cells (H&E, x20).

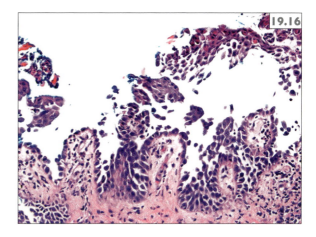

CHAPTER 20

Miscellaneous Dermatoses

Electra Nicolaidou, MD, Christina Stefanaki, MD, and Andreas D. Katsambas, MD

- **Vitiligo**
- **Psoriasis**
- **Lichen planus**
- **Adamandiades–Behçet disease**
- **Lichen sclerosus**

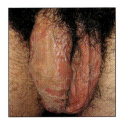
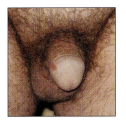
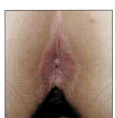
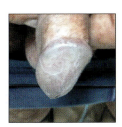

Vitiligo

DEFINITION, ETIOLOGY, AND EPIDEMIOLOGY

Vitiligo is an acquired disease characterized by well-circumscribed, depigmented macules and patches. Vitiligo affects approximately 0.5–2% of the population worldwide. Disease onset in childhood (<12 years of age) has been reported in 25–30% of cases[1].

It is generally agreed that there is an absence of functional melanocytes in lesional skin. Various theories have been suggested for the pathogenesis of vitiligo, such as the autoimmune destruction of melanocytes, an intrinsic defect in the structure and function of melanocytes, a defective defense system against free radicals, and destruction of melanocytes by autocytotoxic metabolites or neurochemical substances[2].

CLINICAL PRESENTATION

Vitiligo is characterized by the presence of uniformly amelanotic macules and patches with fairly discrete borders. Lesions are usually found in areas that are normally hyperpigmented, such as the face, axillae, groins, areolae, and genitalia (**20.1–20.3**), or subjected to repeated friction and trauma, such as the dorsa of hands, feet, elbows, knees, and ankles. Leukotrichia may be present in vitiligo patches (**20.2**). The distribution of the lesions is usually symmetric, but it can also be unilateral or dermatomal. The Koebner phenomenon could be present.

LABORATORY STUDIES

There is an absence of dopa-positive melanocytes in lesional skin.

COURSE, PROGNOSIS, AND COMPLICATIONS

The course of vitiligo is unpredictable. The lesions may enlarge centrifugally over time and new lesions can appear. The disease may stabilize for a long period of time or exacerbate rapidly. Some patients develop autoimmune endocrinopathies, particularly thyroid dysfunction.

DIAGNOSIS

The diagnosis is usually clinical. The differential diagnosis of genital lesions includes mostly lichen sclerosus et atrophicus and postinflammatory hypopigmentation.

TREATMENT

Narrow band ultraviolet B phototherapy, psoralen + ultraviolet A (PUVA), topical corticosteroids, topical calcineurin inhibitors, excimer (exciplex) laser, and surgical therapies have been used with variable results for the treatment of vitiligo[3,4]. Most genital lesions are managed with topical corticosteroids and topical calcineurin inhibitors (tacrolimus and pimecrolimus). Phototherapy is contraindicated in the genital area.

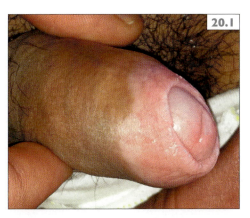

20.1 Vitiligo involving the prepuce and glans penis.

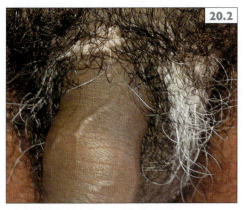

20.2 Vitiligo patches and leukotrichia.

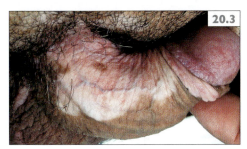

20.3 Vitiligo involving the prepuce and shaft of the penis.

Psoriasis

DEFINITION, ETIOLOGY, AND EPIDEMIOLOGY

Psoriasis is a chronic inflammatory disease that affects the skin and joints. Psoriasis affects approximately 2% of the population worldwide. Although it can appear at any age, two peaks in age of onset have been identified: one at 16–22 years and another at 57–60 years. Patients with early disease onset have, in general, more severe disease and are much more likely to have an affected first-degree relative.

Psoriasis is a polygenic disease caused by polymorphisms in genes involved both in immune function and in keratinocyte biology. Triggering factors, both external (trauma, sunburn) and systemic (infections, drugs, stress) can elicit the disease in genetically predisposed patients.

CLINICAL PRESENTATION

Chronic plaque psoriasis is the most common variant of the disease and it is characterized by sharply-demarcated, erythematous plaques with silvery scale. The body surface area affected can be limited or extensive. Sites of predilection include the scalp, elbows, knees, and presacrum.

The genitalia are involved in 30–40% of psoriasis patients[5]. The genital region is rarely the exclusive site of involvement. Lesions on the male genitalia can have less or no scale and they usually appear as barely raised erythematous plaques or patches. However, the color of the lesions and their well-defined borders are usually distinctive (**20.4, 20.5**).

Flexural psoriasis can affect the groin, vulva, gluteal cleft, as well as other body folds. Scaling is again greatly reduced or absent, but the lesions retain the characteristic psoriatic color and well-defined edges. Fissuring at the depth of the fold is common, especially at the gluteal cleft (**20.6**). Secondary infections and contact dermatitis are common events.

LABORATORY STUDIES

Acanthosis with elongated bulbous rete ridges, hypogranulosis, hyperkeratosis, parakeratosis, dilated blood vessels, and neutrophils singly or within aggregates in the epidermis are found on histology. These characteristics, however, may be more subtle in penile and vulvar lesions.

COURSE, PROGNOSIS, AND COMPLICATIONS

The course of psoriasis is chronic and unpredictable. Relapses are usually common. Bacterial or fungal infection of lesions in the genital area can occur. Psoriasis affecting the genital area may be associated with considerable morbidity and may severely impair the quality of life[6].

DIAGNOSIS

The diagnosis of psoriasis is usually clinical. When a solitary lesion is present on the genitalia, a biopsy may be necessary to exclude erythroplasia of Queyrat and Zoon's plasma cell balanitis. Flexural psoriasis involving the genital area should be distinguished mostly from candidiasis, seborrheic dermatitis, and tinea cruris.

TREATMENT

Low-to-mid-potency topical corticosteroids are the mainstay of therapy for genital psoriasis[7]. Short-term, intermittent use of moderate-to-potent corticosteroids could be used to induce a response in recalcitrant cases. Vitamin D analogs could also be used as monotherapy or in combination with steroids to minimize side-effects. Calcineurin inhibitors (tacrolimus and pimecrolimus) are also potential options for genital and flexural psoriasis.

Systemic therapy, including biologics, is rarely, if ever, indicated for isolated genital psoriasis. Nevertheless, such treatments are beneficial for genital lesions, if prescribed for severe and widespread psoriatic disease.

20.4 Psoriasis. Well-demarcated erythematous plaques with minimal scale on the penis and scrotum.

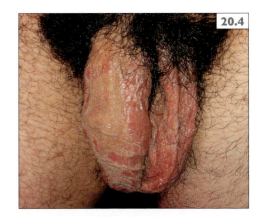

20.5 Psoriasis. Well-demarcated erythematous plaque with minimal scale on the glans penis and prepuce.

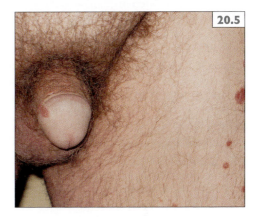

20.6 Flexural psoriasis with fissuring at the depth of the gluteal cleft.

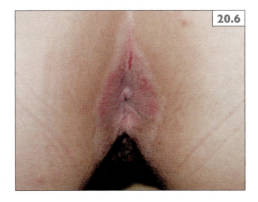

Lichen planus

DEFINITION, ETIOLOGY, AND EPIDEMIOLOGY

Lichen planus is a common inflammatory disorder that affects the skin, mucous membranes, nails, and hair. The exact incidence and prevalence are unknown but the overall prevalence is believed to be less than 1%[8]. Males and females are equally affected between the third and sixth decades; however, males develop the disease at an earlier age.

Immunologic mechanisms mediate the development of lichen planus, with cell-mediated immunity playing the major role. Activated CD8+ T lymphocytes predominate in the cellular infiltrate in lichen planus, leading to keratinocyte apoptosis[9].

CLINICAL PRESENTATION

Lichen planus on fully keratinized skin usually manifests with pruritic, violaceous, flat-topped, well-demarcated, polygonal papules that coalesce[9]. The lesions are usually symmetrically and bilaterally distributed over the extremities, particularly the wrists, although other areas may be involved. Fine whitish puncta or reticulated networks, known as Wickham striae, are present on the surface of many papules and are quite characteristic. Lesions can be distributed on areas of trauma (Koebner phenomenon) and usually heal with hyperpigmentation. Lichen planus can selectively affect the scalp, the nails, the oral mucosa, and the genitalia.

Male genitalia are involved in 25% of cases and the glans penis is most commonly affected, with annular lesions predominating (**20.7**)[9]. Annular lesions develop from arcuate grouping of individual papules (**20.8**). Central clearing and peripheral extension are noted. On the genitalia females develop whitish or erythematous plaques with erosions and occasionally a more generalized desquamative vaginitis, resulting sometimes in vaginal adhesions and labial agglutination[10]. A unique form of lichen planus has been described, involving both the oral mucosa with erythema and erosions of the gingivae and tongue together with desquamation and erosions of the vulva and vagina, associated with burning pain, dyspareunia, and vaginal discharge[11]. Anal lesions usually consist of hyperkeratotic plaques with fissuring and erosions. Inverse lichen planus is a rare form of the disease and is characterized by violaceous discrete papules and plaques affecting flexural areas such as the groin (**20.9**).

LABORATORY STUDIES

Histopathology is a helpful diagnostic tool. The two major findings are epidermal keratinocyte damage and lymphocytic lichenoid interface reaction. The epidermis shows thickening in a saw-toothed pattern. A band-like lymphocytic infiltrate is seen in the papillary dermis, producing some areas of vacuolar degeneration of the basal layer. Dyskeratotic keratinocytes are scattered within the epidermis.

COURSE, PROGNOSIS, AND COMPLICATIONS

Papular lichen planus usually is a self-limited disease and resolution occurs in several years. Erosive forms are more resistant and run a chronic course.

DIAGNOSIS

The diagnosis is made on clinical grounds and is confirmed with histopathology. The papular/annular form of the disease has to be differentiated from erythroplasia of Queyrat, psoriasis, and Zoon's balanitis. Erosive forms have to be distinguished from pemphigus vulgaris, cicatricial pemphigoid, genital herpes, and candidiasis.

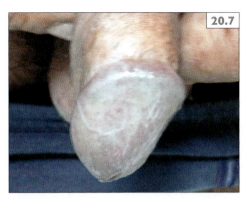

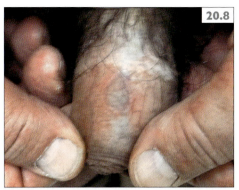

20.7 Lichen planus. Annular lesions on glans penis.

20.8 Lichen planus. Annular lesions on the shaft of the penis.

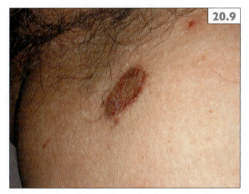

20.9 Inverse lichen planus in the groin of a patient with vulvar lichen planus.

TREATMENT

Potent topical steroids are the first-line treatment in genital lichen planus. Care must be given for the preparations not to spread onto healthy areas because they may cause atrophy. Intralesional steroids or pimecrolimus and tacrolimus can be helpful[12,13]. For recalcitrant cases oral steroids, hydroxychloroquine, oral retinoids, and cyclosporine can be considered.

Adamandiades–Behçet disease

DEFINITION

Adamandiades–Behçet disease is a rare multisystem inflammatory disease classified as systemic vasculitis, affecting all types of blood vessels and clinically manifesting with recurrent oral and genital aphthous ulcers, skin lesions, and iridocyclitis/posterior uveitis, and occasionally with arthritis and vascular, gastrointestinal, and neurologic symptoms[14].

ETIOLOGY AND EPIDEMIOLOGY

Etiology remains unknown. Genetic factors play a role as certain ethnic groups from Japan, the Mediterranean countries, and the Middle East are particularly affected and a significant association exists with HLA-B51. Several environmental factors such as infectious agents triggering autoimmunity have also been implicated. Both genders are equally affected in the second and third decades.

CLINICAL PRESENTATION

Recurrent oral aphthous ulcers (multiple, painful, sharply-demarcated, and 1–3 cm large) are the most frequent presenting sign of the disease[15–18]. Genital ulcers can occur on the penis, scrotum, vagina, labia, anus, perineum, and genital crura. Genital ulcers begin as small vesicles or papules that enlarge to form small, red, punched-out ulcers with a necrotic slough. They may become quite large and deep (**20.10–20.12**) and tend to be more painful in men than in women. Genital ulcers may persist for weeks or months before healing with a characteristic scar. They do not recur as often as oral ones but generally recurrences are unpredictable.

LABORATORY STUDIES

Histopathology of early mucocutaneous lesions is frequently nonspecific but may reveal a neutrophilic vascular reaction or a fully developed leukocytoclastic vasculitis. A positive pathergy test, although not pathognomonic, can be suggestive of the disease. A percentage of patients demonstrates HLA-B51 positivity; however, this only accounts for a minority of sibling risk, as at least 16 genetic loci have been linked with Adamandiades–Behçet disease.

COURSE, PROGNOSIS, AND COMPLICATIONS

Male gender, HLA-B51 positivity and early development of systemic signs predict an unfavorable prognosis. Central nervous system, pulmonary, and large vessel involvement as well as bowel perforation are the major causes of death. Ophthalmic complications are also a major cause of morbidity.

DIAGNOSIS

According to the revised diagnostic criteria of the Behçet's disease Research Committee of Japan, the main symptoms of the disease are:
- Recurrent oral aphthous ulcers.
- Skin lesions (erythema nodosum, superficial thrombophlebitis, papules).
- Ocular lesions (iridocyclitis or posterior uveitis).
- Genital ulcers.

Additional symptoms are:
- Arthritis.
- Epididymitis.
- Gastrointestinal lesions.
- Vascular lesions.
- Central nervous system lesions.

Diagnosis of the complete type of the disease is made if the four main symptoms are fulfilled, whereas it is considered to be of the incomplete type if three main symptoms or two main and two additional are fulfilled.

Genital ulcers have to be differentiated mainly from infectious ones (genital herpes and syphilis) and from ulcus vulvae acutum (Lipschütz ulcer)[19].

TREATMENT

The choice of treatment depends on the site and severity of the clinical manifestations. For painful genital ulcers corticosteroid and antiseptic creams can be applied[20], and for recalcitrant lesions intralesional steroids can be considered.

Patients with mucocutaneous lesions resistant to treatment, with systemic involvement and with markers of poor prognosis are candidates for systemic treatment[21]. Systemic corticosteroids with or without immunosuppressive agents remain the treatment of choice. For genital ulcers, dapsone 100 mg/day, colchicine 1–2 mg/day, interferon-α 2a, thalidomide 100 mg/day, and cyclosporine 3–5 mg/kg/day, or infliximab with or without methotrexate[22] may be considered.

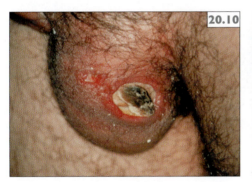

20.10 Adamandiades–Behçet disease. Genital ulcer.

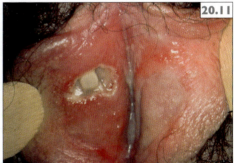

20.11 Adamandiades–Behçet disease. Genital ulcer.

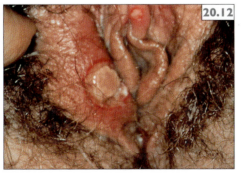

20.12 Adamandiades–Behçet disease. Genital ulcer.

Lichen sclerosus

DEFINITION, ETIOLOGY, AND EPIDEMIOLOGY

Lichen sclerosus (LS) is a chronic inflammatory condition. The causal factors are undetermined. Hormonal and infectious etiologies have been considered. Inflamed areas of LS have a T lymphocyte-dominant inflammatory infiltrate. LS is more common in women, with peaks in incidence in childhood and middle age[13].

CLINICAL PRESENTATION

The most commonly affected areas are the vulva and perianal areas in women[13], sometimes affecting both in a 'figure-of-eight' configuration, which may be a diagnostic clue (**20.13**). In men, the penis is most commonly affected (**20.14**)[13]. Lesions usually begin as an inflamed, well-demarcated plaque and evolve into a white sclerotic one. Sometimes, LS may be dark or blue in coloration and should be distinguished from lesions of abuse. Lesions are often symptomatic with itching or pain. In men, lesions may present as recurrent balanitis (balanitis of Zoon) or phimosis. Blisters are possible within the affected tissue.

DIFFERENTIAL DIAGNOSIS

Morphea, scar, irritant dermatitis, and squamous cell cancer can all occur.

LABORATORY STUDIES (HISTOPATHOLOGY)

The epidermis is thinned with orthohyper–keratosis and vacuolar degeneration of the basal layer. There may be follicular plugging. In early lesions, there is superficial dermal edema and a band-like lymphocytic infiltrate below the dermis. Collagen is homogenized in the dermis. Inflammation may be sparse, especially in long-standing lesions[14].

PROGNOSIS

The chronic nature and the scarring associated with long-standing lesions may be associated with pain, and with urinary, defecation, sexual, and psychological problems. The risk for the development of squamous cell carcinoma (SCC) may be related to the chronic inflammatory nature of the condition; however, the statistics are confounded by treatments associated with the condition, including long-term potent topical steroids and the past use of radiation as treatment. Even then, the risk for developing SCC in LS is estimated to be around 5%[15].

TREATMENT

The first-line treatment is a potent topical steroid[13]. Initial aggressive treatment is often followed by maintenance in order to prevent recurrence. Calcineurin inhibitors have also shown success in treating LS[16].

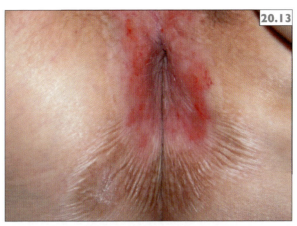

20.13 Lichen sclerosus in the anogential region. (Courtesy of Dr. Tomasz F. Mroczkowski.)

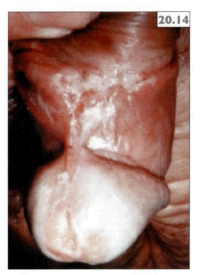

20.14 Lichen sclerosus of the penis. (Courtesy of Dr. Tomasz F. Mroczkowski.)

Bacterial Diseases

Jack M. Bernstein, MD

DEFINITION

This chapter encompasses several bacterial clinical syndromes with multiple etiologies, including folliculitis, furunculosis, perianal streptococcal dermatitis, erysipelas, and impetigo. As much as possible, they will be grouped by commonality and etiologic organism.

Perianal streptococcal dermatitis[1–4] and **erysipelas**[5–7] are relatively superficial infections that are almost invariably caused by *Streptococcus pyogenes*. The syndromes overlap considerably. Perianal streptococcal dermatitis is defined as a bright red, sharply demarcated eruption that is caused by group A beta-hemolytic streptococci, whereas erysipelas is a superficial cutaneous infection that may extend into the lymphatics, almost invariably recognized by a raised red border, sharply demarcating the infected from the uninvolved tissue. Impetigo is an acute, superficial skin infection characterized by exudation and crusting, occasionally involving the dermis but also presenting as a bullous eruption in young children. **Folliculitis** is defined as inflammation/infection of the hair follicle, whereas furunculosis occurs when the infection extends deeper into the dermis, with the formation of an abscess.

ETIOLOGY AND EPIDEMIOLOGY

The etiologic agent of both perianal streptococcal dermatitis and erysipelas is the same, *Streptococcus pyogenes*. The risk factors for contracting perianal streptococcal dermatitis are not known except that many children who contract it have a concurrent streptococcal infection such as 'strep throat'. As such, autoinoculation maybe the mechanism by which the bacteria are introduced to the perianal region. In erysipelas, a small breach in the integument may serve to initiate infection, which then spreads through the subcutaneous tissue; however, no entry wound may be found. In the rare instances in which there is bacteremia associated with erysipelas, the isolate is invariably a streptococcus, usually *S. pyogenes*.

Impetigo has been long recognized as a cause of epidemics among children and within families. Impetigo can be spread by touch, or through fomites such as contaminated toys, blankets, or clothing. Spread may occur to distant body sites by contaminated hands. The major causative organisms are *S. pyogenes* and *Staphylococcus aureus*, as described in the classic paper by

Table 21.1 Presence of *Staphylococcus aureus* and of hemolytic streptococci in lesion swabs of 190 cases of impetigo in south-east Lancashire, UK. One swab from each patient on first attendance at a clinic (1953 and early 1954)[8]

	Number of patients with hemolytic streptococci			No hemolytic streptococci	Total
	Group A	Group C	Group G		
S. aureus present	65	7	2	84	158
S. aureus absent	25	1	0	6	32
Total	90	8	2	90	190

Parker *et al.*[8] (*Table 21.1*), and as described by Shi *et al.*[9]. Impetigo spreads easily from person to person, through close personal contact. Various toxins have been suggested as being causative of the classic syndrome, because the clinical findings are identical in affected persons who are epidemiologically linked. In contradistinction, furunculosis and erysipelas may be seen with the same organisms but are clinically distinct. Bullous impetigo has been associated with *S. aureus* phage type II and staphylococcal exfoliative toxins A and B.

CLINICAL PRESENTATION

The following clinical scenario[7] amply illustrates the presentation of perianal streptococcal dermatitis.

"A 4-year-old boy presented with a complaint of rectal itching and pain. The patient was potty trained but still wore a diaper overnight. Physical examination revealed a bright red, moist eruption that extended approximately 3 cm circumferentially around the perianal area. Several papules located on the peripheral area were observed, and the eruption had spread onto the ventral surface of the penis. The patient was treated for 1 week with a topical ointment (i.e. A&D Ointment) and baby powder, with no improvement of symptoms. A topical antifungal agent was then added to the regimen. The patient showed no improvement in signs after 2 weeks and was referred to a pediatrician for a second opinion. A clinical diagnosis of perianal streptococcal dermatitis was reached and confirmed with a rapid streptococcal (strep) screen of the perianal region. A subsequent culture grew Group A Beta-hemolytic *Streptococcus*. The patient was given oral amoxicillin, and a dramatic improvement was noted within 24 hours.

Several days later, two siblings (2 months and 30 months of age) of the 4-year-old boy in the illustrative case developed similar signs. They experienced a similar, ineffective course of treatment. After physical examination and positive strep tests were performed, treatment with antibiotic therapy was initiated. Clinical improvement again was noted after 24 hours."

Erysipelas presents, typically, with the sudden onset of a painful red eruption. In the pelvic region, prior surgery, with interruption of the lymphatic drainage, is a risk factor for disease. The advancing border of erysipelas shows a sharply demarcated margin (**21.1**). Occasionally, the advancing eruption is accompanied by systemic symptoms of fever and chills. It is rare to see purulence and

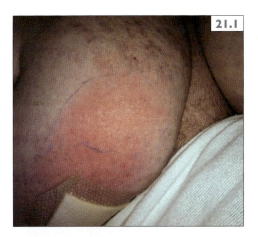

21.1 Erysipelas in the suprapubic region. An infected ulcer is covered by the bandage. The inked line demarcates the edge of the erysipelas.

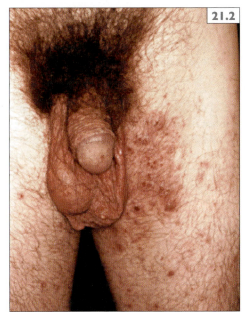

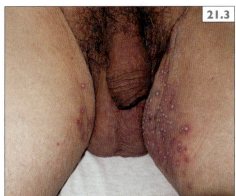

21.3 Pyoderma/furunculosis of the inner aspect of the thighs.

21.2 Folliculitis on the scrotum and inner aspect of the thigh. (Courtesy of Dr. Tomasz F. Mroczkowski.)

the skin is frequently intact; nevertheless, vesicles, bullae, and petechiae may be seen. In some instances, desquamation is seen as the eruption resolves. Regional lymphadenopathy may be seen, and lymphedema may occur as sequela. Occasionally, red lymphangitic streaking may be seen.

Folliculitis presents as an inflammation localized to the hair follicles, which may then progress to a localized pustular eruption and is frequent in the inguinal region (**21.2**). Folliculitis may occur as a result of the hairs turning inwards, as in folliculitis barbae. Folliculitis is usually associated with *S. aureus*, except in outbreaks of *Pseudomonas* folliculitis, which have been associated with exposure to water in hot tubs[10]. The coalescence of several follicular pustules may lead to a deeper infection, as in furunculosis (**21.3**).

LABORATORY STUDIES

Perianal streptococcal dermatitis, folliculitis, furunculosis, and erysipelas: Cultures are rarely useful in perianal streptococcal dermatitis, in which positive cultures are uniformly found, and in erysipelas, where even cultures of the advancing border of the eruption are rarely positive. Due to the increasing prevalence of methicillin-resistant *S. aureus* (MRSA)[11], cultures may be useful in folliculitis and in furunculosis. *S. aureus* strains associated with folliculitis may express virulence factors such as the Panton–Valentine leukocidin[12]. This same leukocidin is associated with infection due to community-acquired methicillin-resistant *S. aureus*. These culture results may guide therapy. Other laboratory tests, such as a complete blood count or erythrocyte sedimentation rate, are not useful.

COURSE, PROGNOSIS, AND COMPLICATIONS

In general, if recognized early, and treated appropriately, all these conditions have a benign outcome. Perianal streptococcal dermatitis, if untreated, may 'fester'. Recurrences are not uncommon. Folliculitis does not usually progress to more serious conditions and may respond to local antiseptics/antibiotics. Furunculosis may worsen and involve deeper structures, forming a carbuncle. If bacteremia ensues, with visceral dissemination, systemic complications, such as osteomyelitis and endocarditis, may occur. Erysipelas is diagnosed by its red, indurated advancing border. Untreated, it may progress and manifest systemic symptoms of fever and chills as well as localized pain. Bacteremia with visceral seeding is a complication of untreated disease.

DIAGNOSIS

In perianal streptococcal dermatitis, erysipelas, folliculitis, and furunculosis, the diagnosis is based upon presentation and history. With perianal streptococcal dermatitis, the differential diagnosis includes 'diaper rash' (**21.4**), perineal candidiasis, psoriasis, seborrheic dermatitis, pinworms, local trauma, and inflammatory bowel disease[7].

Erysipelas and folliculitis have classical presentations which are not usually confused with other syndromes. Necrotizing fasciitis of the inguinal region may be confused with erysipelas, but there is usually much more significant involvement of the deeper skin structure along with significant systemic toxicity. The challenge in folliculitis is to determine the cause, as it may be either infectious or noninfectious. Other syndromes that may appear similar include *Pityrosporum* folliculitis, *Pseudomonas* folliculitis (associated with hot tubs), chemical folliculitis following the use of epilating agents or other chemical agents, Kyrle disease, and, in human immunodeficiency virus (HIV)-infected individuals, eosinophilic folliculitis.

Furunculosis is usually easily recognized as a deep abscess. Potentially, a necrotic tumor could mimic this but this would be very unusual.

TREATMENT

Streptococcal infections, such as perianal streptococcal dermatitis or erysipelas, may be treated with penicillin G or oral cephalosporins. In severe cases, or in the case of penicillin allergy, clindamycin may be used. Animal studies have implied that clindamycin is superior to penicillin in shutting down streptococcal toxin production. In staphylococcal infections, the importance of MRSA must be appreciated. In folliculitis, treatment consists of supportive care of the skin. Pustules should not be unroofed. Warm water soaks may relieve itching and the use of antibacterial soaps, especially chlorhexidene, may be beneficial. In the case of furunculosis, warm water soaks may be useful in encouraging drainage of the abscess. In severe cases with surrounding cellulitis, incision and drainage may be necessary. In these cases, adjunctive antibiotics may be useful. The choice of antibiotic should cover resistant staphylococci. In the author's experience, doxycycline is an excellent choice for staphylococcal infections. Trimethoprim–sulfamethoxazole may also be used but may not be as effective in purulent lesions.

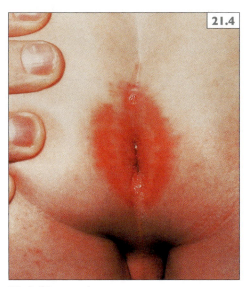

21.4 Diaper rash.

CHAPTER 22

Miscellaneous Viral, Fungal, and Bacterial Diseases

Jack M. Bernstein, MD

- **Herpes zoster**
- **Tinea cruris and candidal intertrigo**
- **Erythrasma**

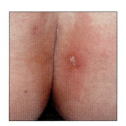
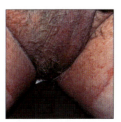
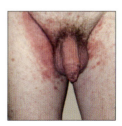
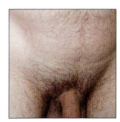

Herpes zoster

DEFINITION

Varicella-zoster virus infections are systemic viral diseases manifest as either primary infections, commonly referred to as chickenpox (varicella), or as a dermatomal recurrence due to the same virus, referred to as shingles (herpes zoster)[1,2].

ETIOLOGY AND EPIDEMIOLOGY

Both chickenpox and zoster are manifestations of the same viral infection. Chickenpox represents the primary infection with varicella-zoster virus and is acquired by seronegative persons. This infection may occur as early as *in utero* or, rarely, in elderly seronegative persons. Infection is acquired by the airborne route. Infectivity is very high and virtually all seronegative persons in close, prolonged, contact with someone who is infected will contract the illness. Herpes zoster may occur as early as in a neonate, in the case of *in utero* infection, or may manifest itself with increasing frequency with age or with immunosuppression due to either endogenous or exogenous causes.

CLINICAL PRESENTATION

The initial manifestation of chickenpox is of a diffuse macular eruption which rapidly evolves to include a vesicular component. The incubation period for chickenpox is usually 14–21 days, frequently associated with prodromal symptoms such as fever and malaise. The vesicles, referred to as 'dewdrops on rose petals', initially contain clear fluid. Over 1–2 days the fluid becomes cloudy, the vesicle ruptures, and a scab will form. Successive generations of vesicles occur over about 4 days. Once all the vesicles have dried, the disease resolves. Varicella is not a genital disease.

Zoster differs from chickenpox in that it usually only manifests in a single dermatome derived from a spinal nerve root. Patients occasionally describe prodromal symptoms such as tingling and dysesthesia in the affected dermatome. When zoster manifests itself in the inguinal region, it is usually due to reactivation of latent virus from the spinal roots of L1, L2 and, occasionally, S2. Zoster DOES NOT manifest itself bilaterally, except in the case of disseminated zoster. A symmetrical, bilateral, eruption in the absence of evidence of disseminated vesicular lesions, is not consistent with zoster. Herpes simplex infection may occur on the buttocks and initially can be confused with zoster (**22.1, 22.2**).

LABORATORY STUDIES AND DIAGNOSIS

The diagnosis of both chickenpox and zoster is primarily clinical. There is no role for serology in the diagnosis of either chickenpox or zoster; seropositivity is merely indicative of previous infection. In cases where the diagnosis is in dispute, a Tzanck smear may be useful in demonstrating intranuclear inclusions consistent with a herpes virus infection. The polymerase chain reaction (PCR) of vesicular fluid may also be useful in confirming the diagnosis.

COURSE, PROGNOSIS, AND COMPLICATIONS

In the majority of cases, both varicella and zoster have benign courses. As noted above, disseminated zoster occurs in immunocompromised individuals and may be associated with serious complications, such as zoster pneumonia or encephalitis. Dermatomal zoster may be followed by relatively intractable pain in the affected dermatome.

TREATMENT

In general, chickenpox requires no treatment. Dermatomal zoster, superficially, has a benign course but postzoster neuralgia is a significant concern. For this reason, early treatment with drugs directed against zoster such as famciclovir and valaciclovir may both shorten the course and decrease the pain. In cases of disseminated zoster, intravenous acyclovir is indicated[3]. There is no role for topical antiviral medications.

22.1 Herpes zoster infection is manifest by crops of vesicles, usually in a unilateral dermatomal distribution. These vesicles coalesce, eventually unroofing and forming an eschar. This illustration shows reactivation herpes zoster from the S1 or S2 dorsal root ganglia.

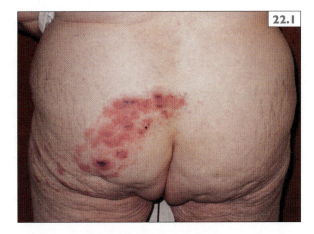

22.2 Herpes simplex infection in the genital region is manifest by small clear vesicles which may become confluent and turn cloudy. The vesicular exanthema is frequently surrounded by an erythematous rim. In this case, the vesicles are a manifestation of reactivation herpes from the sacral ganglion.

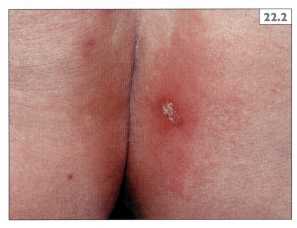

Tinea cruris and candidal intertrigo

DEFINITION

Tinea cruris is the manifestation of tinea corporis involving the crural folds and anogenital region[4]. Candidal intertrigo may be indistinguishable from tinea cruris; however, it is usually located between folds of adjacent skin, both in the inguinal region and under the breasts.

ETIOLOGY AND EPIDEMIOLOGY

Tinea cruris is most commonly caused by *Trichophyton rubrum*. A few cases are caused by *Epidermophyton floccosum* and occasionally *T. mentagrophytes*. Candidal intertrigo is usally caused by *Candida albicans*. Both syndromes are not age limited and may be seen in both infancy and in the elderly. Risk factors include immunosuppression or immunodeficiencies, diabetes, use of corticosteroids, and obesity.

CLINICAL PRESENTATION

Tinea cruris usually presents as the classic 'jock itch'. It is surmised that physical activity and, potentially, tightfitting clothing, allow for the creation of an environment suitable for these opportunistic dermatophytes. It is more common in men than women. Tinea cruris is seen more often in obese, diabetic, and immunocompromised populations. An erythematous patch is seen on the inner aspect of the thighs, spreading outwards. Lesions have a slightly elevated, demarcated border with some central clearing. In severe cases, the disease may spread to the perianal and gluteal regions. The scrotum is usually spared, which distinguishes this from candidal intertrigo[4] (**22.3, 22.4**).

The eruption of candidal intertrigo is more erythematous, appears 'wetter', and may involve the penis. Candidal intertrigo may also be recognized under the breasts, especially in women whose breasts are pendulous. Under these conditions, the apposition of the skin provides ideal conditions for growth of the *Candida* (**22.5**).

LABORATORY STUDIES AND DIAGNOSIS

In general, tinea cruris may be recognized clinically. Other syndromes that may be confused with it include erythrasma and candidal intertrigo. A potassium hydroxide (KOH) examination of a skin scraping reveals segmented hyphae and arthrospores, distinguishing it from candidal infection. Culture may confirm the diagnosis but is rarely needed. When the eruption is under the breast, no specific diagnostic test is needed.

The differential diagnosis includes contact dermatitis, erythrasma, bacterial intertrigo (of the groin) – usually caused by either *Staphylococcus aureus* or *Streptococcus pyogenes* – inverse psoriasis, and herpetic infections which are usually more limited in extent and present with classical vesicles.

COURSE, PROGNOSIS, AND COMPLICATIONS

Without treatment, the dermatitis may spread beyond its initial focus and involve the buttocks, perianal region, and inner thighs.

TREATMENT

Topical antifungal agents are the treatments of choice in this syndrome[5]. These include topical azoles, such as clotrimazole and econazole, as well as the allylamines naftifine and terbinafine. Griseofulvin 250 mg tid or terbinafine 250 mg daily may be used for 2–4 weeks, if systemic therapy is desired. Nystatin has no effect on dermatophyte infections although it may prove effective against candidal intertrigo. It is also important to remedy any physical/clinical factors allowing for the development of these syndromes. These may include obesity and occlusive clothing. Drying powders may be useful, as well as keeping the opposing folds of skin/breast and chest wall, apart.

22.3 Tinea cruris is, by definition, a dermatophytic infection involving the perigenital or perianal region. Shown is the classic rash, demonstrating raised red, scaly plaques with sharply defined borders. The central areas may clear somewhat and become less scaly.

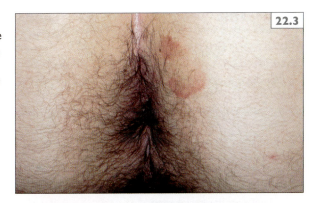

22.4 As tinea cruris advances down the thigh, the border remains prominent with a less prominent rash in the central area.

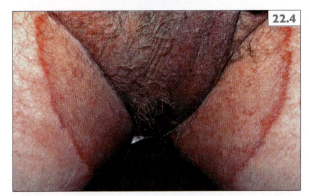

22.5 Candidal intertrigo of the groin, manifest by a moist, macular, erythematous rash. Note the satellite lesions surrounding the confluent rash.

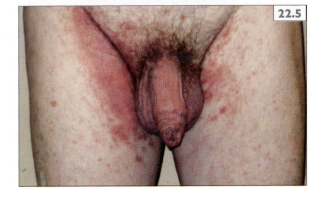

Erythrasma

DEFINITION, ETIOLOGY, AND EPIDEMIOLOGY

Erythrasma is a superficial infection of the skin caused by *Corynebacterium minutissimum*, a gram-positive, nonspore-forming bacillus.

Erythrasma was first described in 1859. Until 50 years ago, it was assumed that erythrasma was caused by a fungus; however, in 1961, the etiologic agent was shown to be *C. minutissimum*, which could be successfully treated with antibacterial agents[6].

Erythrasma may occur in healthy adults, but it is more frequently seen in the elderly, the immunocompromised, or in persons with diabetes. In diabetics, erythrasma may be seen prior to the recognition of diabetes. Obesity, hyperhidrosis, and living in areas with high humidity (e.g. tropical countries) may predispose to the condition.

CLINICAL PRESENTATION

The disorder typically presents as macerated, scaly plaques between the toes or erythematous to brown patches or thin plaques in intertriginous areas. Erythrasma may be seen wherever skin folds are in close apposition. It is frequently seen in the genitocrural region (**22.6**) and in the intergluteal region, where it may be associated with pruritus ani[7]. Nongenital manifestations may also appear in the submammary region as well as in the axillae.

LABORATORY DIAGNOSIS

C. minutissimum produces porphyrin pigments, which fluoresce under the ultraviolet light produced by the Wood's light (**22.7**). Fluorescence may be seen in other disorders, such as porphyria, vitiligo, and tinea versicolor; however, the clinical presentation of erythrasma is usually distinctive enough to distinguish it from these other disorders[8].

Because *C. minutissimum* is a gram-positive rod, Gram stain of skin scrapings may show gram-positive rods and filaments. Culture requires selective media and is rarely useful. KOH preps are NOT useful in the diagnosis of erythrasma but may substantiate coincident infection with dermatophytes.

The differential diagnosis is similar to that of tinea cruris.

TREATMENT

Because erythrasma is caused by a bacterium, it would be expected that drugs directed against gram-positive rods would be most efficacious. In this regard, topical therapy with clindamycin or erythromycin may be effective. For unclear reasons, topical antifungal therapy with azole agents may also clear the infection.

Systemic therapy may be achieved with either erythromycin or one of the newer macrolide antibiotics, such as clarithromycin[9].

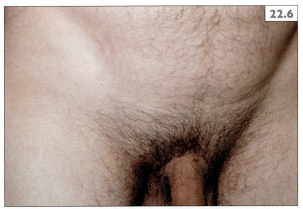

22.6 Erythrasma is manifest by a reddish- brown, slightly scaly rash which is, in this case, partially hidden by the pubic hair. The rash occurs in moist areas such as the groin, axillae, and in skin folds.

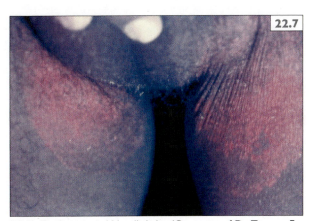

22.7 Erythrasma in Wood's light. (Courtesy of Dr. Tomasz F. Mroczkowski.)

CHAPTER 23

Pediatric Problems in the Anogenital Region

Maryam Piram, MD, and Danielle Marcoux, MD

- **Labial adhesion**
- **Phimosis in children**
- **Lichen sclerosus et atrophicus in children**
- **Genital ulcers in children**
- **Pediatric anogenital warts**
- **Perineal streptococcal dermatitis in children**
- **Infantile perianal pyramidal protrusion**
- **Child sexual abuse**
- **Infantile hemangiomas**
- **Diaper dermatitis and nutritional deficiencies**
- **Candidiasis in children**

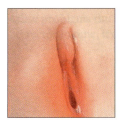
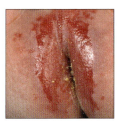
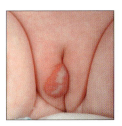
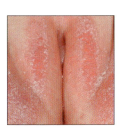

Lichen sclerosus et atrophicus in children

DEFINITION
Lichen sclerosus et atrophicus (LSA) is a chronic inflammatory dermatosis that results in the development of thin, white atrophic plaques. It is also reported as balanitis xerotica obliterans and kraurosis vulvae for glans penis or vulvar presentation, respectively.

ETIOLOGY AND EPIDEMIOLOGY
The cause of inflammation, altered fibroblast function, microvascular changes, and hyaluronic acid accumulation in the papillary dermis in LSA, is unknown. A genetic predisposition, based on family clustering, is apparent. Some studies have linked *Borrelia* or other infections with LSA. Autoimmunity plays a role, as indicated by the presence of autoantibodies to the glycoprotein extracellular matrix protein 1 (ECM1) and by the coexistence of lichen sclerosus and scleroderma and other autoimmune disorders (thyroid, diabetes, or pernicious anemia). Vasculitis and duplication of the basement membrane of blood vessel walls may contribute to hypoxia and ischemia, causing the initial cellular and vascular damage, as supported by increased glut-1 and decreased vascular endothelial growth factor (VEGF) expression in affected skin and mucosa. Local irritation or other inflammatory conditions and an altered hormonal status are also considered contributory factors.

The male-to-female ratio is 1:6. Although LSA occurs most often in postmenopausal women and in uncircumcised men, up to 15% of cases occur in children, the majority in girls, as well as in uncircumcised or incompletely circumcised boys. LSA, both genital and extragenital, has no racial predilection. The population prevalence is unknown, but the rate of circumcision in a given group is influential. A study of foreskins, submitted after therapeutic circumcision for phimosis, revealed many cases of unrecognized lichen sclerosus.

CLINICAL PRESENTATION
Genital presentations, both vulvar and penile, outnumber rarer extragenital involvement by more than 5:1. Extragenital LSA is even rarer in children. LSA usually begins as white, polygonal papules that coalesce into plaques. Evenly spaced dells or comedo-like plugs correspond to obliterated appendicular ostia, easily identified with dermatoscopy. The plugs and dells eventually disappear leaving a smooth, shiny, porcelain-white plaque. Telangiectases and purpura may be present. Vulvar LSA may be confined to the labia majora but usually progresses to gradual obliteration of the labia minora and stenosis of the introitus. Severe inflammation may result in vesicular or large, occasionally hemorrhagic, bullae. It may be confused with the trauma of sexual abuse or other genital ulcerative diseases. Anal fissures and rectorrhagias may be present (**23.2**).

Genital LSA usually presents with progressive pruritus, pain, dysuria, encopresis, and dyspareunia or genital bleeding in older girls. Often, an hourglass, butterfly, or figure of 8 pattern involves the perivaginal and perianal areas, with minimal involvement of the perineum in-between.

Penile LSA is usually preceded by pruritus and may present with a sclerotic ring at the prepuce edge or with a sudden phimosis of previously retractable foreskin; urinary obstruction can result. Male genital lesions are usually confined to the glans penis and the prepuce or foreskin remnants. Penile shaft and scrotal involvement is rare.

Rare oral cases can be seen in patients with generalized LSA. Some cases of clinically diagnosed oral lichen planus may actually be oral LSA. Asymptomatic or pruritic extragenital lesions may occur anywhere, but the back and shoulders are most frequently affected. Distribution along Blaschko lines and the isomorphic (Koebner) phenomenon have been reported.

COURSE, PROGNOSIS, AND COMPLICATIONS

Pediatric cases usually improve with puberty, although vulvodynia may persist. The rate of spontaneous resolution is reported to be lower than 25%. Severe cases, especially those associated with erosion or progressive scarring, may result in urinary problems and severe sexual dysfunction. There is an increased risk of developing squamous cell carcinoma in affected areas, but its rate and cofactors (human papillomavirus infection or prior radiotherapy) are not known. Cancer arising in extragenital presentations is described only rarely.

DIAGNOSIS

The diagnosis of LSA relies on a thorough medical history and physical examination focusing not only on the affected skin but also on the whole body skin surface. A biopsy is confirmatory. In pediatric patients, biopsy and blood work are usually not required.

TREATMENT

Potent topical corticosteroid ointments, applied nightly for 6–8 weeks, followed by maintenance therapy with less potent topical corticosteroids and/or topical calcineurin inhibitors usually bring symptomatic relief and halt tissue destruction[3].

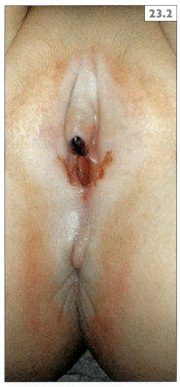

23.2 Lichen sclerosus et atrophicus.

Genital ulcers in children

DEFINITION, ETIOLOGY, AND EPIDEMIOLOGY

The etiology of genital ulceration[4] is variable: causes can be infectious, autoimmune, drug-induced, neoplastic, or traumatic. Infectious causes include: herpes simplex infection, syphilis, chancroid, donovanosis, granuloma inguinale, lymphogranuloma venereum (LGV), Epstein–Barr virus (EBV) infection[5], influenza, candidiasis, mycobacteria infection, cytomegalovirus and herpes zoster/varicella infections (in immunocompromised hosts), and histoplasmosis (in acquired immunodeficiency syndrome [AIDS] patients). Herpes simplex infection is more prevalent in North America, while in other parts of the world syphilis, chancroid, LGV, and human immunodeficiency virus (HIV) will be more frequent.

The Lipschütz ulcer (ulcus vulvae acutum) occurs mainly in teenage girls in whom vulvar ulcerations are associated with acute infectious manifestations, associated with influenza[6], EBV infection, mycoplasma pneumonia, or paratyphoid infection. Autoimmune causes include Behçet's disease, pyoderma gangrenosum, inflammatory bowel diseases, lichen planus, erosive lichen sclerosus et atrophicus, lupus erythematosus, bullous dermatoses (cicatricial pemphigoid, pemphigus vulgaris, and linear IgA dermatosis).

Drug-induced causes include fixed drug eruption, possibly due to nonsteroidal anti-inflammatory agents (NSAIDs, acetaminophen), metronidazole, sul-fonamides, tetracyclines, phenytoin, or oral contraceptives; erythema multiforme, or toxic epidermal necrolysis.

Neoplastic etiologies include lymphoma, leukemia, squamous cell carcinoma, basal cell carcinoma, Paget disease, Bowen disease, and erythroplasia of Queyrat. Traumatic causes include caustic burns, foreign body insertion, facticial creation. Erythema multiforme due to herpes simplex infection and hydradenitis suppurativa may also present with vulvar ulceration. Unfortunately, the cause of 50% of vulvar ulcerations is not found.

CLINICAL PRESENTATION

Unique or multiple ulcerations over the clitoris, vaginal introitus, and friction areas can be exquisitely painful and may be associated with vaginal secretions, painful lymphadenopathy, or oral ulcers (**23.3**, **23.4**).

LABORATORY STUDIES

Complete blood count, erythrocyte sedimentation rate, C-reactive protein (CRP) and antinuclear antibody (ANA) titers should be obtained. Potassium hydroxide (KOH) and fungal culture, as well as cultures for *Haemophilus ducreyi*, should be performed, as well as polymerase chain reaction (PCR) for *Chlamydia trachomatis* and immune-fluorescence studies, viral cultures and serology for herpes simplex, fluorescent treponemal antibody (FTA) and rapid plasma reagin (RPR) for syphilis, EBV serology and immunoglobulin (Ig)M and IgG for viral capsid antigen (VCA) and HIV testing. Histology is specific in only one-quarter of cases.

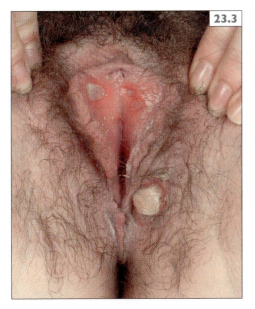

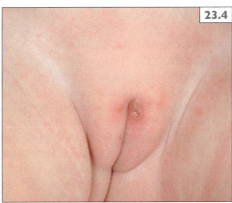

23.3, 23.4 Genital ulcers.

COURSE, PROGNOSIS, AND COMPLICATIONS

Genital ulcers of infectious origins will heal with appropriate anti-infective therapy. Genital ulcers of inflammatory cause may run a protracted, chronic, or recurrent course.

DIAGNOSIS

Age of onset, sexual activity, progression, recurrences, symptoms, general health, immune status, and drug intake are all information that can help to determine the etiology.

TREATMENT

Avoidance of irritants or of tight clothing and sexual abstinence are important. Sitz baths or wet compresses with Burow's solution 1:40 for 15 minutes three to four times daily may help. Petrolatum jelly or zinc oxide ointment can be applied locally. Analgesia is often required and includes NSAIDs, acetaminophen, or even opiates. Oral prednisone for severe ulcerations due to EBV may be helpful, as well as azithromycin orally in one dose, possibly along with acyclovir, famciclovir, or valacyclovir BID for 10 days.

Pediatric anogenital warts

DEFINITION, ETIOLOGY, AND EPIDEMIOLOGY

Anogenital warts (AGWs) are due to HPV infection of the perianal and genital areas. It remains very difficult to assess with certainty the source of HPV contamination in children with AGW, as neither HPV typing nor the clinical characteristics permits identification of the mode of transmission as sexual or not. Careful clinical history, including age at onset, duration prior to first visit, presence of warts on the child or caretakers, presence or history of AGW in the mother or father, abnormal maternal cervical findings and, most importantly, careful assessment of the family situation and of the child's behavior remain of prime importance in trying to identify the source of transmission.

The reported prevalence and mode of transmission of AGW in children vary with the socio-demographic profile (countries, socio-economic classes, or sources of referrals) of the pediatric populations studied. In children, HPV contamination of the genital and perineal area extends from infection with external warts to the mere presence of viral deoxyribonucleic acid (DNA), often short-lived and reversible. Genital HPV carriage in nonabused prepubertal children is not a rare occurrence. Vertical transmission of HPV has been reported to be responsible for at least 20% of AGW in children, and occurs by contamination of the newborn descending through the birth canal, by viral ascent through the membranes *in utero*, or by hematogenous transplacental transmission. Congenital cases of AGW support an ascending vertical mode of transmission.

Horizontal transmission by caregivers or caretakers from the first days of life is another modality of HPV contamination in neonates. Autotransmission in older children is also frequent. Infants and children can also acquire HPV infections by exposure to contaminated fomites such as underwear. Sexual abuse as a mode of transmission of AGW has been reported from all over the world.

CLINICAL PRESENTATION

Verrucous papules may take the appearance of flat warts or cauliflower-like lesions. They localize more often on the perianal area or buttocks and less often on the penis or vulva (**23.5–23.7**).

LABORATORY STUDIES

The role of HPV typing for identifying the mode of transmission is limited. Biopsies and HPV typing of chronic, recurrent, or recalcitrant lesions may be useful to identify children who might be infected with oncogenic types or to exclude other pathologies.

COURSE, PROGNOSIS, AND COMPLICATIONS

Confounding questions relating to HPV genital infection concern carriage status, autoresolution, and latency, which can exceed 2 years prior to overt infection. The persistence of HPV for more than 6 months appears to be related to the older age group, as well as infection with multiple types of HPV and oncogenic types. The role of age, hormonal immaturity, and immunity remains unclear.

There is a concern that the acquisition of HPV during the perinatal period could induce some form of immunological tolerance to HPV and increase the risk of intraepithelial neoplasia in later life. Due to this and due to possible recurrence, as well as to potential long-term risks associated with oncogenic types and frequent delayed unveiling of sexual abuse, follow-up of children with AGW is recommended.

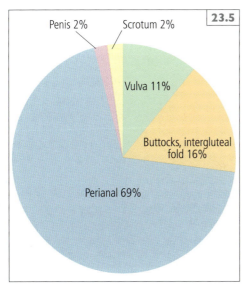

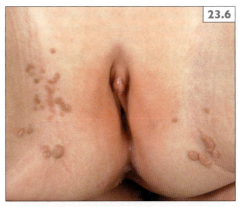

23.5 Distribution of presentation of pediatric genital warts.

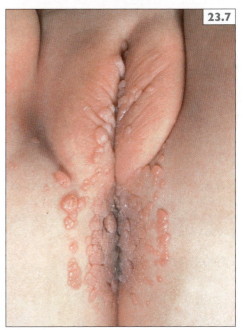

DIAGNOSIS

A detailed physical examination should search for any sign of abuse and microbiological assessment of other sexually transmitted diseases should be done if appropriate. It has to be kept in mind that a negative questionnaire and examination never totally rule out such a possibility.

TREATMENT

Podophyllin 25% or imiquimod can be treatment options in the pediatric age group. Cryosurgery may not be well tolerated[7].

23.6, 23.7 Anogenital warts of the vulva.

Perineal streptococcal dermatitis in children

DEFINITION, ETIOLOGY, AND EPIDEMIOLOGY

This perineal disease is caused by group A β-hemolytic streptococci. Several cases of group B and group G *Streptococcus* or *Staphylococcus aureus*-induced perineal streptococcal dermatitis have been documented.

Perineal streptococcal infection is common and affects primarily children in the first decade with a peak between 3 and 6 years old. A seasonal distribution similar to patterns of streptococcal pharyngitis (spring) suggests an association with respiratory infection.

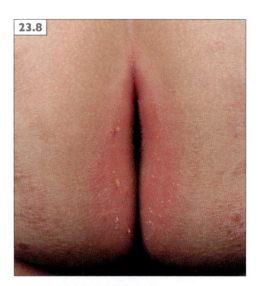

CLINICAL PRESENTATION

A sharply-demarcated perianal or vulvovaginal erythema is characteristic, often accompanied by superficial edema. Pruritus and tenderness are the most common symptoms. Other clinical manifestations include dysuria, constipation, discharge, bleeding at defecation, abdominal pain, and signs known to be related to streptococcal infection, such as a scarlatiniform eruption or guttate psoriasis (**23.8, 23.9**).

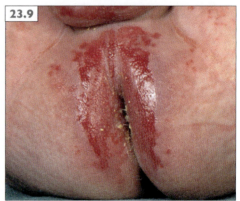

LABORATORY STUDIES

Swab sample for bacterial culture from affected tissues should be useful.

23.8, 23.9 Streptococcal perianal cellulitis.

COURSE, PROGNOSIS, AND COMPLICATIONS

This disease is successfully treated by oral antimicrobials with rapid relief of signs and symptoms. In some cases, a second course of antimicrobials may be necessary. The most common complication is delay in diagnosis and treatment, which leads to prolonged discomfort, increases the risk of dissemination of the infection, and adds to the risk of spread to close contacts.

DIAGNOSIS AND TREAMENT

Culture of β-hemolytic streptococci from an affected tissue will confirm the diagnosis. Oral antibiotic therapy with penicillin V or a macrolide for 14–21 days is recommended. Additional topical therapy with antiseptics or antibiotics may accelerate bacterial clearance[8,9].

Infantile perianal pyramidal protrusion

DEFINITION, ETIOLOGY, AND EPIDEMIOLOGY

Infantile perianal pyramidal protrusion, also referred to as infantile perineal protrusion, was originally reported as skin tags or skin folds. It occurs in three settings: constitutional (sometimes genetic or familial); functional (after constipation, diarrhea, or other irritant exposure); or associated with LSA. Some protrusions are congenital, but mechanical irritation or weeping after defecation has been recognized as trigger factors. It is not rare and presents typically in prepubertal children, especially girls.

CLINICAL PRESENTATION

Infantile perianal pyramidal protrusion appears on the perineal median raphe of prepubertal girls as a pyramidal soft tissue swelling, covered by smooth red or rose-colored skin (**23.10**).

COURSE, PROGNOSIS, AND COMPLICATIONS

Infantile perianal pyramidal protrusion is, at least in some patients, a peculiar form of LSA that can precede other more characteristic manifestations.

DIAGNOSIS AND TREATMENT

Infantile perianal pyramidal protrusion may easily be mistaken for condyloma acuminatum or as a sign of trauma, leading to an investigation of sexual abuse. This may be avoided with awareness of this entity, a thorough history, and a classic clinical presentation.

No treatment is required unless LSA is present[10,11].

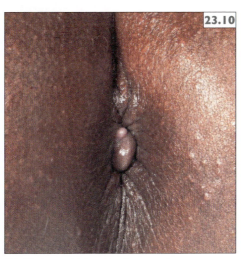

23.10 Pyramidal perianal protrusion.

Infantile hemangiomas

DEFINITION, ETIOLOGY, AND EPIDEMIOLOGY

Infantile hemangiomas (IHs) are the most common benign vascular tumor of infancy. Less than 10% of IHs are localized in the perineal area.

CLINICAL PRESENTATION

IHs are usually absent or barely noticeable at birth (telangiectasias, pallor, red macule, and even ulceration) and proliferate during the first months of life. They present as bright red nodules or plaques or can even be subcutaneous, making them less noticeable (**23.13**).

LABORATORY STUDIES

None are required. Abdominoperineal magnetic resonance imaging (MRI) may be indicated if there is a lumbosacral IH.

COURSE, PROGNOSIS, AND COMPLICATIONS

IHs appear during the first month of life. After a proliferative phase that lasts about 6–8 months, most IHs undergo slow, spontaneous involution without complications; however, ulcerations along with pain and sometimes bleeding and infection and risk of permanent scarring are very common in the diaper area, especially in large plaque-like hemangiomas (**23.14–23.16**). Perineal hemangiomas can also be part of a poly-malformation syndrome: PELVIS syndrome (perineal hemangiomas, external genital malformations, lipomyelomeningocele, vesicorenal abnormalities, imperforate anus, and skin tags)[15].

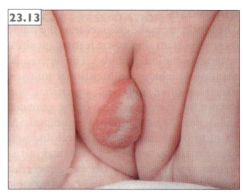

23.13 Hemangiomas of the vulva.

DIAGNOSIS AND TREATMENT

The diagnosis is made clinically; however, a Doppler ultrasound study in subcutaneous IH may be warranted. With uncomplicated IH, observation or propranolol (topical or systemic) administration may be recommended. With ulcerating IH, wound care, pain management, topical or oral antimicrobials, and systemic propranolol might be the treatment of choice[15,16].

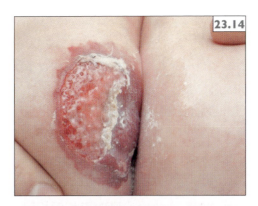

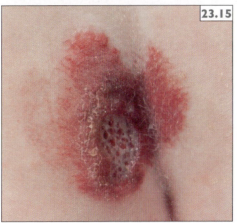

23.14, 23.15 Ulcerated infantile hemangiomas.

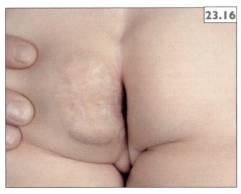

23.16 Residual scarring of an ulcerated infantile hemangioma.

Diaper dermatitis and nutritional deficiencies

syn: napkin rash, nappy rash

DEFINITION

Diaper dermatitis is an acute inflammatory skin reaction in the area covered by the diaper. Frictional dermatitis, irritant contact dermatitis, and diaper candidiasis are the most common types. Seborrheic dermatitis, psoriasis, and intertrigo also have to be considered. Some nutritional deficiencies may mimic a severe irritant contact dermatitis in the diaper area.

ETIOLOGY AND EPIDEMIOLOGY

Diaper dermatitis is a very common disorder of infancy with a peak incidence between 9 and 12 months of age. The most common nutritional deficiencies causing diaper dermatitis are zinc deficiency (**23.17, 23.18**), biotin deficiency, and essential fatty acid deficiency. These conditions result from inadequate dietary intake or genetic defects and are more prevalent in developing countries.

CLINICAL PRESENTATION

Diaper dermatitis may present as frictional or irritant contact dermatitis with redness of the convex surfaces (thighs, genitalia, buttocks, or abdomen), along with sparing of intertriginous creases. Diaper candidiasis will show widespread bright red erythema with raised edge, sharp marginization with white scale at the border, and pinpoint pustulovesicular satellite lesions.

In the case of zinc deficiency, the eruption will appear around the body orifices and acral sites (hands, feet, elbows, knees), along with diarrhea and alopecia. With biotin deficiency, there are periorificial eruption, alopecia, developmental delay, seizure and hypotonia, and ophthalmologic abnormalities. With an essential fatty acid deficiency, there are periorificial dermatitis and weeping intertriginous areas, alopecia, increased susceptibility to infections, increased capillary fragility, and impaired wound healing.

LABORATORY STUDIES

If a nutritional deficiency is suspected and the clinical presentation is suspicious the following studies should be considered: serum zinc level, alkaline phosphatase, serum albumin, serum biotin, plasma linoleic, arachidonic, and eicosatrienoic acid levels.

COURSE, PROGNOSIS, AND COMPLICATIONS

Frictional or irritant diaper dermatitis responds to frequent diaper changes and good diaper hygiene. Infections need specific topical antifungal or antimicrobial treatment. In addition, all diaper dermatitis may be complicated by ulceration, pain, and infection. Failure to thrive and systemic complications are suggestive of nutritional deficiency.

DIAGNOSIS

The etiology of diaper dermatitis relies on a thorough medical history and physical examination, focusing not only on the affected skin but also on the entire skin surface. A skin swab for bacterial and/or fungal culture may be useful, as well as blood tests when there is suspicion of nutritional deficiency.

TREATMENT

For frictional or irritant contact dermatitis, frequent diaper changes and good diaper hygiene are in order. Zinc oxide and petrolatum-based creams should be used at every diaper change. In addition, a low-potency corticosteroid may be added to the regimen.

For diaper candidiasis, a topical antifungal agent is in order, while for a nutritional deficiency, oral supplementation will be needed[17, 18].

There are several basic designs for pubic hair removal:

- Basic bikini design removes hair from the sides and top of the line where a bikini or briefs come to. The basic bikini design may be further modified by hair also being removed from the labia or penis and scrotum, perineum, perianal regions, and natal cleft.
- Brazilian design involves leaving a small 'landing strip' of hair about the mons pubis or it may be removed. The hair of the buttocks may also be eliminated at the same time.
- Rising sun design similarly involves the landing strip area.

Hair grows rapidly. Within 3 weeks, the selected procedure may be needed again. Secondary infection of the follicles and pili incarnati tortii may complicate the styling.

Body paint

Actors and artists have always used theatrical make-up for effect. Painted buttocks, often employing very crude designs, may be created, perhaps with the idea in mind of 'mooning', a temporary sport of adolescent males.

Temporary tattoo

Modern temporary transfer tattoos are made of ink and glue and sold through many commercial concerns with instructions on how to apply them[6]. They usually last up to 5 days or can be removed by washing. There is no reason why they should not be applied to the genital area for instant, albeit temporary, appeal.

Henna (mehndi) tattoos are originally from India. The henna paste comes from henna (*Lawsonia inermis*), which is applied in delicate designs to the skin, binding with keratin. The paste is left on the skin for several hours to stain. As the skin sheds, so does the design disappear. It was never intended for the genitals but usually for the back of the hands. Occasional contact dermatitis develops from the paraphenylene diamine (PPD) that is associated with this type of tattoo.

Permanent genital adornment[7,8]
Permanent tattoo

Designs of tattoos elsewhere on the trunk or legs but ending on the lower abdomen or genitals or buttocks are well recognized and often masterpieces of the skill of the tattooist. The famous British Royal Navy design of a fox chasing hounds down the back is one such example, and ends somewhere about the natal cleft.

Whole body tattoos, which at least cover the buttocks as well as the face, from Polynesia have long been known. There are some multicolored whole body tattoos from Japan, often indicating masculinity and with significance to those in the know. More recently western ideas of Polynesian tattoos, often covering the trunk as well as the pubic and buttocks area, have become popular in trendy male circles.

Some tattoos in both sexes that descend to the genitals have sexual connotations and often the proud owner will be found also to have various types of genital piercings. It seems that only a minority of those with genital tattoos wish to get rid of them and consult dermatologists or plastic surgeons.

There are some small tattoos which are placed on the buttocks of both sexes, more as a pleasant decoration than anything else, with designs such as small stars, angels, slogans, or bluebirds. Occasionally, with men, there are arrows pointing to the anus, signifying willingness to take the passive role. Sometimes, patients who participate in fist fornication (FF)[9] will have a tattoo circumferentially around the anus or a guiche piercing in the perineum. FF is more frequently performed than many might imagine. It involves the insertion of the fist in 'le main d'accoucher position' into the anorectal canal.

Tattoos are found on the penis, occasionally very amateur ones, but often small miniatures of the tattooist's art. They may well signify either naval service or just the result of drunken revels when 'boys will be boys'. They may also be found on the shaft, prepuce, glans, and scrotum.

Popular tattoos in the vernacular refer to the ability to gain an erection; the tattooist often reverted to the Latin, 'resurgam'. At present there is a group of hyper-masculine gay men who have various tattoos with designs on their genitals, again often with multiple genital piercings.

Piercings on and around the genitals

There is evidence from ancient images that fish bones were used for genital adornment[10]. Genital piercings may be found alone or with multiple piercings at other body sites such as the ears, eyebrows, nose, lips, tongue, nipples (**24.1**), and umbilicus[11].

Genital piercing in men has been noticed to cause urinary tract infections, especially if sexual intercourse starts before the healing process. Ruptures of the skin in both sexes have occurred in sexual foreplay and intercourse. If a cock ring is too tight or too small, it is likely to cause complications during erection[9]. Genital piercing in men includes:

- Ampallang – horizontal through the glans penis.
- Apadravyas – vertical through the glans penis.
- Deep – through the shaft of the penis or scrotum.
- Dolphin – through the penis but does not go out of the glans.

- Dydoes – through the glans and coronal ridge.
- Frenal – through the frenulum (**24.2**).
- Guiche – variable sites in the perineum and frequently fitted with a ring or barbell; often found in those who like to be fisted.
- Penile and scrotal ladders – multiple ones in a line, hence the term; in the scrotum may be around the medial raphe or laterally (hafada).
- 'Prince Albert' – transurethral, exiting underneath the glans penis (**24.3, 24.4**).
- Prince's wand – a small tube extending into the urethra and attached to the Prince Albert.
- Pubic.
- Reverse Prince Albert – the same but exiting on the superior surface of the glans penis.

In women piercing includes[12]:
- Christina – piercing of the mons pubis.
- Labia – usually through the labia minora.
- Labret – piercing with jewelry inserted into the lower lip; similarly may be placed in the male or female genitals; often multiple.
- Triangle – piercing through the clitoral hood passing posterior to the body of the clitoris and anterior to the urethra (**24.5**).

Scrotal infusion with normal saline[13]

Scrotal infusion or inflation is a practice made popular for several years, in which normal saline is infused slowly via a butterfly needle into the scrotal sac to make the contents larger and heavier (**24.6**). Some pleasure must be obtained from it, although there is always the danger of self-inflicted infection.

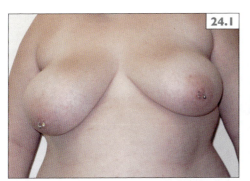

24.1 Nipple piercing.

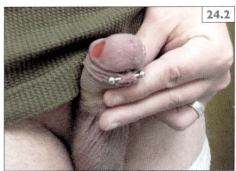

24.2 Frenal Piercing. (Courtesy of Dr. Tomasz F. Mroczkowski.)

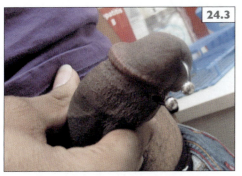

24.3 Piercing Prince Albert. (Courtesy of Dr. Tomasz F. Mroczkowski.)

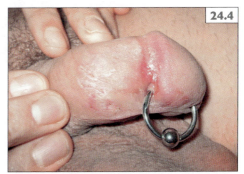

24.4 Prince Albert inserted in the penis of a patient with herpes progenitalis. (Courtesy of Dr. Darren Russell, Cairns, Australia.)

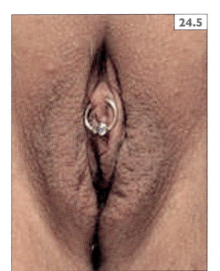

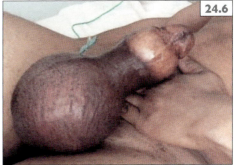

24.6 Scrotal saline infusion.

24.5 Piercing of the clitoris.

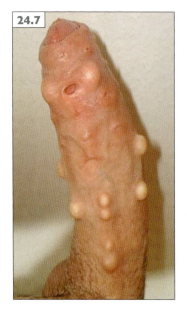

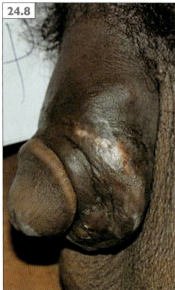

24.7 Pearling of the penis, with loss at the distal end.

24.8 Paraffin injected into the penile shaft to enhance the size. (Courtesy of Dr. Kelwyn Browne, Port Moresby, Papua New Guinea.)

Scarification and self-mutilation

Scarification is not as unknown to Western society as may be thought[12]. Recent events in body arts show that raised designs caused by scar tissue (almost a keloid) on the arms, legs, and back are considered by some to be beautiful. Implantation of coral or pearls and self-injections of dangerous foreign matter, such as industrial silicone oil, paraffin, and cooking oil, under the skin of the penis to facilitate more pleasure in sex is found worldwide (**24.7**).

Within recent decades, implantation of stainless steel, Teflon, titanium, niobium, and other objects has been employed to cause tactile designs. The Japanese criminal group, Yakuza, has been known to insert a pearl for each year in prison. The lateral or dorsal slitting of the skin of the penis to insert such objects as pearls is a common practice, especially in South East Asia.

The dangers are manifold. They include breakdown and rejection with infection; abscess and cyst formation; degrees of mutilation; and nonfunctional anatomy.

In nonindustrialized societies such as Papua New Guinea, the following have been used for the purposes of sexual enhancement: small shells, paraffin (**24.8**), melted plastic, bone, horn, mineral oil injection (vaseline), rubber bands with plastic bottle tops (**24.9**), and more or less anything which will cause a raised bump, including modifications utilizing porcupine quills and nylon fishing line (**24.10**). These usually have complications such as localized infection leading to abscess and fistula formation; these in turn lead to quite unwished-for penile modification.

Self-mutilation may involve some degree of genital change, i.e. cutting the suspensory ligament. There are sects in India who castrate themselves, in the end removing their penis, scrotum, and testicles. The web has shown this sort of activity is not as rare as may be imagined in industrialized societies. Severe body modification with self-amputation of the penis has been documented (**24.11**).

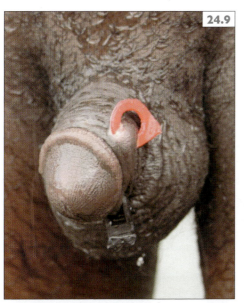

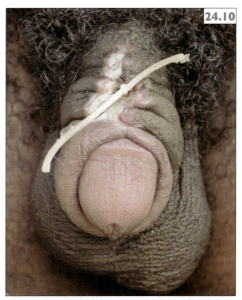

24.9 Plastic bottle injected into the penile shaft. (Courtesy of Dr. Kelwyn Browne, Port Moresby, Papua New Guinea.)

24.10 Nylon fishing line inserted into the penile shaft that was knotted, leading to pyoderma. (Courtesy of Dr. Kelwyn Browne, Port Moresby, Papua New Guinea.)

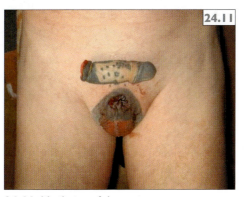

24.11 Mutilation of the penis.

COMPLICATIONS

Genital piercing

Knowledge is increasing all the time about body piercing[14]. It is widespread and is found across all socioeconomic groups. The major concentration is among adolescents and young adults under 30 years. As would be expected, common physical risks are bleeding, tissue trauma (**24.12**), and bacterial infections, but psychosocial risks such as unhappiness, low self-esteem, and disappointment need also to be taken into consideration.

In industrialized countries regulations to try to enforce basic health precautions have been attempted, usually after outbreaks of hepatitis B and C from tattoo parlors. The regulations implemented in The Netherlands[15] after June 2006 for all skin procedures performed by nonmedical persons may be taken as a practical model to minimize the infectious and physical complications of tattooing and piercing.

Genital piercing is an invasive procedure with almost every puncture releasing serosanguinous fluid that predisposes the client to local infections and more serious systemic disease such as blood-borne infections, hepatitides, human immunodeficiency virus (HIV), syphilis, and a variety of bacterial and viral infections[14]. Lay people perform the procedures with virtually no knowledge of anatomy, sanitation, or procedural precautions.

A recent study on genital piercing on students attending 18 universities in the USA and 1 in Australia showed infections at the site occurred in 45%, while skin irritation occurred in 39%[16]. There were few verbal or written instructions. Hepatitis B was the most common long-term viral complication. In some groups hepatitis C and HIV must be considered, especially where these are frequent, as in drug users and men who have sex with men (MSM). Although most genital bacterial infections are localized, endocarditis has also been reported.

It should be realized that keloid formation as the result of piercing is more frequent in black skin.

Tattooing

In addition to all the complications that may arise from genital piercing, there are specific complications that may develop from tattooing the genitals[17]. Urticaria may be provoked, particularly by rubbing the blue-black tattooed areas made by cobalt and carbon pigments. In the dyes used in tattooing, there are metal components that may cause dermatitides. These may occur from any of the red, yellow, green, blue, and black pigments used and have been described in detail[17]. Unless the subject is unclothed, photodermatitis is unlikely to occur on the genitals. The Koebner phenomenon may be observed occasionally in patients with psoriasis and lichen planus.

Temporary henna tattoos are popular world wide and may cause dermatitis[18]. It is in fact the components put into some of the temporary tattoos that may cause problems. There is little evidence to show that pure henna causes much trouble, but PPDs are well known in causing allergic contact dermatitis, which needs to be considered where dermatitis ensues after temporary tattoos on the genitals.

Ideally, the decision-making process before piercing and tattooing should be of the 'Health Belief Model'[14], where consideration has been given to the various risks and rewards before undertaking either procedure. Unfortunately, tattooing and piercing are often undertaken without appropriate consideration, often on young people under the influence of alcohol or street drugs, and often in locales where basic health provision regulations are not applied.

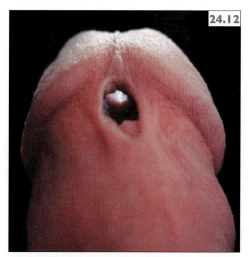

24.12 Urethral fistula after removal of a Prince
Albert piercing.

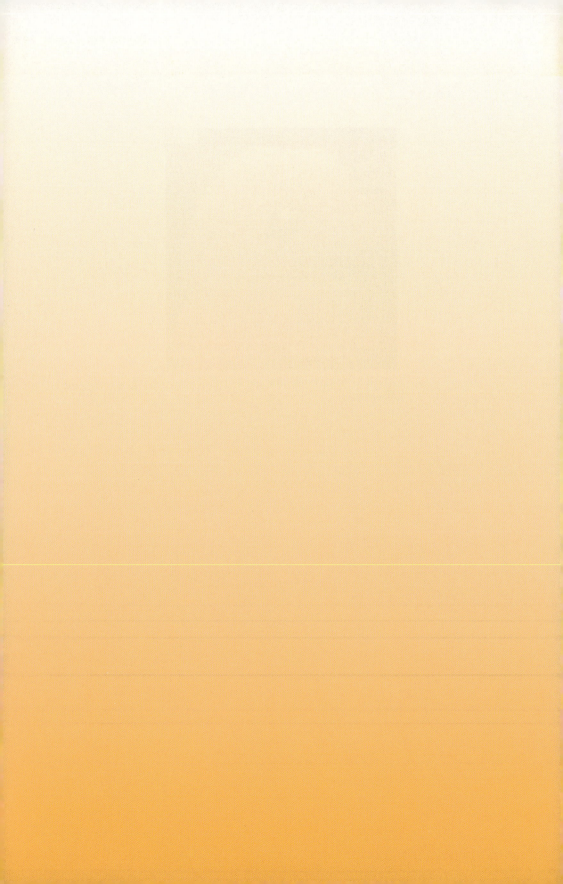

Genital Mutilation

Ngianga-Bakwin Kandala, PhD

DEFINITION

Female genital mutilation (FGM), also referred to as female circumcision, is the intentional partial or total removal of the female genitalia for nonmedical reasons (**25.1**). The procedure is usually carried out on young girls under the age of 15 years, although on the rare occasion adult women are also subjected to it. Between 100 million and 140 million girls and women around the world are living with the consequences of FGM. In Africa, about 92 million girls 10 years of age and above are estimated to have undergone FGM. The procedure is most common in Africa; in particular it occurs in the East, West, and North-east areas, especially Somalia and Sudan. It is also found in certain parts of Asia and the Middle-East and among migrants from these areas located in North America and Europe, as they are not yet accustomed to the ways of their foreign land[1]. This chapter will focus on practices common in Sudan, Senegal, Egypt, Somalia, Ethiopia, and some other African countries.

25.1 Normal uncircumcised female anatomy in comparison with different types of female genital mutilation.

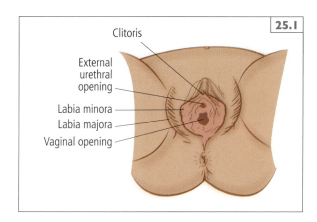

25.1

Clitoris

External urethral opening

Labia minora

Labia majora

Vaginal opening

ETIOLOGY

The reason FGM exists is due to religious, cultural, and socially acceptable norms within a community. In some locales, it is a social convention making it difficult for those who dare to defy it. This leads to the practice being perpetuated within the community. FGM is considered the 'proper' way of raising a female child, as it prepares her for adulthood and marriage. Such communities hold a negative view on premarital relations and believe that this is a way of reducing such promiscuity[1,2].

Many of the community and religious leaders could be partially responsible for this process still taking place. While some do try to demote it, there is no doubt that the voice that advocates it is stronger and thus upholds this tradition. Much more needs to be done if there is to be an end to this form of maltreatment of women[2].

EPIDEMIOLOGY

FGM results from a range of different factors dependent on the country from which the victim comes and her religion. The victims are girls usually 2 months to 18 years of age.

FGM is said to have no health benefits for those directly subjected to it. Immediate complications may include bleeding, severe pain, tetanus or other bacterial sepsis, shock, urinary retention, genital ulcerations, and additional injury to nearby genital tissue. Later in life, it can cause parturition complications, and newborn deaths. It can also lead to infertility, and genitourinary complications, requiring future surgical intervention; an example of this situation could be the FGM procedure that seals or narrows a vaginal opening (Type III) and needs to be cut open later to allow for sexual intercourse and childbirth. Sometimes, it is stitched again several times, including after childbirth; hence, the woman goes through repeated opening and closing procedures, further increasing and repeating both immediate and long-term risks[1]. In addition, this will adversely affect society, with fewer births occurring[1,2].

CLINICAL PRESENTATION

The patient may present as a woman with delayed puberty. In western countries, physicians see predominantly type III FGM, although overall type II FGM (excision) is more common where FGM is practiced (West Africa). The reasons are, first, that no barrier is created at the introitus, and women surviving type II and I FGM are usually asymptomatic – thus, even if mutilation is present, it may be overlooked. Second, even in most areas with traditionally high levels of FGM, only about 45% of women have been mutilated and the long-term morbidity is low[2].

In countries where FGM is predominant, late complications affecting the vulva may be the cause of hospital admission. In the western world, FGM presents mainly in one of two ways. Either the woman has just married and it has proved impossible to consummate the marriage due to the barrier of scar tissue, or she has become pregnant despite the barrier at the introitus, which will complicate delivery.

In Somalia, if penetrative sex is impossible, deinfibulation (opening up) is carried out by a local midwife or traditional birth attendant immediately after marriage (especially in Northern Somalia, where the residual opening tends to be very small – 0.2 inch [0.5 cm] or less). If the opening permits, the opening may be widened by forceful penile penetration.

LABORATORY STUDIES

Examination of the external genitalia can show the type of FGM. Laboratory examinations can include: per rectum examination, hormonal studies, and cytogenetic analysis.

Relatively little research has been conducted on the effect female genital alteration may have on human immunodeficiency virus (HIV) prevalence[3]. Some studies have found increased risk of HIV among women who have undergone FGM[4]. Other studies have found no statistically significant associations[5] or have identified more complex patterns[6]. Two reports have revealed that FGM is associated with a decreased risk of HIV[7,8].

Recent reviews have suggested that FGM may increase the risk of HIV[9,10]. Several mechanisms have been proposed by which FGM would expose women to greater risk of HIV. These include: nonsterile procedures (because the same instrument is frequently used); an increase in blood transfusions due to blood loss during the procedure itself, intercourse, or childbirth; increased anal intercourse due to difficult or painful vaginal intercourse; tearing of the vagina during intercourse; and increased susceptibility to infectious conditions that are recognized risk factors for HIV, such as genital ulcers[11].

COURSE

FMG is performed using a sharp instrument, usually a razor blade, to cut or remove part of the female genitalia. The World Health Organization recognizes three types of mutilation that are performed[1,2]. This practice is often carried out without any anesthetic/ antiseptics or pain medication.

Type I FGM (clitoridectomy)

This is described as being the removal of the clitoris, including partial removal[1,2,12].

Type I FGM, often termed clitorectomy, involves excision of the skin surrounding the clitoris with or without excision of part of or the entire clitoris (25.2). When this procedure is performed in infants and young girls, a portion of or all of the clitoris and surrounding tissues may be removed. If only the clitoral prepuce is removed, the physical manifestation of Type I FGM may be subtle, necessitating a careful examination of the clitoris and adjacent structures for recognition.

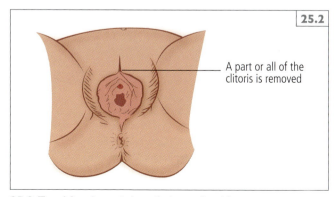

25.2

A part or all of the clitoris is removed

25.2 Type I female genital mutilation – clitoridectomy.

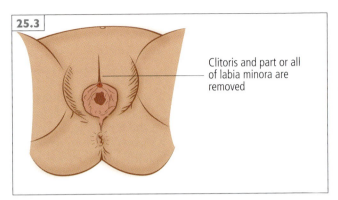

Clitoris and part or all of labia minora are removed

25.3 Type II female genital mutilation – excision.

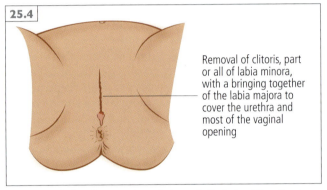

Removal of clitoris, part or all of labia minora, with a bringing together of the labia majora to cover the urethra and most of the vaginal opening

25.4 Type III female genital mutilation – infibulation. The clitoris and labia are removed and the vagina is sewn up, leaving only a small opening for urine and menstrual blood.

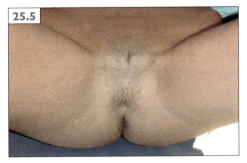

25.5 Type IV female genital mutilation – Pharaonic circumcision. (Courtesy of Ellaithi M, et al. [2006]. Female genital mutilation of a karyotypic male presenting as a female with delayed puberty. *BMC Women's Health* 6:6; © 2006 Ellaithi et al; licensee BioMed Central Ltd.)

Type II FGM (excision)

This is the practice of clitoridectomy whilst also removing the labia minora (**25.3**)[1,2,12].

Type II FGM, referred to as excision, is the removal of the entire clitoris and part or all of the labia minora. Crude stitches of catgut or thorns may be used to control bleeding from the clitoral artery and raw tissue surfaces, or mud poultices may be applied directly to the perineum. Patients with Type II FGM do not have the typical contour of the anterior perineal structures, as a result of the absence of the labia minora and clitoris. The vaginal opening is not covered in the Type II procedure.

Type III FGM (infibulation)

Type III FGM, known as infibulation, is the most severe form in which the entire clitoris and some or all of the labia minora are excised, and incisions are made in the labia majora to create raw surfaces. The labial raw surfaces are stitched together to cover the urethra and vaginal introitus, leaving a small posterior opening for urinary and menstrual flow (**25.4**). In Type III FGM, the patient will have a firm band of tissue replacing the labia and obliteration of the urethra and vaginal openings.

Type IV FGM (Pharaonic circumcision)

Type IV includes different practices of variable severity including pricking, piercing, or incision of the clitoris and/or labia; stretching of the clitoris and/or labia; cauterization of the clitoris; and scraping or introduction of corrosive substances into the vagina (**25.5**)[13].

PROGNOSIS

FGM, also commonly referred to as 'female circumcision', has no health benefits for the individual. This is in contrast to male circumcision, which has been proven to reduce the likelihood of catching sexually transmitted diseases. Despite the practice being performed for reasons such as tradition/religion or the belief that it curbs promiscuity in women, FGM has no such effects. Instead, it can and usually does lead to discomfort, scar tissue, and shock[2,4,13]. Due to the unsanitary nature of the practice, FGM can cause mild to severe complications for the individual affected.

COMPLICATIONS

The physical complications associated with FGM may be acute or chronic. Because the practice is often carried out by spiritual or authoritative leaders without any safety precautions, early, life-threatening risks include hemorrhage, shock secondary to blood loss or pain, local infection and failure to heal, septicemia, tetanus, trauma to adjacent structures, and urinary retention. Infibulation (Type III) is often associated with long-term gynecologic or urinary tract difficulties. Common gynecologic problems involve the development of painful subcutaneous dermoid cysts and keloid formation along excised tissue edges. More serious complications include pelvic infection, dysmenorrhea, hematocolpos, painful intercourse, infertility, recurrent urinary tract infection, and urinary calculus formation. Pelvic examination is difficult or impossible for women who have been infibulated, and vaginal childbirth requires an episiotomy to avoid serious vulvar lacerations[1,2].

Less well-understood are the psychological, sexual, and social consequences of FGM, because little research has been conducted in countries where the practice is endemic. Personal accounts by women who have had a ritual genital procedure recount anxiety before the event, terror at being seized and forcibly held during the event, great difficulty during childbirth, and lack of sexual pleasure during intercourse[2,14].

The practice thus removes sexual pleasure from the victim in an attempt to fulfill these four customs.

TREATMENT

For many victims of FGM, treatment is available to help amend what has been damaged in order to give the victim a better standard of living. There are two popular types of treatment that victims of FGM can undergo; deinfibulation and genital reconstructive surgery.

- Deinfibulation. This attempts to reverse the effects of infibulation by opening up the stitched scar tissue and leaving the normal vaginal opening. This is usually done at the time of childbirth if the opening is not sufficient. This surgery is usually carried out at around 20 weeks of gestation or later and is performed using local anesthetics[1].
- Reconstructive surgery. Also known as FGM corrective surgery, this involves recreating the clitoris for the victim using techniques similar to that of cosmetic penis enlargement. Physiotherapy may then be used to stimulate the nerves again[1].

Vaginal closure

Closure of the vagina involves surgery for an older woman whose uterus has moved from its natural position, pressing uncomfortably into the vagina (uterine prolapse). This procedure may also be done if an older woman's vagina severely sags or drops into the vaginal canal (vaginal vault prolapse). In this surgery, the vagina is sewn shut, so it is only done if the woman no longer desires sexual intercourse.

Vaginal obliteration is performed by removing the entire vaginal lining except for 1–1.5 inch (2.5–3.8 cm). The vagina is then sewn shut. If the uterus is still present, a small opening is left in the vagina to allow fluids to drain from the uterus. Because vaginal obliteration is a relatively brief surgical procedure, it may be performed when a woman has one or more severe long-term (chronic) medical conditions, such as asthma or heart disease, that make a longer procedure more of a risk.

ACKNOWLEDGMENT
Adeola Chetachi Adesola and Olukorede O. Korede, two students from the Department of Law, University of Warwick, UK, contributed to this chapter as part of the Undergraduate Research Scholarship Scheme.

CHAPTER 26

Genital and Perianal Diseases of Psychogenic Origin

Adam Reich, MD, and Jacek C. Szepietowski, MD

- **Urogenital pain syndromes**
- **Vulvodynia (vestibulodynia)**
- **Other urogenital pain syndromes**
- **Pruritus ani**
- **Venereophobia**
- **Genital self-inflicted lesions**

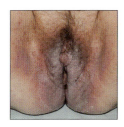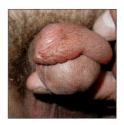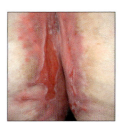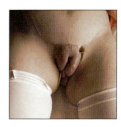

Urogenital pain syndromes

Cutaneous dysesthesias or pain syndromes associated with psychological factors are characterized by pain, which is a predominant manifestation of the disease and is reported by the patient as clinically significant and causes suffering or professional and social detriment. However, the pain cannot be explained by a somatic disease or a psychiatric disorder[1]. Among them, vulvodynia has been most widely studied.

Vulvodynia (vestibulodynia)

DEFINITION
Vulvodynia is defined as a vulvar pain syndrome of uncertain etiology characterized by intermittent or constant pain or discomfort (burning, stinging, rawness) within the vulva, lasting for at least 6 months[2]. Vulvodynia can be localized (limited to a specific area of the vulva) or generalized (involving the entire vulva). Symptoms of vulvodynia can be either provoked (by stimuli that are usually not painful, like touch or pressure) or spontaneous[2].

ETIOLOGY AND EPIDEMIOLOGY
The etiology of vulvodynia remains elusive. There is no relationship between vulvodynia and sexually transmitted diseases (STDs)[3]. In the past, it has been suggested that this condition might be of psychogenic origin; however, more recent data have demonstrated that women with vulvodynia have normal marital satisfaction, are psychologically comparable with women without this problem, and are not more likely to have been abused[3]. On the other hand, it has been reported that adult-onset vulvodynia is strongly associated with frequent abuse as a child, either physically or sexually.

Interestingly, women with vulvodynia showed increased neuronal proliferation and branching in the vulva in comparison with tissue specimens of healthy controls.

Affected women are also more likely to have altered contractile function of the pelvic floor muscles. Not only are women with vulvodynia more sensitive to touch in the vestibular region but, in addition, they show a decreased pain threshold at the periphery. These alterations in the pathogenesis of vulvodynia still warrant further investigation, but it seems that vulvodynia may be considered a form of neuropathic pain syndrome. Recently, it has also been suggested that an altered immunoinflammatory response to environmentally-induced allergic reactions may predispose women to the development of vulvodynia.

The exact prevalence of vulvodynia is difficult to establish, as this ailment is a diagnosis of exclusion and there is no specific test that would confirm the disease; however, based on several studies assessing the symptoms of vulvodynia, it can be estimated that it is present in about 4–7% of female patients at the time of investigation, whereas the lifetime prevalence is approximately 9–18%[4,5]. Vulvodynia may begin at any age, but most women with this disorder are between 20 and 50 years of age[3]. Women with vulvodynia more frequently suffer from other psychogenic-related conditions, like chronic fatigue syndrome (odds ratio [OR]: 2.78–3.19), fibromyalgia (OR: 2.15–3.84), depression (OR: 1.46–2.99), and irritable bowel syndrome (OR: 1.86–3.11)[6].

CLINICAL PRESENTATION
In some women, symptoms of vulvodynia begin in childhood or at the time of first intercourse, while in others complaints emerge after several years of painless sex[3]. The pain is often described as burning, but it may also be sharp, prickly, or even pruritic[3]. Most women report pain on contact at the time of tampon insertion, intercourse, or pelvic examination, and many of them declare that pain limits or prevents sexual intercourse. The pain can begin suddenly when provoked, and then it tends to dissipate gradually. Sometimes, women with vulvodynia

complain of pain or discomfort for several hours to days after intercourse or a pelvic examination. The degree may vary from mild to severe. Clinically, the region of pain looks normal but, occasionally, slight erythema or edema may be present.

Many women have associated urinary symptoms (frequency and bladder irritability) in the absence of infection. Usually, the symptoms of vulvodynia are aggravated by sexual intercourse, tight clothes, partner's touch, bicycle riding, use of tampons, or prolonged sitting. The following measures may improve vulvodynia: loose clothing, not wearing underwear, application of ice to the painful area, distraction, or rest[3].

DIAGNOSIS

The diagnosis of vulvodynia depends on a consistent history, lack of a documented infectious or dermatologic cause of symptoms, and in most women, tenderness when gentle pressure is applied by a cotton swab to the vulva, introitus, or hymenal area[2]. Importantly, vulvodynia is a diagnosis of exclusion. It must be differentiated from allergic vulvitis (signs of irritation and/or erythema, burning or pruritus of the vulva after exposure to allergens), chronic candidal vulvovaginitis (erythema, edema, and/or white discharge with positive mycological examination from the vulva), lichen planus (white reticulate lesions on the mucous membrane), lichen sclerosus, pudendal canal syndrome (unilateral genital pain, often increased with sitting), vaginismus (pelvic floor muscle spasm present and accentuated by examination), vulvar atrophy (pale, thinned mucosa), and vulvar intraepithelial neoplasia[3].

A cotton swab test may be helpful in making the proper diagnosis. A cotton swab is used to gently indent (about 5 mm [0.2 inch]) several locations within the vulvar vestibule[3]. The pressure will provoke discomfort or pain in nearly all women with vulvodynia[3]. The cotton swab test is considered positive if the tested woman scores the pain equal to or more

than 4 points on a 10-point visual analog scale[7]. Recently, a standardized insertion and removal tampon test has also been proposed as a helpful tool in examining patients with vulvodynia, as it provides an alternative to sexual intercourse pain[7]. The 'tampon test' was shown to be a reliable instrument with good construct validity and may be used as the primary endpoint in future clinical trials assessing treatments for vulvodynia[7].

TREATMENT

To date, there are only limited data on the effectiveness of various treatment options in vulvodynia. Some authors consider tricyclic antidepressants in combination with local lignocaine gel as the first-choice therapy; however, a recent randomized prospective clinical trial failed to confirm the efficacy of low-dose amitriptyline, a classic tricyclic antidepressant, in reducing pain in women with vulvodynia. Alternatively, pregabalin or gabapentin may be tried to alleviate or reduce pain in vulvodynia, as there are several case reports documenting their efficacy and they are also commonly used in the treatment of neuropathic pain[3,8].

Patients with vulvodynia may also benefit from psychosocial treatments. Cognitive behavioral therapy, especially a directed treatment approach that involves the learning and practice of specific pain-relevant coping and self-management skills, has been shown to provide durable improvement in vulvar pain with intercourse. In addition, biofeedback and physical therapy should be considered to help patients regain control of the pelvic floor musculature[3]. Some positive effect was also noted after acupuncture. Perineoplasty or vestibulectomy with removal of hypersensitive tissue and replacement with vaginal mucosa should be reserved for women with severe vulvodynia, unresponsive to other therapies[3].

Other urogenital pain syndromes

Genital pain in men usually affects the testicles and perineum; less frequently, isolated penile pain may occur[1]. Patients often complain of the feeling of pressure, pulling pain, sometimes radiating to the testicles, burning in the distal urethra or a feeling of pressure in the sacrum[1]. These symptoms may be related to impaired sexuality, neuroticism, compulsive personality, or spousal conflicts. Differential diagnosis includes prostate inflammation, testicular neoplasia (if the pain is unilateral), or affliction of nerve roots L1 and L2. In addition, penile erysipelas, balanoposthitis, cavernitis, urethritis, and Peyronie's disease must be excluded[1].

Anodynia (anorectal pain) most frequently occurs together with other pain syndromes, like vulvodynia or phallodynia, but sometimes it may be isolated. The predominant symptom is a persistent, severe pain that cannot be explained by an underlying physical condition. A psychogenically-caused rectal pain may persist even during diagnostic spinal or epidural anaesthesia[1].

Pruritus ani

DEFINITION, ETIOLOGY, AND EPIDEMIOLOGY

Pruritus ani is defined as an intense chronic itching affecting the perianal area. The etiology of pruritus ani is multifactorial and includes perianal fecal contamination, various dermatologic conditions (lichen sclerosus, atopic dermatitis, lichen planus, contact dermatitis, seborrheic dermatitis, psoriasis, or acne inversa), dietary factors (coffee, chocolate, tomatoes, citrus fruits, cow milk, alcohol, peanuts, or spices), infections and infestations (e.g. enterobiasis, scabies, pediculosis pubis, candidiasis, dermatophytosis, beta-hemolytic streptococcal infections, *Staphyloccocus aureus*

infections, erythrasma, genital warts, or genital herpes), drugs (caffeine, colchicine, gemcitabine, or quinidine), gastrointestinal problems (rectal prolapse, chronic diarrhea, chronic constipation, soiling and anal incontinence, hemorrhoids, anal papilloma, anal fissure, anal fistula, or abscesses), excessive cleaning or local application of irritative agents, systemic diseases (diabetes mellitus, celiac disease, hyperbilirubinemia, leukemia, iron deficiency anemia, aplastic anemia, or hyperthyroidism), neoplasms (Bowen's disease, extramammary Paget's disease, squamous cell carcinoma, or colorectal cancer), as well as psychological factors (depression, anxiety, or stress)[9-13]. In total, more than 100 causative factors have been described in the literature[9]; however, the underlying condition cannot be determined in about one-quarter of patients, and pruritus ani is considered as idiopathic[9]. Importantly, regardless of the etiology, the itch–scratch cycle becomes self-propagating and results in chronic pathologic changes that persist even if the initiating factor is removed[12].

It is estimated that about 1–5% of the general population may suffer from pruritus ani. It is approximately four times more frequent in men and most commonly appears between the ages of 40 and 60 years[9]. Pruritus ani has been found to be the second (after hemorrhoids) most frequently observed benign anal disease[10].

CLINICAL PRESENTATION

Examination of the perineum may reveal a wide range of abnormalities depending on the etiology, but even in patients experiencing severe pruritus, the perineum and anus may sometimes look quite normal. When pruritus ani becomes chronic, the perianal area usually becomes lichenified and appears white with fine fissures (*Table 26.1*)[10].

DIAGNOSIS

The diagnosis of pruritus ani is based on patients' complaints. Every patient with anal pruritus has to undergo a thorough history and physical examination in order to detect the underlying factors. The medical history should include data about concomitant diseases, medicines, diet, and cleaning habits. A detailed inspection of the anal and perianal areas may reveal anal abnormalities, skin diseases, infections, or infestations. A full body examination may help to diagnose skin diseases or infections of other areas. In many patients, more specific examinations are necessary to establish the proper diagnosis[10]. Microscopic examination and cultures on specific media of bacterial and fungal specimens should confirm the infectious etiology of pruritus ani. Wood's lamp examination may facilitate the diagnosis of erythrasma. Anoscopy is of help in the detection of deeper anal lesions. If needed, a biopsy should be performed from affected, as well as neighboring normal, skin[10,13]. In addition, many patients with pruritus ani show positive patch tests to various contact allergens.

TREATMENT

If possible, the underlying factors should be treated first. The patient must be informed about the necessity of regular defecation, proper cleaning after defecation, and avoiding the use of cleansing materials that may produce irritation (e.g. bleached or perfumed toilet paper, soaps). The anal area should be kept dry (e.g. patted dry with a soft cloth or dried with a hair dryer). Rubbing or scrubbing the area is to be discouraged[13]. Patients should be advised to wear loose, natural fiber clothing and to avoid prolonged sitting.

More specific treatments usually include emollients, corticosteroids, and capsaicin[14]. Skin barriers such as topical zinc oxide or emollients can themselves provide pruritus relief, but are often used as a sustained measure. Topical corticosteroids may help to break the vicious itch–scratch cycle[13,15]. Use of a perianal cleaner is helpful.

Table 26.1 Clinical stages of pruritus ani (adapted from Kuehn et al.[10])

Stage 1 – mild	No lesions seen at inspection of anal verge but the patient finds the palpation or anoscopy painful (other anal conditions have to be excluded)
Stage 2 – moderate	Red dry skin, occasionally transient weeping skin with superficial round splits and longitudinal superficial fissures
Stage 3 – severe	Reddened, weeping skin, with superficial ulcers and excoriations disrupted by pale, whitish areas with no hair
Stage 4 – chronic	Pale, whitened, thickened, dry, leathery, scaly skin with no hair and no superficial ulcers or excoriations

Venereophobia

DEFINITION
Venereophobia comprises persistent, excessive preoccupation with the fear or conviction of suffering from an STD, without sufficient physical findings[1]. Sometimes, the fear may be restricted to one particular infection, e.g. acquired immunodeficiency syndrome (AIDS) phobia or syphilis phobia.

CLINICAL PRESENTATION
The patient demonstrates a fear of or conviction of having an STD. The fear or conviction persists despite negative medical diagnostic tests and assurance from the physician about the absence of the infection. The disease may be elicited by a traumatizing life event, e.g. death of a close relative.

DIAGNOSIS
The diagnosis is based on a thorough history and physical examination. If necessary, STDs should be excluded using standard procedures. A psychiatric consultation is recommended for definite diagnosis of venereophobia.

TREATMENT
Therapy depends on the concomitant psychiatric symptoms. The treatment includes psychotherapy, sometimes in combination with selective serotonin reuptake inhibitors or tricyclic antidepressants, if depression or anxiety is present, or neuroleptics when psychotic symptoms are the prominent disturbances[1].

Genital self-inflicted lesions

DEFINITION
Self-inflicted lesions include all self-mutilating actions that lead directly or indirectly to clinically relevant damage of the organism, without the direct intention of committing suicide[1]. Detailed characteristics of various forms of self-mutilations are presented in *Table 26.2*.

ETIOLOGY AND EPIDEMIOLOGY
Most frequently the injuries are mechanical, although self-inflicted infections and toxic damage may also occur (**26.1, 26.2**). A number of psychiatric disorders have been recognized in subjects with self-mutilation: personality disorders, emotionally unstable personality disorders of the borderline type, narcissistic personality disorders, histrionic personality disorders, antisocial personality disorders, dependency personality disorders, depressive disorders, anxiety disorders, compulsive disorders, and post-traumatic stress disorders[1]. The prevalence of factitious disorders, also including genital self-inflicted injuries, is estimated at 0.05–0.4% in the general population[1].

Table 26.2 Various forms of self-inflicted lesions in the genital area

Type of self-inflicted lesion	Definition	Symptoms
Dermatologic factitious disorders (formerly: dermatitis artefacta)	Self-inflicted lesions are regarded as 'an appeal for help' when the patient is confronted with various everyday-life stressors	Patients typically deny the self-inflicted nature of their lesions Typical history: sudden appearance of fully developed lesions without any prodromal symptoms
Obsessive–compulsive excoriations (formerly neurotic excoriations)	Lesions created by patients having a perfectionistic personality, obsessive–compulsive disorder, or depression	The lesions (most frequently various forms of excoriation) may be triggered by some cutaneous dysesthesia (e.g. itch) or an urge to excoriate even the slightest irregularity found on the skin
Munchausen's syndrome (hospital addiction)	Lesions created to receive help of health care professionals	Patients notoriously visit different hospitals with dramatic and untrue stories of various diseases (skin lesions are only one of the possible presentations, other complaints include recurrent abdominal pain, neurological symptoms, hemorrhages of different origin, etc) Patients usually present an antisocial personality
Malingering	A fully consciously created lesion in order to obtain certain external profit (financial compensation, early retirement, etc)	Various morphology of lesions, usually not fitting with the patient's description of the disease course and not in accordance with any well-known disease Sometimes patients may intentionally worsen a pre-existing condition (e.g. psoriasis, atopic eczema)
Dermatologic pathomimicry	Intentional or unconscious mimicry of a skin disease (could be a form of factitious disorder or malingering)	Patients mimic their original dermatologic disease by reproducing the original mechanisms of disease or by interfering with therapy

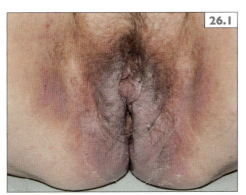

26.1 Self-inflicted dermatitis with thickening of the vulva due to chronic rubbing provoked by psychogenic pruritus.

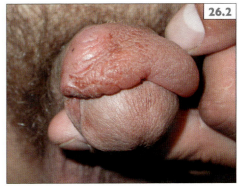

26.2 Eczematous skin lesions in a man with a washing compulsion. (Courtesy of Dr. Uwe Gieler, Giessen, Germany.)

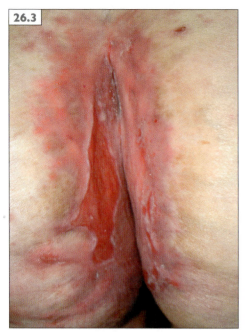

26.3 Obsessive–compulsive excoriations with profound scarring in the perianal region. (Courtesy of Dr. Uwe Gieler, Giessen, Germany.)

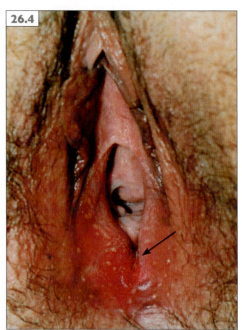

26.4 Self-inflicted injury presenting as a small ulcer (arrow) mimicking infectious genital ulcer. (Courtesy of Dr. Alina Ilie, Bucharest, Romania.)

CLINICAL PRESENTATION

As underlined by Harth *et al.*[1], a 'typical' is what is atypical – usually patients may have lesions in atypical locations, with atypical morphology and histology, or may not respond to the treatment that should be helpful (**26.3**). Self-inflicted lesions may also morphologically mimic most skin or mucosal diseases (**26.4**). Patients with dermatologic factitious disorder appear to be astonished by the skin lesions and cannot give a clear explanation of how the skin changes appeared and developed. In malingering, the lesions may be similar, but are done intentionally and fully consciously. Sometimes the lesions may resemble a well-defined dermatologic condition, if the patient is able to reproduce the original mechanism of the disease (dermatologic pathomimicry).

DIAGNOSIS

Diagnosis is based on clinical presentation and detailed history. In most cases of self-inflicted injuries, a psychiatric or psychological consultation is needed to diagnose the underlying psychiatric disorder. Sometimes, the patient must be followed for a longer time to document the self-mutilating behavior objectively.

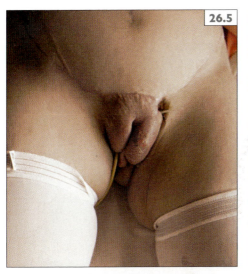

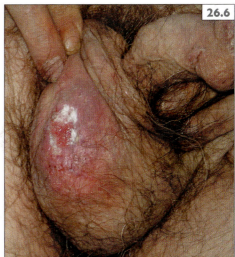

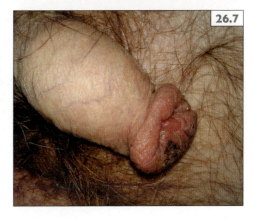

26.5 Permanent mutilation of female genitalia due to multiple, repeated injections of various liquids into the labia majora in a patient with a body dysmorphic disorder. (Courtesy of Dr. Uwe Gieler, Giessen, Germany.)

26.6 An abscess due to chronic compulsive manipulation within the male genitalia.

26.7 Same patient as in **26.6**: mutilation of the foreskin due to compulsive manipulation.

COMPLICATIONS

Self-inflicted injuries within the genital area are connected with a number of long-lasting complications. Many patients experience difficulties with sexual intercourse, including dyspareunia in women, and may have recurrent urinary tract infections or dysuria. Women may also suffer from difficulties with menstruation and dysmenorrhea, or may have serious obstetric complications, including injury of the sphincter ani and infections (**26.5**). In some patients, self-inflicted injuries may result in the formation of profound scarring, cysts, or abscesses (**26.6**, **26.7**).

TREATMENT

The most important issue is to diagnose the underlying psychiatric disorder and to start psychiatric therapy. Therapy includes various psychotropic drugs, psychotherapy, and relaxation therapy[1]. If successful, the treatment results in cessation of the self-mutilating behavior, which in milder forms usually leads to spontaneous healing of the lesions. Mild disinfectants or antimicrobial agents may be helpful in accelerating the healing process. In more severe cases, various reconstructive surgical procedures may be indicated; however, it must be emphasized that in some patients with factitious disorders, all treatment options may be unsuccessful.

References

Preface

1 Gensini GF, Conti AA, Lippi D (2007). The contributions of Paul Ehrlich to infectious disease. *J Infect* **54**:221–4.
2 Kampmeier RH (1976). Syphilis therapy: an historical perspective. *J Am Vener Dis Assoc* **3**:99–108.
3 O'Leary P (1955). Editorial. *AMA Arch Dermatol Syphilol* **71**:1.
4 Mroczkowski TF (1990). *Sexually Transmitted Diseases*. Igaku-Shoin, New York, vii, 404 pp.
5 Mroczkowski TF (2006). Choroby Przenoszone Droga Płciowa, Wydawnictwo Czelej, Lublin, Poland, 584 pp.
6 Parish LC, Gschnait F (1989). *Sexually Transmitted Diseases: a Guide for Clinicians*. Springer-Verlag, New York, xiv, 388 pp.
7 Parish LC, Sehgal VN, Buntin DM (1991). *Color Atlas of Sexually Transmitted Diseases*. Igaku-Shoin, New York, vii, 173 pp.

Section 1 Sexually Transmitted Diseases

CHAPTER 1 SYPHILIS

1 Crissey JT, Denenholz DA (1984). Syphilis. *Clin Dermatol* **2**(1):1–166.
2 Stary A (2008). Sexually transmitted infections. In: Bolognia J, Jorizzo J, Rapini R (eds). *Dermatology*. Mosby Elsevier, St. Louis, pp. 1239–50.
3 Golden MR, Marra CM, Holmes KK (2003). Update on syphilis: resurgence of an old problem. *JAMA* **290**:1510–14.
4 Peterman TA, Furness BW (2007). The resurgence of syphilis among men who have sex with men. *Curr Opin Infect Dis* **20**:54–9.
5 Su JR, Beltrami JF, Zaidi AA, *et al.* (2011). Primary and secondary syphilis among black and Hispanic men who have sex with men: case report data from 27 States. *Ann Intern Med* **155**:145–51.
6 Mroczkowski TF (1990). Syphilis. In: *Sexually Transmitted Diseases*. Igaku-Shoin, New York, pp. 164–227.
7 Dourmishev LA, Dourmishev AL (2005). Syphilis: uncommon presentations in adults. *Clin Dermatol* **23**:555–64.
8 Gregory N (1991). Clinical problems of syphilis in the presence of HIV. *Clin Dermatol* **9**:71–4.

9 Stokes JH, Beerman H, Ingraham NR (1944). *Modern clinical syphilology diagnosis, treatment*, case study. vii. WB Saunders, Philadelphia, 1332 pp.
10 Domantay-Apostol GP, Handog EB, Gabriel MT (2008). Syphilis: the international challenge of the great imitator. *Dermatol Clin* **26**:191–202, v.
11 Zeltser R, Kurban AK (2004). Syphilis. *Clin Dermatol* **22**:461–8.
12 Sanchez M (2010). Syphilis. In: Lebwohl M, Heyman W, Berth-Jones J, *et al.* (eds). *Treatment of Skin Diseases: Comprehensive Therapeutic Strategies*. Saunders Elsevier, Philadelphia, pp. 730–5.
13 Goh BT (2005). Syphilis in adults. *Sex Transm Infect* **81**:448–52.
14 Blank LJ, Rompalo AM, Erbelding EJ, *et al.* (2011). Treatment of syphilis in HIV-infected subjects: a systematic review of the literature. *Sex Transm Infect* **87**:9–16.

CHAPTER 2 GONORRHEA

1 http://www.cdc.gov/std/stats10/gonorrhea.htm.
2 Ching B (2011). The porcelain terror: can a toilet give you gonorrhea? http://www.clinicalcorrelations.org/?p=4206.
3 Centers for Disease Control and Prevention (1997). Gonorrhea among men who have sex with men – selected sexually transmitted diseases clinics, 1993–1996. *MMWR* **46**:889–92.
4 Rothman KJ, Lanza L, Lal A, Peskin EG, Dreyer NA (1996). Incidence of pelvic inflammatory disease among women treated for gonorrhea or chlamydia. *Pharmacoepidemiol Drug Saf* **5**:409–14.
5 McCormack WM (1994). Pelvic inflammatory disease. *N Engl J Med* **330**:115–19.
6 Jarusintanakorn S, Chalermchockcharoenkit A (2008). Prevalence of gonorrhoeal and/or chlamydial infection in hospitalized patients with pelvic inflammatory disease. *Thai J Obst Gyn* **16**:234–42.
7 Lee JS, Choi HY, Lee JE, Lee SH, Oum BSS (2002). Gonococcal keratoconjunctivitis in adults. *Eye* **16**:646–9.
8 Alexander ER (1984). Maternal and infant sexually transmitted diseases. *Urol Clin North Am* **11**:131–9.

9 Scott MJ Jr, Scott MJ Sr (1982). Primary cutaneous *Neisseria gonorrhoeae* infections. *Arch Dermatol* **118**:351–2.

10 Spencer SE, Bash MC (2006). Extragenital manifestations of *Neisseria gonorrhoeae*. *Curr Infect Dis Rep* **8**: 132–8.

11 Wolff CB, Goodman HV, Vahrman J (1970). Gonorrhoea with skin and joint manifestations. *Br Med J* **2**:271–3.

12 Driessen CM, de Jong SA, Bastiaens MT, *et al*. (2011). [Dermatitis or arthritis as a sign of gonorrhoea]. *Ned Tijdschr Geneeskd* **155**:A2250.

13 Suzaki A, Hayashi K, Kosuge K, *et al*. (2011). Disseminated gonococcal infection in Japan: a case report and literature review. *Intern Med* **50**:2039–43.

14 Densen P, Mackeen LA, Clark RA (1982). Dissemination of gonococcal infection is associated with delayed stimulation of complement-dependent neutrophil chemotaxis *in vitro*. *Infect Immun* **38**:563–72.

15 O'Brien JP, Goldenberg DL, Rice PA (1983). Disseminated gonococcal infection: a prospective analysis of 49 patients and a review of pathophysiology and immune mechanisms. *Medicine* **62**:395–406.

16 Van Dyck E, Ieven M, Pattyn S, *et al*. (2001). Detection of *Chlamydia trachomatis* and *Neisseria gonorrhoeae* by enzyme immunoassay, culture, and three nucleic acid amplification tests. *J Clin Microbiol* **39**:1751–6.

17 Alcorn, TM, Cohen, MS (1994). Gonococcal pathogenesis: adaptation and immune evasion in the human host. *Curr Opin Infect Dis* **7**:310–16.

CHAPTER 3 CHANCROID

1 WHO (1995). Global prevalence and incidence of selected curable sexually transmitted diseases: overview and estimates. WHO, Geneva (unpublished document WHO/GPA/STD/95.1).

2 Trees DL, Morse SA (1995). Chancroid and *Haemophilus ducreyi*: an update. *Clin Microbiol Rev* **8**:357–75.

3 Steen R (2001). Eradicating chancroid. *Bull WHO* **79**:818–26.

4 D'Costa LJ, Plummer, FA, Bowmer I, *et al*. (1985). Prostitutes are a major reservoir of sexually transmitted diseases in Nairobi, Kenya. *Sex Transm Dis* **12**:64–7.

5 Centers for Disease Control and Prevention (2011). Sexually transmitted diseases surveillance. www.cdc.gov/std/stats11/

6 Morse SA (1989). Chancroid and *Haemophilus ducreyi*. *Clin Microbiol Rev* **2**:137–57.

7 Jessamine PG, Ronald AR (1990). Chancroid and the role of genital ulcer disease in the spread of human retrovirus. *Med Clin North Am* **74**:1417–31.

8 Al-Tawfiq A, Spinola S (2002). *Haemophilus ducreyi*: clinical disease and pathogenesis. *Curr Opin Infect Dis* **15**:43–7.

9 Spinola SM, Bauer ME, Munson RS (2002). Immunopathogenesis of *Haemophilus ducreyi* (chancroid). *Infect Immun* **70**:1667–76.

10 Lewis DA (2003). Chancroid: clinical manifestations, diagnosis, and management. *Sex Transm Infect* **79**:68–71.

11 Lewis DA (2000). Diagnostic tests for chancroid. *Sex Transm Infect* **76**:137–41.

12 Orle KA, Gates CA, Martin DH, *et al*. (1996). Simultaneous PCR detection of *Haemophilus ducreyi*, *Treponema pallidum*, and herpes simplex virus Types 1 and 2 from genital ulcers. *J Clin Microbiol* **34**:49–54.

13 Patterson K, Olsen B, Thomas C, *et al*. (2002). Development of a rapid immunodiagnostic test for *Haemophilus ducreyi*. *J Clin Microbiol* **40**:3694–702.

14 Elkins C, Yi K, Olsen B, *et al*. (2000). Development of a serological test for *Haemophilus ducreyi* for seroprevalence studies. *J Clin Microbiol* **38**:1520–6.

15 Workowski KA, Berman SM; Centers for Disease Control and Prevention (2010). Sexually transmitted diseases treatment guidelines. *MMWR Recomm Rep* **59**(RR-12):1–110.

CHAPTER 4 LYMPHOGRANULOMA VENEREUM

1 Mabey D, Peeling RW (2002). Lymphogranuloma venereum. *Sex Transm Infect* **78**:90–2.

2 Burgoyne RA (1990). Lymphogranuloma venereum. *Prim Care* **17**:153–7.

3 Papagrigoriadis S, Rennie JA (1998). Lymphogranuloma venereum as a cause of rectal strictures. *Postgrad Med J* **74**:168–9.

4 Schachter J, Moncada J (2005). Lymphogranuloma venereum: how to turn an endemic disease into an outbreak of a new disease? Start looking. *Sex Transm Dis* **32**:331–2.

5 Savage EJ, van de Laar MJ, Gallay A, *et al*. (2009). Lymphogranuloma venereum in Europe, 2003–2008. *Euro Surveill* **14**(pii):19428.

6 Sethi G, Allason-Jones E, Richens J, *et al*. (2009). Lymphogranuloma venereum presenting as genital ulceration and inguinal syndrome in men who have sex with men in London, United Kingdom. *Sex Transm Infect* **85**:165–70.

7 Schachter J, Osoba AO (1983). Lymphogranuloma venereum. *Br Med Bull* **39**:151–4.

8 Greaves AB (1963). The frequency of lymphogranuloma venereum in persons with perirectal abscesses, fistulae in ano, or both. *Bull World Health Organ* **29**:797.

9 Van Dyck E, Meheus AZ, Piot P (1999). *Laboratory Diagnosis of Sexually Transmitted Diseases*. World Health Organization, Geneva, p. 135.
10 Wang S-P, Grayston JT (1970). Immunologic relationship between genital TRIC, lymphogranuloma venereum, and related organisms in a new microtiter indirect immunofluorescence test. *Am J Ophthalmol* **70**:367–74.
11 Maurin M, Raoult D (2000). Isolation in endothelial cell cultures of *Chlamydia trachomatis* LGV (Serovar L2) from a lymph node of a patient with suspected cat scratch disease. *J Clin Microbiol* **38**:2062-4.
12 Schaeffer A, Henrich B (2008). Rapid detection of *Chlamydia trachomatis* and typing of the lymphogranuloma venereum-associated L-serovars by TaqMan PCR. *BMC Infect Dis* **8**:56.
13 van Nieuwkoop C, Gooskens J, Smit VT, *et al.* (2007). Lymphogranuloma venereum proctocolitis: mucosal T cell immunity of the rectum associated with chlamydial clearance and clinical recovery. *Gut* **56**:1476–7.
14 Workowski KA, Berman SM; Centers for Disease Control and Prevention (2010). Sexually transmitted diseases treatment guidelines. *MMWR Recomm Rep* **59**(RR-12):1–110.

CHAPTER 5 DONOVANOSIS

1 Galarza C (2000). Donovanosis. *Dermatol Peru* **10**:35–8.
2 Fonseca A, Souza EM (1984). Donovanose. *Dermatologia Clínica*. 1st edn. Guanabara Koogan, Rio de Janeiro, p. 167.
3 Donovan C (1905). Ulcerating granuloma of the pudenda. *Indian Med Gaz* **40**:414–15.
4 Aragão HB, Vianna G (1913). Pesquisas sobre o granuloma venéreo. *Mem Inst Oswaldo Cruz* **5**:211–38.
5 Veeranna S, Raghu TY (2003). A clinical and investigational study of donovanosis. *Indian J Dermatol Venereol Leprol* **69**:159-62.
6 O'Farrell N (2001). Donovanosis: an update. *Int J STD AIDS* **12**:423–37.
7 Morrone A, Toma L, Franco G, *et al.* (2003). Donovanosis in developed countries: neglected or misdiagnosed disease? *Int J STD AIDS* **14**:288–9.
8 O'Farrell N (2002). Donovanosis. *Sex Transm Infect* **78**:452–7.
9 Sehgal VN, Jain MK (1988). Pattern of epidemics of donovanosis in the 'nonendemic' region. *Int J Dermatol* **27**:396–9.
10 Sehgal VN (2012). *Donovanosis*, 2nd edn. Jaypee Brothers Medical Publishers, New Delhi, India.
11 O'Farrell N, Hoosen AA, Coetzee K, *et al.* (1990). A rapid stain for the diagnosis of granuloma inguinale. *Genitourin Med* **66**:200–1.
12 Kharsany AB, Hoosen AA, Kiepiela P, *et al.* (1997). Growth and cultural characteristics of *Calymmatobacterium granulomatis* – the aetiological agent of granuloma inguinale (donovanosis). *J Med Microbiol* **46**:579–85.
13 Carter J, Hutton S, Sriprakash KS, *et al.* (1997). Culture of the causative organism of donovanosis (*Calymmatobacterium granulomatis*) in HEp2 cells. *J Clin Microbiol* **35**: 2915–17.
14 Bastian I, Bowden FJ (1996). Amplification of *Klebsiella*-like sequences from biopsy samples from patients with donovanosis. *Clin Infect Dis* **23**: 1328–30.
15 Carter JS, Kemp DJ (2000). A colorimetric detection system for *Calymmatobacterium granulomatis*. *Sex Transm Inf* **76**:134–6.
16 Mackay IM, Harnett G, Jeoffreys N, *et al.* (2006). Detection and discrimination of herpes simplex viruses, *Haemophilus ducreyi, Treponema pallidum*, and *Calymmatobacterium (Klebsiella) granulomatis* from genital ulcers. *Clin Infect Dis* **42**:1431–8.

CHAPTER 6 NONGONOCOCCAL URETHRITIS

1 Centers for Disease Control and Prevention (2006). Sexually Transmitted Diseases Treatment Guidelines. *MMWR Recomm Rep* **55**(RR-11).
2 Schwartz MA, Hooton TM (1998). Etiology of nongonococcal nonchlamydial urethritis. *Dermatol Clin* **16**:727–33, xi.
3 Aral SO, Holmes KK (1999). Social and behavioral determinants of the epidemiology of STDs: industrialized and developing countries. In: Holmes KK, Sparling PF, Mardh P-A, *et al. Sexually Transmitted Diseases*, 3rd edn. McGraw-Hill, New York, pp. 39–76.
4 Bradshaw CS, Tabrizi SN, Read TR, *et al.* (2006). Etiologies of nongonococcal urethritis: bacteria, viruses, and the association with orogenital exposure. *J Infect Dis* **193**:336–45.
5 Shahmanesh M, Moi H, Lassau F, *et al.* IUSTI/WHO (2009). 2009 European guideline on the management of male nongonococcal urethritis. *Int J STD AIDS* **20**:458–64.
6 Miller WC, Ford CA, Morris M, *et al.* (2004). Prevalence of chlamydial and gonococcal infections among young adults in the United States. *JAMA* **291**:2229–36.
7 Burstein GR, Zenilman JM (1999). Nongonococcal urethritis – a new paradigm. *Clin Infect Dis* **28** (Suppl 1):S66–73.
8 Horner PJ, Thomas B, Gilroy CB, *et al.* (2002). Do all men attending departments of genitourinary medicine need to be screened for nongonococcal urethritis? *Int J STD AIDS* **13**:667–73.

9   Horner P, Thomas B, Gilroy CB, Egger M, Taylor-Robinson D (2001). Role of *Mycoplasma genitalium* and *Ureaplasma urealyticum* in acute and chronic nongonococcal urethritis. *Clin Infect Dis* **32**:995–1003.

10 Corey L, Adams HG, Brown ZA, *et al.* (1983). Genital herpes simplex virus infections: clinical manifestations, course, and complications. *Ann Intern Med* **98**:958–72.

11 Nacey JN, Tulloch GS, Ferguson AF (1985). Catheter-induced urethritis: a comparison between latex and silicone catheters in a prospective clinical trial. *Br J Urol* **57**:325–8.

12 Centers for Disease Control and Prevention (2010). Sexually transmitted diseases treatment guidelines. *MMWR Recomm Rep* **59**(RR-12):1–110.

13 Smith R, Copas AJ, Prince M, *et al.* (2003). Poor sensitivity and consistency of microscopy in the diagnosis of low-grade nongonococcal urethritis. *Sex Transm Infect* **79**:487–90.

14 Chernesky MA, Martin DH, Hook EW, *et al.* (2005). Ability of new APTIMA CT and APTIMA GC assays to detect *Chlamydia trachomatis* and *Neisseria gonorrhoeae* in male urine and urethral swabs. *J Clin Microbiol* **43**:127–31.

15 Ainbinder SW, Ramin SM (2003). Sexually transmitted diseases and pelvic infections. In: DeCherney AH, Nathan L. *CURRENT Diagnosis & Treatment Obstetrics & Gynecology*, 9th edn. McGraw-Hill Medical, New York, pp. 716–50.

16 Galadari I, Galadari H (2004). Nonspecific urethritis and reactive arthritis. *Clin Dermatol* **22**:469–75.

17 Kanerva L, Kousa M, Niemi KM, *et al.* (1982). Ultrahistopathology of balanitis circinata. *Br J Vener Dis* **58**:188–95.

CHAPTER 7 GENITAL HERPES

1   Marques AR, Straus SE (2008). Herpes simplex. In: Wolff K, Goldsmith LA, Katz SI, *et al. Fitzpatrick's Dermatology in General Medicine*, 7th edn. McGraw-Hill Medical, New York. Vol 2, pp. 1873–1885.

2   Xu F, Sternberg MR, Kottiri BJ, *et al.* (2006). Trends in herpes simplex virus type 1 and type 2 seroprevalence in the United States. *JAMA* **296**:964–73.

3   Ryder N, Jin F, McNulty AM, *et al.* (2009). Increasing role of herpes simplex virus type 1 in first-episode anogenital herpes in heterosexual women and younger men who have sex with men, 1992–2006. *Sex Transm Infect* **85**:416–19.

4   Roberts CM, Pfister JR, Spear SJ (2003). Increasing proportion of herpes simplex virus type 1 as a cause of genital herpes infection in college students. *Sex Transm Dis* **30**:797–800.

5   Fleming DT, McQuillan GM, Johnson RE, *et al.* (1997). Herpes simplex virus type 2 in the United States, 1976 to 1994. *N Engl J Med* **337**:1105–11.

6   Mertz GJ, Benedetti J, Ashley R, *et al.* (1992). Risk factors for the sexual transmission of genital herpes. *Ann Intern Med* **116**:197–202.

7   Centers for Disease Control and Prevention (2010). Seroprevalence of herpes simplex virus type 2 among persons aged 14–49 years: United States, 2005–2008. *MMWR* **59**(15):456–9.

8   Wolff K, Johnson RA (2009). Section 30: Sexually transmitted infections. In: Wolff K, Johnson RA. *Fitzpatrick's Color Atlas & Synopsis of Clinical Dermatology*, 6th edn. McGraw-Hill Medical, New York, pp. 896–941.

9   Leone P (2007). Genital herpes. In: Klausner JD, Hook EW III. *Current Diagnosis & Treatment of Sexually Transmitted Diseases*. Lange Medical Books/McGraw-Hill Medical, New York.

10 Corey L (2008). Herpes simplex viruses. In: Fauci AS, Braunwald E, Kasper DL, *et al. Harrison's Principles of Internal Medicine*, 17th edn. Vol 1. McGraw-Hill, New York, Vol 1, pp. 1095–102.

11 Gupta R, Warren T, Wald A (2007). Genital herpes. *Lancet* **370**:2127–37.

12 Kimberlin DW, Rouse DJ (2004). Genital herpes. *N Engl J Med* **350**:1970–7.

13 Wolff K, Johnson RA (2009). Viral infections of skin and mucosa. In: Wolff K, Johnson RA. *Fitzpatrick's Color Atlas & Synopsis of Clinical Dermatology*, 6th edn. McGraw-Hill Medical, New York, pp. 770–853.

14 Centers for Disease Control and Prevention (2010). Sexually Transmitted Diseases Treatment Guidelines, *MMWR Recomm Rep* **59**(RR-12):1–110. http://www.cdc.gov/std/treatment/2010/default.htm

CHAPTER 8 GENITAL WARTS

1   Giuliano AR, Anic G, Nyitray AG (2010). Epidemiology and pathology of HPV disease in males. *Gynecol Oncol* **117**:S15–19.

2   Forcier M, Musacchio N (2010). An overview of human papillomavirus infection for the dermatologist: disease, diagnosis, management, and prevention. *Dermatol Ther* **23**:458–76.

3   Stanley M (2010). Pathology and epidemiology of HPV infection in females. *Gynecol Oncol* **117**:S5–10.

4   Mayeaux EJ, Jr, Dunton C (2008). Modern management of external genital warts. *J Low Genit Tract Dis* **12**:185–92.

5   Winer RL, Hughes JP, Feng Q, *et al.* (2006). Condom use and the risk of genital human papillomavirus infection in young women. *N Engl J Med* **354**:2645–54.

6   Moscicki AB, Ellenberg JH, Farhat S, *et al.* (2004). Persistence of human papillomavirus infection in HIV-infected and -uninfected adolescent girls: risk factors and differences, by phylogenetic type. *J Infect Dis* **190**:37–45.

7 Beutner KR, Wiley DJ, Douglas JM, *et al*. (1999). Genital warts and their treatment. *Clin Infect Dis* **28**(Suppl 1):S37–56.
8 McCutcheon T (2009). Anal condyloma acuminatum. *Gastroenterol Nurs* **32**:342–9.
9 Mayeaux EJ, Jr, Harper MB, Barksdale W, *et al*. (1995). Noncervical human papillomavirus genital infections. *Am Fam Physician* **52**:1137–46, 1149–50.
10 Pomfret TC, Gagnon JM, Jr, Gilchrist AT (2011). Quadrivalent human papillomavirus (HPV) vaccine: a review of safety, efficacy, and pharmacoeconomics. *J Clin Pharm Ther* **36**:1–9.
11 Fairley CK, Hocking JS, Gurrin LC, *et al*. (2009). Rapid decline in presentations of genital warts after the implementation of a national quadrivalent human papillomavirus vaccination programme for young women. *Sex Transm Infect* **85**:499–502.

CHAPTER 9 MOLLUSCUM CONTAGIOSUM
1 Braue A, Ross G, Varigos G, *et al*. (2005). Epidemiology and impact of childhood molluscum contagiosum: a case series and critical review of the literature. *Pediatr Dermatol* **22**; 287–94.
2 Nakamura J, Muraki Y, Yamada M, *et al*. (1995). Analysis of molluscum contagiosum virus genomes isolated in Japan. *J Med Virol* **46**:339–48.
3 Niizeki K, Kano O, Kondo Y (1984). An epidemic study of molluscum contagiosum. Relationship to swimming. *Dermatologica* **169**:197–8.
4 Perna AG, Tyring SK (2002). A review of the dermatologic manifestations of poxvirus infections. *Dermatol Clin* **20**:343–6.
5 Schwartz J, Myskowski P (1992). Molluscum contagiosum in patients with human immunodeficiency virus infection. *J Am Acad Dermatol* **27**:583–8.
6 Mansur AT, Goktay F, Gunduz S, *et al*. (2004). Multiple giant molluscum contagiosum in a renal transplant recipient. *Transpl Infect Dis* **6**:120–3.
7 Cronin TA, Resnik BI, Elgart G, *et al*. (1996). Recalcitrant giant molluscum contagiosum in patient with AIDS. *J Am Acad Dermatol* **35**:266–7.
8 Fife KH, Whitfield M, Faust H, *et al* (1996). Growth of molluscum contagiosum virus in a human foreskin xenograft model. *Virology* **226**:95–101.
9 Fox R, Thiemann A, Everest D, Steinbach F, Dastjerdi A, Finnegan C (2012). Molluscum contagiosum in two donkeys. *Vet Rec* **170**:649.
10 Thompson CH, de Zwart-Steffe RT, Donovan B (1992). Clinical and molecular aspects of molluscum contagiosum infection in HIV-1 positive patients. *Int J STD AIDS* **3**:101–6.
11 Cribier B, Scrivener Y, Grosshans E (2001). Molluscum contagiosum histologic patterns and associated lesions. A study of 578 cases. *Am J Dermatopathol* **23**:99–103.
12 Weller R, O'Callaghan CJ, MacSween RM, *et al*. (1999). Scarring in molluscum contagiosum: comparison of physical expression and phenol ablation. *BMJ* **319**:1540.
13 Dohil M, Prendiville JS (1996). Treatment of molluscum contagiosum with oral cimetidine: clinical experience in 13 patients. *Pediatr Dermatol* **13**:310–12.
14 Syed TA, Lundin S, Ahmad M (1994). Topical 0.3% and 0.5% podophyllotoxin cream for self-treatment of molluscum contagiosum in males. *Dermatology* **189**:65–8.
15 Coloe J, Morrell DS (2009). Cantharidin use among pediatric dermatologists in the treatment of molluscum contagiosum. *Pediatr Dermatol* **26**:405–8.
16 Nelson MR, Chard S, Barton SE (1995). Intralesional interferon for the treatment of recalcitrant molluscum contagiosum in HIV antibody positive individuals – a preliminary report. *Int J STD AIDS* **6**:351–2.

CHAPTER 10 HIV INFECTION/AIDS
1 Centers for Disease Control and Prevention (1981). Pneumocystis pneumonia – Los Angeles. *MMWR* **5**:250–2.
2 Lansky A, Brooks JT, DiNenno E, *et al*. (2010). Epidemiology of HIV in the United States. *J Acquir Immune Defic Syndr* **55**(Suppl 2):S64–8.
3 Schacker T, Collier AC, Hughes J, *et al*. (1997). Clinical and epidemiologic features of primary HIV infection. *Ann Intern Med* **125**:257–64. Erratum in: *Ann Intern Med* 1997;**126**:174.
4 Cooper DA, Gold J, Maclean P, *et al*. (1985). Acute AIDS retrovirus infection. Definition of a clinical illness associated with seroconversion. *Lancet* **1**:537–40.
5 Centers for Disease Control and Prevention (2010). Sexually transmitted diseases treatment guidelines. *MMWR Recomm Rep* **59**(RR-12):1–110.
6 Moore RD, Chaisson RE (1996). Natural history of opportunistic disease in an HIV-infected urban clinical cohort. *Ann Intern Med* **124**:633–42.
7 Kalichman SC, Pellowski J, Turner C (2011). Prevalence of sexually transmitted coinfections in people living with HIV/AIDS: systematic review with implications for using HIV treatments for prevention. *Sex Transm Infect* **87**:183–90.
8 Centers for Disease Control and Prevention (2007). Symptomatic early neurosyphilis among HIV-positive men who have sex with men: four cities, United States, January 2002–June 2004. *MMWR* **56**:625–8.
9 Centers for Disease Control and Prevention (2004). Lymphogranuloma venereum among men who have sex with men – Netherlands, 2003–2004. *MMWR* **53**:985–8.

10 Taniguchi T, Nurutdinova D, Grubb JR, *et al*. (2012). Transmitted drug-resistant HIV type 1 remains prevalent and impacts virologic outcomes despite genotype-guided antiretroviral therapy. *AIDS Res Hum Retrovirus* **28**:259–64.
11 Buchacz K, Baker RK, Palella FJ, Jr, *et al*., HOPS Investigators (2010). AIDS-defining opportunistic illnesses in US patients, 1994–2007: a cohort study. *AIDS* **24**:1549–59.
12 Sackoff JE, Hanna DB, Pfeiffer MR, Torian LV (2006). Causes of death among persons with AIDS in the era of highly active antiretroviral therapy: New York City. *Ann Intern Med* **145**:397–406.
13 CDC (2010). HIV in the United States. July 2010.
14 Panel on Antiretroviral Guidelines for Adults and Adolescents (2013). Guidelines for the use of antiretroviral agents in HIV-1-infected adults and adolescents. Department of Health and Human Services. Available at http://aidsinfo.nih.gov/contentfiles/lvguidelines/AdultandAdolescentGL.pdf Accessed March 3, 2013.

CHAPTER 11 VULVOVAGINITIS

1 Centers for Disease Control and Prevention (2010). Sexually Transmitted Disease Surveillance 2009. US Department of Health and Human Services, Atlanta.
2 Holland J, Young M, Lee O, Chen S (2003). Vulvovaginal carriage of yeasts other than *Candida albicans*. *Sex Trans Infect* **79**:249–50.
3 Lindner J, Plantema F, Hoogkamp K (1978). Quantitative studies of vaginal flora of healthy women and of obstetric and gynaecological patients. *J Med Microbiol* **11**:233–41.
4 Sutton M, Sternberg M, Koumans E, *et al*. (2007). The prevalence of *Trichomonas vaginalis* infection among reproductive-age women in the United States 2001–2004. *Clin Infec Dis* **45**:1319–26.
5 Koumans EH, Sternberg M, Bruce C, *et al*. (2007). The prevalence of bacterial vaginosis in the United States, 2001–2004: associations with symptoms, sexual behaviors, and reproductive health. *Sex Trans Dis* **34**:864–9.
6 Wolner-Hanssen P, Kreiger J, Stevens C, *et al*. (1989). Clinical manifestations of vaginal trichomoniasis. *JAMA* **264**:571–6.
7 Bickley L, Krisher K, Punsalang A, *et al*. (1989). Comparison of direct fluorescent antibody, acridine orange and wet mount and culture for detection of *Trichomonas vaginalis* in women attending a public sexually transmitted disease clinic. *Sex Trans Dis* **16**(3): 127–31.
8 Ison I, Hay P (2002). Validation of a simplified grading of Gram stained vaginal smears for use in genitourinary medicine clinics. *Sex Trans Infect* **78**:413–15.
9 Van Der P, Kraft C, Williams J (2006). Use of an adaptation of a commercially available PCR assay aimed at diagnosis of chlamydia and gonorrhea to detect *Trichomonas vaginalis* in urogenital specimens. *J Clin Microbiol* **44**:366–73.
10 Nye M, Schwebke J, Body B (2009). Comparison of APTIMA *Trichomonas vaginalis* transcription-mediated amplification to wet mount microscopy, culture, and polymerase chain reaction for diagnosis of trichomoniasis in men and women. *Am J Obstet Gynecol* **200**:188–9.
11 Goldenberg R, Hauth J, Andrews W (2000). Intrauterine infection and preterm delivery. *N Engl J Med* **342**:1500–7.
12 Cotch M, Pastorek J, Nugent R, *et al*. (1997). *Trichmonas vaginalis* associated with low birth weight and preterm delivery. *Sex Trans Dis* **24**:353–60.
13 Sorvillo F, Kernott P (1998). *Trichomonas vaginalis* and amplification of HIV-1 transmission. *Lancet* **351**:213–14.

OTHER GUIDELINES USED:
Clinical Effectiveness Group (Association for Genitourinary Medicine and the Medical Society for the Study of Venereal Diseases), United Kingdom National Guideline on the Management of Vulvovaginal Candidiasis, 2007, http://www.bashh.org/guidelines
Clinical Effectiveness Group (Association for Genitourinary Medicine and the Medical Society for the Study of Venereal Diseases), United Kingdom National Guideline on the Management of *Trichomonas vaginalis*, 2007, http://www.bashh.org/guidelines
Clinical Effectiveness Group (Association for Genitourinary Medicine and the Medical Society for the Study of Venereal Diseases), United Kingdom National Guideline on the Management of Bacterial Vaginosis, 2012, http://www.bashh.org/guidelines
Clinical Effectiveness Group (Association for Genitourinary Medicine and the Medical Society for the Study of Venereal Diseases), United Kingdom National Guideline on the Management of Vulval Conditions, 2007, http://www.bashh.org/guidelines
Centers for Disease Control and Prevention (2010). Sexually Transmitted Diseases Treatment Guidelines. US Department of Health and Human Services, Atlanta. http://www.cdc.gov/std/treatment/2010/STD-Treatment-2010-RR5912.pdf
Sherrard J, Donders G, White D, Skov Jensen J (2011). European (IUSTI/WHO) Guideline on the Management of Vaginal Discharge. *Int J STD AIDS* **22**:421–9.

CHAPTER 12 ECTOPARASITOSIS

1 Meinking TL, Burkhart CN, Burkhart CG, Elgart G (2007). Infestations. In: Bolognia J, Jorizzo JL, Rapini RP, *et al*. (eds). *Dermatology*, Vol. 1. Mosby, St. Louis, pp. 1291–301.

2 Meinking TL, Burkhart CG, Burkhart CN (1999). Ectoparasitic diseases in dermatology: reassessment of scabies and pediculosis. In: James W (ed). *Advances in Dermatology*, Vol. 15. Mosby, St. Louis, pp. 67–108.
3 Centers for Disease Control and Prevention (2010). Sexually Transmitted Diseases Treatment Guidelines. *MMWR Recomm Rep* **59**(RR-12):1–110. http://www.cdc.gov/std/treatment/2010/default.htm.
4 Chosidow O (2000). Scabies and pediculosis. *Lancet* **355**:819–26.
5 Burkhart CG, Burkhart CN (2000). An epidemiological and therapeutic reassessment of scabies. *Cutis* **65**: 233–40.
6 Bezold G, Lange M, Schiener R, *et al*. (2001). Hidden scabies: diagnosis by polymerase chain reaction. *Br J Dermatol* **144**:614–18.
7 Kristjansson AK, Smith MK, Gould JW, Gilliam AC (2007). Pink pigtails are a clue for the diagnosis of scabies. *J Am Acad Dermatol* **57**:174–5.
8 Prins C, Stucki L, French L, *et al*. (2004). Dermoscopy for the *in vivo* detection of *Sarcoptes scabiei*. *Dermatology* **208**:241–3.
9 Popescu CM, Popescu R (2012). Efficacy and safety of spinosad cream rinse for head lice. *Arch Dermatol* **148**:1065–9.

CHAPTER 13 SEXUAL ABUSE
1 Centers for Disease Control and Prevention (2010). Sexual violence surveillance: uniform definitions and recommended data elements, Version 1.0. Accessed December 13, 2010 at: http://www.cdc.gov/ViolencePrevention/pub/SV_surveillance.html.
2 Lahoti SL, McClain N, Girardet R, McNeese M, Cheung K (2001). Evaluating the child for sexual abuse. *Am Fam Physician* **63**:883–93.
3 Centers for Disease Control and Prevention (2010). Injury prevention and control: Violence prevention; Sexual violence. Accessed December 13, 2010, at: http://www.cdc.gov/ViolencePrevention/sexualviolence/index.html.
4 Berkoff MC, Zolotor AJ, Makoroff KL, *et al*. (2008). Has this prepubertal girl been sexually abused? *JAMA* **300**(23):2779–92.
5 Swerdlin A, Berkowitz C, Craft N (2000). Cutaneous signs of child abuse. *J Am Acad Dermatol* **57**: 371–92.
6 Jones JS, Dunnuck C, Rossman L, Wynn BN, Nelson-Horan C (2004). Significance of toluidine blue positive findings after speculum examination for sexual assault. *Am J Emerg Med* **22**:201–3.
7 American College of Emergency Physicians (2011). Evaluation and management of the sexually assaulted or sexually abused patient. Accessed Jan 8, 2011, at: http://www.acep.org/search.aspx?searchtext=sexual.

8 Sugar NF, Fine DN, Eckert LO (2004). Physical injury after sexual assault: findings of a large case series. *Am J Obstet Gynecol* **190**:71–6.
9 Riggs N, Houry D, Long G, Markovchick V, Feldhaus KM (2000). Analysis of 1,076 cases of sexual assault. *Ann Emerg Med* **35**:358–62.
10 Centers for Disease Control and Prevention (2010). 2010 STD Treatment guidelines. Accessed Jan 10, 2010 at: http://www.cdc.gov/std/treatment/2010/STD-Treatment-2010-RR5912.pdf.

Section 2 Cutaneous Diseases of the Anogenital Region

CHAPTER 14 ANATOMIC ABNORMALITIES
1 McGregor TB, Pike JG, Leonard MP (2007). Pathologic and physiologic phimosis: approach to the phimotic foreskin. *Can Fam Physician* **53**:445–8.
2 Gairdner D (1949). The fate of the foreskin, a study of circumcision. *Br Med J* **2**:1433–7.
3 Berdeu D, Sauze L, Ha-Vinh P, *et al*. (2001). Cost-effectiveness analysis of treatments for phimosis: a comparison of surgical and medicinal approaches and their economic effect. *BJU Int* **87**:239–44.
4 Kiss A, Kiraly L, Kutasy B, *et al*. (2005). High incidence of balanitis xerotica obliterans in boys with phimosis: prospective 10-year study. *Pediatr Dermatol* **22**:305–8.
5 Maden C, Sherman KJ, Beckmann AM, *et al*. (1993). History of circumcision, medical conditions, and sexual activity and risk of penile cancer. *J Natl Cancer Inst* **85**:19–24.
6 Albers N, Ulrichs C, Gluer S, *et al*. (1997). Etiologic classification of severe hypospadias: implications for prognosis and management. *J Pediatr* **131**:386–92.
7 Baskin LS, Himes K, Colborn T (2001). Hypospadias and endocrine disruption: is there a connection? *Environ Health Perspect* **109**:1175–83.
8 Brouwers MM, Van Der Zanden LF, De Gier RP, et al. (2010). Hypospadias: risk factor patterns and different phenotypes. *BJU International* **105**:254–62.
9 Soomro NA, Neal DE (1998). Treatment of hypospadias: an update of current practice. *Hosp Med* **59**:553–6.
10 Khuri FJ, Hardy BE, Churchill BM (1981). Urologic anomalies associated with hypospadias. *Urol Clin North Am* **8**:565–71.
11 Kramer SA, Kelalis PP (1982). Assessment of urinary continence in epispadias: review of 94 patients. *J Urol* **128**:290–3.
12 Duckett JW, Jr (1978). Epispadias. *Urol Clin North Am* **5**:107–26.

13 Agrawal SK, Bhattacharya SN, Singh N (2004). Pearly penile papules: a review. *Int J Dermatol* **43**:199–201.

14 Ackerman AB, Kronberg R (1973). Pearly penile papules. Acral angiofibromas. *Arch Dermatol* **108**: 673–5.

15 Glicksman JM, Freeman RG (1966). Pearly penile papules. A statistical study of incidence. *Arch Dermatol* **93**:56–9.

16 Sonnex C, Dockerty WG (1999). Pearly penile papules: a common cause of concern. *Int J STD AIDS* **10**:726–7.

17 Neri I, Bardazzi F, Raone B, *et al*. (1997). Ectopic pearly penile papules: a paediatric case. *Genitourin Med* **73**:136.

18 O'Neil CA, Hansen RC (1995). Pearly penile papules on the shaft. *Arch Dermatol* **131**:491–2.

19 Ozeki M, Saito R, Tanaka M (2008). Dermoscopic features of pearly penile papules. *Dermatology* **217**:21–2.

20 Ferenczy A, Richart RM, Wright TC (1991). Pearly penile papules: absence of human papillomavirus DNA by the polymerase chain reaction. *Obstet Gynecol* **78**:118–22.

21 McKinlay JR, Graham BS, Ross EV (1999). The clinical superiority of continuous exposure versus short-pulsed carbon dioxide laser exposures for the treatment of pearly penile papules. *Dermatol Surg* **25**:124–6.

22 Baumgartner J (2012). Erbium: yttrium-aluminum-garnet (Er:YAG) laser treatment of penile pearly papules. *J Cosmet Laser Ther* **14**:155–8.

23 Hyman AB, Brownstein MH (1969). Tyson's 'glands'. Ectopic sebaceous glands and papillomatosis penis. *Arch Dermatol* **99**:31–6.

24 Goldberg JM, Bedaiwy MA (2007). Recurrent umbilical endometriosis after laparoscopic treatment of minimal pelvic endometriosis: a case report. *J Reprod Med* **52**:551–2.

25 Moen MH, Muus KM (1991). Endometriosis in pregnant and nonpregnant women at tubal sterilization. *Hum Reprod* **6**:699–702.

26 Agarwal A, Fong YF (2008). Cutaneous endometriosis. *Singapore Med J* **49**: 704–9.

27 Terada S, Miyata Y, Nakazawa H, *et al*. (2006). Immunohistochemical analysis of an ectopic endometriosis in the uterine round ligament. *Diagn Pathol* **1**:27.

28 De Giorgi V, Massi D, Mannone F, *et al*. (2003). Cutaneous endometriosis: noninvasive analysis by epiluminescence microscopy. *Clin Exp Dermatol* **28**: 315–17.

29 Reddy S, Rock JA (1998). Treatment of endometriosis. *Clin Obstet Gynecol* **41**:387–92.

30 Otsuka T, Ueda Y, Terauchi M, *et al*. (1998). Median raphe (parameatal) cysts of the penis. *J Urol* **159**:1918–20.

31 Nagore E, Sanchez-Motilla JM, Febrer MI, *et al*. (1998). Median raphe cysts of the penis: a report of five cases. *Pediatr Dermatol* **15**:191–3.

32 Nishida H, Kashima K, Daa T, *et al*. (2012). Pigmented median raphe cyst of the penis. *J Cutan Pathol* **39**:808–10.

33 Dini M, Baroni G, Colafranceschi M (2001). Median raphe cyst of the penis: a report of two cases with immunohistochemical investigation. *Am J Dermatopathol* **23**:320–4.

34 Shibagaki N, Ohtake N, Furue M (1996). Spontaneous regression of congenital multiple median raphe cysts of the raphe scroti. *Br J Dermatol* **134**:376–8.

35 Golitz LE, Robin M (1981). Median raphe canals of the penis. *Cutis* **27**:170–2.

36 Asarch RG, Golitz LE, Sausker WF, *et al*. (1979). Median raphe cysts of the penis. *Arch Dermatol* **115**:1084–6.

CHAPTER 15 BENIGN TUMORS

1 Kamino H, Meehan SA, Pui J (2008). Fibrous and fibrohistiocytic proliferations of the skin and tendons. In: Bolognia JL, Jorizzo JL, Rapini RP (eds). *Dermatology*, 2nd edn. Mosby, London, pp. 1813–14.

2 Prieto MA, Guitierrez JV, Sambucety PS (2004). Vestibular papillae of the vulva. *Int J Dermatol* **43**:143–4.

3 Moyal-Barracco M, Leibowitch M, Orth G (1990). Vestibular papillae of the vulva. Lack of evidence for human papillomavirus etiology. *Arch Dermatol* **126**:1594–8.

4 Kim S, Seo S, Ko H, *et al*. (2009). The use of dermatoscopy to differentiate vestibular papillae, a normal variant of the female external genitalia, from condyloma acuminata. *J Am Acad Dermatol* **60**:353–5.

5 Cockerell CJ, Larsen F (2008). Benign epidermal tumors and proliferations. In: Bolognia JL, Jorizzo JL, Rapini RP (eds). *Dermatology*, 2nd edn. Mosby, London, pp. 1661–4.

6 Thakur JS, Thakur A, Chauhan C, *et al*. (2008). Giant pedunculated seborrheic keratosis of penis. *Indian J Dermatol* **53**:37–8.

7 Vun Y, De'Ambrosis B, Spelman L, *et al*. (2006). Seborrheic keratosis and malignancy: collision tumour or malignant transformation? *Australas J Dermatol* **47**:106–8.

8 James WD, Berger TG, Elston DM (2006). Dermal and subcutaneous tumors. In: *Andrews' Diseases of the Skin: Clinical Dermatology*, 10th edn. WB Saunders, Philadelphia, pp. 623–4.

9 Greeley DJ, Sullivan JG, Wolfe GR (1995). Massive primary lipoma of the scrotum. *Am Surg* **61**:954–5.

10 Kim SO, Im, CM, Joo JS, *et al*. (2009). Scrotal primary lipoma with unusual clinical appearance in newborn. *Urology* **73**:1024–5.

11 Argenyi ZB (2008). Neural and neuroendocrine neoplasms. In: Bolognia JL, Jorizzo JL, Rapini RP (eds). *Dermatology*, 2nd edn. Mosby, London, pp. 1801–2.

12 Kousseff BG, Hoover DL (1999). Penile neurofibromas. *Am J Med Genet* **87**:1–5.

13 Stone, MS (2008). Cysts. In: Bolognia JL, Jorizzo JL, Rapini RP (eds). *Dermatology*, 2nd edn. Mosby, London, pp. 1681–2.

14 Eilber KS, Raz S (2003). Benign cystic lesions of the vagina: A literature review. *J Urol* **170**:717–22.

15 Stone MS (2008). Cysts. In: Bolognia JL, Jorizzo JL, Rapini RP (eds). *Dermatology*, 2nd edn. Mosby, London, pp. 1688–9.

16 Hwang JH, Oh MJ, Lee NW, *et al.* (2009). Multiple vaginal müllerian cysts: a case report and review of the literature. *Arch Gynecol Obstet* **280**:137–9.

17 Pradhan S, Tobon H (1986). Vaginal cysts: a clinicopathological study of 41 cases. *Int J Gynecol Pathol* **5**:35–46.

18 Omole F, Simmons BJ, Hacker Y (2003). Management of Bartholin's duct cyst and gland abscess. *Am Fam Physician* **68**:135–40.

19 James WD, Berger TG, Elston DM (2006). Epidermal nevi, neoplasms, and cysts. In: *Andrews' Diseases of the Skin: Clinical Dermatology*, 10th edn. WB Saunders, Philadelphia, pp. 667–8; 679–80.

20 Smith FJD, Corden LD, Rugg EL, *et al.* (1997). Missense mutations in keratin 17 cause either pachyonychia congenita type 2 or a phenotype resembling steatocystoma multiplex. *J Invest Dermatol* **108**:220–3.

21 Rongioletti F, Cattarini G, Romanelli P (2002). Late onset vulvar steatocystoma multiplex. *Clin Exp Dermatol* **27**:445–7.

22 Cunningham SC, Kao GF, Moore GW, Napolitano LM (2004). Steatocystoma simplex. *Surgery* **136**:95–7.

23 Schmook T, Burg G, Hafner J (2001). Surgical pearl: mini-incisions for the extraction of steatocystoma multiplex. *J Am Acad Dermatol* **44**:1041–2.

24 O'Grady TC (2003). Pigmented lesions in specific anatomic sites. *Curr Probl Dermatol* **15**:189–96.

25 Rock B, Hood AF, Rock JA (1990). Prospective study of vulvar nevi. *J Am Acad Dermatol* **22**:104–6.

26 Ribe A (2008). Melanocytic lesions of the genital area with attention given to atypical genital nevi. *J Cutan Pathol* **35**(Suppl. 2):24–7.

27 Rudolf RI (1990). Vulvar melanosis. *J Am Acad Dermatol* **23**:982–4.

28 Revuz J, Clerici T (1989). Penile melanosis. *J Am Acad Dermatol* **20**: 567–70.

29 Lenane P, Keane CO, Connell BO, *et al.* (2000). Genital melanotic macules: clinical, histologic, immunohistochemical, and ultrastructural features. *J Am Acad Dermatol* **42**:640–4.

30 Sarma DP, Weilbaecher TG (1984). Scrotal calcinosis: calcification of epidermal cysts. *J Surg Oncol* **27**:76–9.

31 James WD, Berger TG, Elston DM (2006). Errors in metabolism. In: *Andrews' Diseases of the Skin: Clinical Dermatology*, 10th edn. WB Saunders, Philadelphia, p. 528.

32 Saladi RN, Persaud AN, Phelps RG, Cohen SR (2004). Scrotal calcinosis: is the cause still unknown? *J Am Acad Dermatol* **51**:S97–101.

33 Yahya H, Rafindadi AH (2005). Idiopathic scrotal calcinosis: a report of four cases and review of the literature. *Int J Dermatol* **44**:206–9.

34 Ozcan A, Senol M, Aydin NE, *et al.* (2003). Fox–Fordyce disease. *J Eur Acad Dermatol Vener* **17**:244–9.

35 James WD, Berger TG, Elston DM (2006). Diseases of the skin appendages. In: *Andrews' Diseases of the Skin: Clinical Dermatology*, 10th edn. WB Saunders, Philadelphia, pp. 779–80.

36 Kao PH, Hsu CK, Lee JY (2009). Clinicopathological study of Fox–Fordyce disease. *J Dermatol* **36**:485–90.

37 Ghislain PD, van Der Endt JD, Delescluse J (2002). Itchy papules of the axillae. *Arch Dermatol* **138**: 259–64.

38 Haley JC, Mirowski GW, Hood AF (1998). Benign vulvar tumors. *Semin Cutan Med Surg* **17**:196–204.

39 Scurry J, Van der Putte SCJ, Pyman J, *et al.* (2009). Mammary-like gland adenoma of the vulva: review of 46 cases. *Pathology* **41**:372–8.

40 Veerana S, Vijaya (2009). Solitary nodule over the labia majora. Hidradenoma papilliferum. *Indian J Dermatol Venereol Leprol* **75**:327–8.

41 Miranda JJ, Shahabi S, Salih S, Bahtiyar OM (2002). Vulvar syringoma: report of a case and review of the literature. *Yale J Biol Med* **75**:207–10.

42 Kavala M, Can B, Zindanci I, *et al.* (2008). Vulvar pruritus caused by syringoma of the vulva. *Int J Dermatol* **47**:831–2.

43 Olson JM, Robles DT, Argenyi AB, *et al.* (2008). Multiple penile syringomas. *J Am Acad Dermatol* **59**:S46–7.

44 Petersson F, Mjornber P, Kazakov DV, Bisceglia M (2009). Eruptive syringoma of the penis: a report of 2 cases and a review of the literature. *Am J Dermatopathol* **31**:436–8.

45 Wu CY (2009). Multifocal penile syringoma masquerading as genital warts. *Clin Exp Dermatol* **34**:290–1.

CHAPTER 16 SKIN CANCER OF THE GENITALIA

1 Dittmer C, Fischer D, Diedrich K, Thill M (2011). Diagnosis and treatment options of vulvar cancer: a review. *Arch Gynecol Obstet* **285**:183–93. Epub 2011/09/13.

2 Micali G, Nasca MR, Innocenzi D, Schwartz RA (2006). Penile cancer. *J Am Acad Dermatol* **54**:369–91; quiz 91–4. Epub 2006/02/21.

3 Crispen PL, Mydlo JH (2010). Penile intraepithelial neoplasia and other premalignant lesions of the penis. *Urol Clin North Am* **37**:335–42. Epub 2010/08/03.

4 Heller DS, van Seters M, Marchitelli C, *et al.* (2010). Update on intraepithelial neoplasia of the vulva: proceedings of a Workshop at the 2009 World Congress of the International Society for the Study of Vulvovaginal Diseases, Edinburgh, Scotland, September 2009. *J Low Genit Tract Dis* **14**:363–73. Epub 2010/10/05.

5 Brady KL, Mercurio MG, Brown MD (2013). Malignant tumors of the penis. *Dermatol Surg* **39**:527–47. Epub 2012/11/16.

6 Pizzocaro G, Algaba F, Horenblas S, *et al.* (2010). EAU penile cancer guidelines 2009. *Eur Urol* **57**:1002–12. Epub 2010/02/19.

7 Leijte JA, Kirrander P, Antonini N, Windahl T, Horenblas S (2008). Recurrence patterns of squamous cell carcinoma of the penis: recommendations for follow-up based on a two-centre analysis of 700 patients. *Eur Urol* **54**:161–8. Epub 2008/04/29.

8 Brown MD, Zachary CB, Grekin RC, Swanson NA (1987). Penile tumors: their management by Mohs micrographic surgery. *J Dermatol Surg Oncol* **13**:1163–7. Epub 1987/11/01.

9 Shindel AW, Mann MW, Lev RY, *et al.* (2007). Mohs micrographic surgery for penile cancer: management and long-term follow-up. *J Urol* **178**:1980–5. Epub 2007/09/18.

10 Gibson GE, Ahmed I (2001). Perianal and genital basal cell carcinoma: a clinicopathologic review of 51 cases. *J Am Acad Dermatol* **45**:68–71. Epub 2001/06/26.

11 De Simone P, Silipo V, Buccini P, *et al.* (2008). Vulvar melanoma: a report of 10 cases and review of the literature. *Melanoma Res* **18**:127–33. Epub 2008/03/14.

12 van Geel AN, den Bakker MA, Kirkels W, *et al.* (2007). Prognosis of primary mucosal penile melanoma: a series of 19 Dutch patients and 47 patients from the literature. *Urology* **70**:143–7. Epub 2007/07/28.

13 Omholt K, Grafstrom E, Kanter-Lewensohn L, Hansson J, Ragnarsson-Olding BK (2011). KIT pathway alterations in mucosal melanomas of the vulva and other sites. *Clin Cancer Research* **17**:3933–42. Epub 2011/06/18.

14 Kanitakis J (2007). Mammary and extramammary Paget's disease. *J Eur Acad Dermatol Venereol* **21**:581–90. Epub 2007/04/24.

15 Petrie MS, Hess S, Benedetto AV (2011). Automated 15-minute cytokeratin 7 immunostaining protocol for extramammary Paget's disease in Mohs micrographic surgery. *Dermatol Surg* **37**:1811–15. Epub 2011/11/19.

16 Green JS, Burkemper NM, Fosko SW (2011). Failure of extensive extramammary Paget disease of the inguinal area to clear with imiquimod cream, 5%: possible progression to invasive disease during therapy. *Arch Dermatol* **147**:704–8.

17 Cohen PR, Schulze KE, Tschen JA, *et al.* (2006). Treatment of extramammary Paget disease with topical imiquimod cream: case report and literature review. *South Med J* **99**:396–402.

18 Lam C, Funaro D (2010). Extramammary Paget's disease: summary of current knowledge. *Dermatol Clin* **28**:807–26. Epub 2010/10/05.

19 Micali G, Nasca MR, De Pasquale R, Innocenzi D (2003). Primary classic Kaposi's sarcoma of the penis: report of a case and review. *J Eur Acad Dermatol Venereol* **17**:320–3. Epub 2003/04/19.

20 Ibekwe PU, Ogunbiyi OA, Ogun GO, George OA (2011). Kaposi's sarcoma in HIV-infected women and men in Nigeria. *AIDS Patient Care STDs* **25**:635–7. Epub 2011/10/05.

21 Antman K, Chang Y (2000). Kaposi's sarcoma. *New Engl J Med* **342**:1027–38. Epub 2000/04/06.

22 Maurer T, Ponte M, Leslie K (2007). HIV-associated Kaposi's sarcoma with a high CD4 count and a low viral load. *New Engl J Med* **357**:1352–3. Epub 2007/09/28.

23 Dewdney S, Kennedy CM, Galask RP (2005). Leiomyosarcoma of the vulva: a case report. *J Reprod Med* **50**:630–2.

24 McAdams AJ Jr, Kistner RW (1958). The relationship of chronic vulvar disease, leukoplakia, and carcinoma in situ to carcinoma of the vulva. *Cancer* **11**:740–57.

CHAPTER 17 ANOGENITAL HEMANGIOMAS

1 Mattassi R, Loose DA, Vaghi M, Villavicencio JL (FRW) (2009). *Hemangiomas and Vascular Malformations: An Atlas of Diagnosis and Treatment*. Springer, Milan.

2 Drolet BA, Esterly NB, Frieden IJ (1999). Hemangiomas in children. *New Engl J Med* **341**:173–81.

3 Hochman M, Adams DM, Reeves TD (2011). Current knowledge and management of vascular anomalies: I. Hemangiomas. *Arch Facial Plastic Surg* **13**:145–51.

4 Barnés CM, Christison-Lagay EA, Folkman J (2007). The placenta theory and the origin of infantile hemangioma. *Lymphat Res Biol* **5**:245–55.

5 Haggstrom AN, Drolet BA, Baselga E, *et al.* (2007). Prospective study of infantile hemangiomas: demographic, prenatal, and perinatal characteristics. *J Pediatr* **150**:291–4.

6 Halbert AR, Chan JJ (2002). Anogenital and buttock ulceration in infancy. *Australas J Dermatol* **43**:1–6; quiz 7–8.

7 Boon LM, Enjolras O, Mulliken JB (1996). Congenital hemangioma: evidence of accelerated involution. *J Pediatr* **128**:329–35.

8 Stockman A, Boralevi F, Taieb A, Leaute-Labreze C (2007). SACRAL syndrome: spinal dysraphism, anogenital, cutaneous, renal and urologic anomalies, associated with an angioma of lumbosacral localization. *Dermatology* **214**:40–5.
9 Girard C, Bigorre M, Guillot B, Bessis D (2006). PELVIS syndrome. *Arch Dermatol* **142**:884–8.
10 Morelli JG, Tan OT, Yohn JJ, Weston WL (1994). Treatment of ulcerated hemangiomas infancy. *Arch Pediatr Adolesc Med* **148**:1104–5.
11 Lacour M, Syed S, Linward J, Harper JI (1996). Role of the pulsed dye laser in the management of ulcerated capillary haemangiomas. *Arch Dis Child* **74**:161–3.
12 Witman PM, Wagner AM, Scherer K, Waner M, Frieden IJ (2006). Complications following pulsed dye laser treatment of superficial hemangiomas. *Lasers Surg Med* **38**: 116–23.

CHAPTER 18 ALLERGIC DERMATITIS, IRRITANT DERMATITIS, AND DRUG REACTIONS

1 Belsito DV (2009). Contact dermatitis: allergic and irritant. In: Gaspar AA, Tyring SK. *Clinical and Basic Immunodermatology*. Springer, Heidelberg pp. 171–92.
2 Green CM, Holden CR, Gawkrodger DJ (2007). Contact allergy to topical medicaments becomes more common with advancing age: an age-stratified study. *Contact Dermatitis* **56**:229–31.
3 Jacobs JJ, Lehe CL, Hasegawa H, Elliott GR, Das PK (2006). Skin irritants and contact sensitizers induce Langerhans cell migration and maturation at irritant concentration. *Exp Dermatol* **15**:432–40.
4 Novak N, Baurecht H, Schafer T, *et al.* (2008). Loss-of-function mutations in the filaggrin gene and allergic contact sensitization to nickel. *J Invest Dermatol* **128**:1430–5.
5 Aydogan K, Karadogan S, Balaban AS, Tunali S (2005). Lupus erythematosus associated with erythema multiforme: report of two cases and review of the literature. *J Eur Acad Dermatol Venereol* **19**:621–7.
6 Carducci M, Latini A, Acierno F, *et al.* (2004). Erythema multiforme during cytomegalovirus infection and oral therapy with terbinafine: a virus–drug interaction. *J Eur Acad Dermatol Venereol* **18**:201–3.
7 Grosber M, Alexandre M, Poszepczynska-Guigne E, *et al.* (2007). Recurrent erythema multiforme in association with recurrent *Mycoplasma pneumoniae* infections. *J Am Acad Dermatol* **56**(5 Suppl):S118–19.
8 Huff JC, Weston WL, Tonnesen MG (1983). Erythema multiforme: a critical review of characteristics, diagnostic criteria, and causes. *J Am Acad Dermatol* **8**:763–75.

9 Lee AY (2000). Fixed drug eruptions. Incidence, recognition, and avoidance. *Am J Clin Dermatol* **1**: 277–85.
10 Ozkaya-Bayazit E (2003). Specific site involvement in fixed drug eruption. *J Am Acad Dermatol* **49**:1003–7.
11 Shiohara T (2009). Fixed drug eruption: pathogenesis and diagnostic tests. *Curr Opin Allergy Clin Immunol* **9**:316–21.
12 Zawar V, Chuh A (2006). Fixed drug reaction may be sexually induced. *Int J Dermatol* **45**:1003–4.
13 Foureur N, Vanzo B, Meaume S, Senet P (2006). Prospective aetiological study of diaper dermatitis in the elderly. *Br J Dermatol* **155**:941–6.
14 Visscher MO (2009). Recent advances in diaper dermatitis: etiology and treatment. *Pediatr Health* **3**:81–98.
15 Wolf R, Wolf D, Tüzün B, Tüzün Y (2000). Diaper dermatitis. *Clin Dermatol* **18**:657–60.

CHAPTER 19 BULLOUS DISEASES

1 Akhyani M, Chams-Davatchi C, Naraghi Z, *et al.* (2008). Cervicovaginal involvement in pemphigus vulgaris: a clinical study of 77 cases. *Br J Dermatol* **158**:478–82.
2 Malik M, Ahmed AR (2005). Involvement of the female genital tract in pemphigus vulgaris. *Obstet Gynecol* **106**:1005–12.
3 Batta K, Munday PE, Tatnali FM (1999). Pemphigus vulgaris localized to the vagina presenting as chronic vaginal discharge. *Br J Dermatol* **140**:945–7.
4 Sami N, Ahmed AR (2001). Penile pemphigus. *Arch Dermatol* **137**:756–8.
5 Malik M, El Tal AK, Ahmed AR (2006). Anal involvement in pemphigus vulgaris. *Dis Colon Rectum* **49**:500–6.
6 Mazzi G, Raineri A, Zanolli FA, *et al.* (2003). Plasmapheresis therapy in pemphigus vulgaris and bullous pemphigoid. *Transfus Apher Sci* **28**:13–18.
7 El Tal AK, Posner MR, Spigelman Z, *et al.* (2006). Rituximab: a monoclonal antibody to CD20 used in the treatment of pemphigus vulgaris. *J Am Acad Dermatol* **55**:449–59.
8 Gürcan HM, Jeph S, Ahmed AR (2010). Intravenous immunoglobulin therapy in autoimmune mucocutaneous blistering diseases: a review of the evidence for its efficacy and safety. *Am J Clin Dermatol* **11**:315–26.
9 Zaraa I, Sellami A, Bouguerra C, *et al.* (2011). Pemphigus vegetans: a clinical, histological, immunopathological and prognostic study. *J Eur Acad Dermatol Venereol* **25**:1160–7.
10 Ichimiya M, Yamamoto K, Muto M (1998). Successful treatment of pemphigus vegetans by addition of etretinate to systemic steroids. *Clin Exp Dermatol* **23**:178–80.

11 Sehgal VN, Srivastava G (2009). Paraneoplastic pemphigus/paraneoplastic autoimmune multiorgan syndrome. *Int J Dermatol* **48**:162–9.

12 Farrell AM, Kirtschig G, Dalziel KL, *et al.* (1999). Childhood vulval pemphigoid: a clinical and immunopathological study of five patients. *Br J Dermatol* **140**:308–12.

13 Saad RW, Domloge-Hultsch N, Yancey KB, *et al.* (1992). Childhood localized vulvar pemphigoid is a true variant of bullous pemphigoid. *Arch Dermatol* **128**:807–10.

14 Levine V, Sanchez M, Nestor M (1992). Localized vulvar pemphigoid in a child misdiagnosed as sexual abuse. *Arch Dermatol* **128**:804–6.

15 Lebeau S, Mainetti C, Masouye I, Saurat JH, Borradori L (2004). Localized childhood vulvar pemphigoid treated with tacrolimus ointment. *Dermatology* **208**:273–5.

16 Semkova K, Black M (2009). Pemphigoid gestationis: current insights into pathogenesis and treatment. *Eur J Obstet Gynecol Reprod Biol* **145**:138–44.

17 Amato L, Mei S, Gallerani I, *et al.* (2003). A case of chronic herpes gestationis: persistent disease or conversion to bullous pemphigoid? *J Am Acad Dermatol* **49**:302.

18 Egan CA, Lazarova Z, Darling TN, *et al.* (2001). Anti-epiligrin cicatricial pemphigoid and relative risk of cancer. *Lancet* **357**:1850–1.

19 Goldstein AT, Anhalt GJ, Klingman D, Burrows LJ (2005). Mucous membrane pemphigoid of the vulva. *Obstet Gynecol* **105**:1188–90.

20 Chan LS, Ahmed AR, Anhalt GJ, *et al.* (2002). The first international consensus on mucous membrane pemphigoid: definition, diagnostic criteria, pathogenic factors, medical treatment, and prognostic indicators. *Arch Dermatol* **138**:370–9.

21 Bolotin D, Petronic-Rosic V (2011). Dermatitis herpetiformis: Part II. Diagnosis, management, and prognosis. *J Am Acad Dermatol* **64**:1027–33.

22 Gürcan HM, Ahmed AR (2011). Current concepts in the treatment of epidermolysis bullosa acquisita. *Expert Opin Pharmacother* **12**:1259–68.

23 Langenberg A, Berger TG, Cardelli M, *et al.* (1992). Genital benign chronic pemphigus (Hailey–Hailey disease) presenting as condylomas. *J Am Acad Dermatol* **26**:951–5.

24 Holst VA, Fair KP, Wilson BB, Patterson JW (2000). Squamous cell carcinoma arising in Hailey–Hailey disease. *J Am Acad Dermatol* **43**: 368–71.

25 Nanda A, Khawaja F, Harbi R, *et al.* (2010). Benign familial pemphigus (Hailey–Hailey disease) responsive to low dose cyclosporine. *Indian J Dermatol Venereol Leprol* **76**:422–4.

26 Vilarinho C, Ventura F, Brito C (2010). Methotrexate for refractory Hailey–Hailey disease. *J Eur Acad Dermatol Venereol* **24**:106.

CHAPTER 20 MISCELLANEOUS DERMATOSES

1 Nicolaidou E, Antoniou C, Miniati A, *et al.* (2012). Childhood- and later-onset vitiligo have diverse epidemiologic and clinical characteristics. *J Am Acad Dermatol* **66**:954–8.

2 Alikhan A, Felsten LM, Daly M, Petronic-Rosic V (2011). Vitiligo: a comprehensive overview Part I. Introduction, epidemiology, quality of life, diagnosis, differential diagnosis, associations, histopathology, etiology, and work-up. *J Am Acad Dermatol* **65**:473–91.

3 Nicolaidou E, Antoniou C, Stratigos A, Katsambas AD (2009). Narrowband ultraviolet B phototherapy and 308-nm excimer laser in the treatment of vitiligo: a review. *J Am Acad Dermatol* **60**:470–7.

4 Felsten LM, Alikhan A, Petronic-Rosic V (2011). Vitiligo: a comprehensive overview. Part II. Treatment options and approach to treatment. *J Am Acad Dermatol* **65**:493–514.

5 Meeuwis KA, de Hullu JA, Massuger LF, van de Kerkhof PC, van Rossum MM (2011). Genital psoriasis: a systematic literature review on this hidden skin disease. *Acta Derm Venereol* **91**:5–11.

6 Meeuwis KA, de Hullu JA, van de Nieuwenhof HP, *et al.* (2011). Quality of life and sexual health in patients with genital psoriasis. Br J *Dermatol* **164**:1247–55.

7 Menter A, Korman NJ, Elmets CA, *et al.* (2009). Guidelines of care for the management of psoriasis and psoriatic arthritis: Section 3. Guidelines of care for the management and treatment of psoriasis with topical therapies. *J Am Acad Dermatol* **61**:451–85.

8 Ridley M, Neill SM (2004). White lesions. In: Edwards L (ed). *Genital Dermatology Atlas*. Lippincott Williams and Wilkins, Philadelphia pp. 131–48.

9 Pittelkow MR, Daoud MS (2008). In: Wolff K, Goldsmith L, Katz SI, *et al.* (eds). *Fitzpatrick's Dermatology in General Medicine*, 7th edn. McGraw Hill, New York, pp. 244.

10 McPherson T, Cooper S (2010). Vulval lichen sclerosus and lichen planus. *Dermatol Ther* **23**:523–32.

11 Pelisse M (1989). The vulvo-vaginal-gingival syndrome: a new form of erosive lichen *planus. Int J Dermatol* **28**:381–4.

12 Lonsdale-Eccles AA, Velangi S (2005). Topical pimecrolimus in the treatment of genital lichen planus: a prospective case series. *Br J Dermatol* **153**:390–4.

13 Kirtsching G, Vander Meulen AJ, Ion Lipan JW, *et al.* (2002). Successful treatment of erosive vulvovaginal lichen planus with topical tacrolimus. *Br J Dermatol* **147**:625–6.

14 Zouboulis C (2008). Adamandiades Behçets disease. In: Wolff K, Goldsmith L, Katz SI, *et al.* (eds). *Fitzpatrick's Dermatology in General*

Medicine, 7th edn. McGraw Hill, New York, pp. 1620–6.

15 Suzuki Kurokawa M, Suzuki N (2004). Behçet's disease. *Clin Exp Med* **4**:10–20.

16 Altiner A, Mandal R (2010). Behçet syndrome. *Dermatol Online J* **16**:18.

17 McCarty MA, Garton RA, Jorizzo JL (2003). Complex apthosis and Behçet's disease. *Dermatol Clin* **21**:41–8.

18 Magro CM, Crowson AN (1995). Cutaneous manifestations of Behçet's disease. *Int J Dermatol* **34**:159–65.

19 Rosen T, Brown TJ (1998). Genital ulcers: evaluation and treatment. *Dermatol Clin* **16**:673–85.

20 Chams-Davatchi C, Barikbin B, Shahram F, *et al*. (2010). Pimecrolimus versus placebo in genital aphthous ulcers of Behcet's disease: a randomized double-blind controlled trial. *Int J Rheum Dis* **13**:253–8.

21 Pipitone N Olivieri I, Cantini F, *et al*. (2006). New approaches in the treatment of Adamandiades-Behçet disease. *Curr Opin Rheumatol* **18**:3–9.

22 Chan WP, Lee HS (2012). Combination therapy with infliximab and methotrexate in recalcitrant mucocutaneous Behçet disease. *Cutis* **89**:185–90.

CHAPTER 21 BACTERIAL DISEASES

1 Amren DP, Anderson AS, Wannamaker LW (1966). Perianal cellulitis associated with group A streptococci. *Am J Dis Child* **112**:546–52.

2 Barzilai A, Choen HA (1998). Isolation of group A streptococci from children with perianal cellulitis and from their siblings. *Pediatr Infect Dis J* **17**:358–60.

3 Kokx NP, Comstock JA, Facklam RR (1987). Streptococcal perianal disease in children. *Pediatrics* **80**:659–63.

4 Krol A (1990). Perianal streptococcal dermatitis. *Pediatr Dermatol* **7**: 97–100.

5 Bernard P, Bedane C, Mounier M, *et al*. (1989). Streptococcal cause of erysipelas and cellulitis in adults. A microbiologic study using a direct immunofluorescence technique. *Arch Dermatol* **125**:779–82.

6 Bonnetblanc J-M, Bédane C (2003). Erysipelas: recognition and management. *Am J Clin Dermatol* **4**:157–63.

7 Brilliant LC (2000). Perianal streptococcal dermatitis. *Am Fam Physician* **61**:391–3, 397.

8 Parker MT, Tomlinson AJ, Williams RE (1955). Impetigo contagiosa; the association of certain types of *Staphylococcus aureus* and of *Streptococcus pyogenes* with superficial skin infections. *J Hyg* (Lond) **53**:458–73.

9 Shi D, Higuchi W, Takano T, *et al*. (2011). Bullous impetigo in children infected with methicillin-resistant *Staphylococcus aureus* alone or in combination with methicillin-susceptible *S. aureus*: analysis of genetic characteristics, including assessment of exfoliative toxin gene carriage. *J Clin Microbiol* **49**:1972–4.

10 Segna KG, Koch LH, Williams JV (2011). 'Hot tub' folliculitis from a nonchlorinated children's pool. *Pediatr Dermatol* **28**(5):590–1.

11 Nagaraju U, Bhat G, Kuruvila M, *et al*. (2004). Methicillin-resistant *Staphylococcus aureus* in community-acquired pyoderma. *Int J Dermatol* **43**:412–14.

12 Del Giudice P, Bes M, Hubiche T, *et al*. (2011). Panton–Valentine leukocidin-positive *Staphylococcus aureus* strains are associated with follicular skin infections. *Dermatology* **222**:167–70.

CHAPTER 22 MISCELLANEOUS VIRAL, FUNGAL, AND BACTERIAL DISEASES

1 Bjekic M, Markovic M, Sipetic S (2011). Penile herpes zoster: an unusual location for a common disease. *Braz J Infect Dis* **15**:599–600.

2 Whitley RJ (2009). A 70-year-old woman with shingles: review of herpes zoster. *JAMA* **302**:73–80.

3 Bruxelle J, Pinchinat S (2012). Effectiveness of antiviral treatment on acute phase of herpes zoster and development of post herpetic neuralgia: Review of international publications. *Med Mal Infect* **42**:53–8.

4 Otero L, Palacio V, Vázquez F (2002). Tinea cruris in female prostitutes. *Mycopathologia* **153**:29–31.

5 Gupta AK, Cooper EA (2008). Update in antifungal therapy of dermatophytosis. *Mycopathologia* **166**:353–67.

6 Sarkany I, Taplin D, Blank H (1961). Erythrasma – common bacterial infection of the skin. *JAMA* **177**: 130–2.

7 Bowyer A, McColl I (1971). Erythrasma and pruritus ani. *Acta Derm Venereol* (Stockh) **51**:444–7.

8 Ruocco E, Baroni A, Donnarumma G, Ruocco V (2011). Diagnostic procedures in dermatology. *Clin Dermatol* **29**:548–56.

9 Cochran RJ, Rosen T, Landers T (1981). Topical treatment for erythrasma. *Int J Dermatol* **20**:562–4.

CHAPTER 23 PEDIATRIC PROBLEMS IN THE ANOGENITAL REGION

1 Thibaud E, Duflos C (2003). Plea for child: labial agglutination should not be treated. *Arch Pediatr* **10**:465–6.

2 McGregor TB, Pike JG, Leonard MP (2007). Pathologic and physiologic phimosis. Approach to the phimotic foreskin. *Can Fam Physician* **53**:445–8.

3 Loening-Baucker V (1998). Lichen sclerosus et atrophicus in children. *Am J Dis Child* **145**: 1058–61.

4 Bartholomew D (2004). Genital erosions and ulcers in childhood and adolescence. *J Pediatr Adolesc Gynecol* **17**:151–3.

5 Barnes CJ, Alió AB, Cunningham BB, Friedlander SF (2007). Epstein–Barr virus-associated genital ulcers: an under-recognized disorder. *Pediatr Dermatol* **24**:130–4.

6 Wetter DA, Bruce AJ, MachLaughlin KL, Rogers RS 3rd (2008). Ulcus vulvae acutum in a 13-year-old girl after influenza A infection. *Skinmed* **7**:95–8.

7 Marcoux D, Nadeau K, McCuaig C, PowellL J, Oligny LL (2006). Pediatric anogenital warts: a 7-year review of cases referred to a tertiary-care hospital in Montreal, Canada. *Pediatr Dermatol* **23**:199–207.

8 Mogielnicki NP, Schwartzman JD, Elliot JA (2000). Perineal group A streptococcal disease in pediatric practice. *Pediatrics* **106**:276–81.

9 Jongen J, Eberstein A, Peleikis HG, *et al.* (2008). Perianal streptococcal dermatitis: an important differential diagnosis in pediatric patients. *Dis Colon Rectum* **51**:584–7.

10 Fleet SL, Davis LS (2005). Infantile perianal pyramidal protrusion: report of a case and review of the literature. *Pediatr Dermatol* **22**:151–2.

11 Khachemoune A, Guldbakke KK, Ehrsam E (2006). Infantile perineal protrusion. *J Am Acad Dermatol* **54**:1046–9.

12 Swerdlin A, Berkowitz C, Craft N (2007). Cutaneous signs of child abuse. *J Am Acad Dermatol* **57**:371–92.

13 Gilbert R, Widom CS, Browne K, *et al.* (2009). Burden and consequences of child maltreatment in high-income countries. *Lancet* **373**:68–81.

14 Kos L, Shwayder T (2006). Cutaneous manifestations of child abuse. *Pediatr Dermatol* **23**:311–20.

15 Girard C, Bigorre M, Guillot B, Bessis D (2006). PELVIS syndrome. *Arch Dermatol* **142**:884–8.

16 Hermans DJ, van Beynum IM, Schultze Kool LJ, *et al.* (2011). Propranolol, a very promising treatment for ulceration in infantile hemangiomas: a study of 20 cases with matched historical controls. *J Am Acad Dermatol* **64**:833–8.

17 Paller A, Mancini AJ (2011). Cutaneous disorders of the newborn. In: *Hurwitz Clinical Pediatric Dermatology*, 4th edn. Saunders/Elsevier, Philadelphia, Chapter 2.

18 Gehrig KA, Dinulos JGH (2010). Acrodermatitis due to nutritional deficiency. *Curr Opin Pediatr* **22**: 107–12.

19 Paller A, Mancini AJ (2011). Skin disorders due to fungi. In: *Hurwitz Clinical Pediatric Dermatology*, 4th edn. Saunders/Elsevier, Philadelphia, Chapter 17.

20 Banerjee K, Curtis E, San Lazaro C, Graham JC (2004). Low prevalence of genital candidiasis in children. *Eur J Clin Microbiol Infect Dis* **23**:696–8.

CHAPTER 24 GENITAL ADORNMENT

1 Bullough B (1997). *Personal Stories of 'How I got into Sex': leading researchers, sex therapists, educators, prostitutes, sex toy designers, sex surrogates, trans-sexuals, criminologists, clergy, and more*. Prometheus Books, Amherst, 480 pp.

2 Hollander A (2004). *Sex and Suits*. Knopf, New York, 206 pp.

3 Taylor E, Sharkey L, Mount A (2006). *Em & Lo's Sex Toy: an A–Z guide to bedside accessories*. Chronicle Books, San Francisco, 208 pp.

4 Polhemus T (2004). *Hot Bodies, Cool Styles: new techniques in self-adornment*. Thames & Hudson, London, 176 pp.

5 Antoszewski B, Sitek A, Fijalkowska M, *et al.* (2010). Tattooing and body piercing: what motivates you to do it? *Int J Soc Psychiatry* **56**:471–9.

6 Kazandjieva J, Grozdev I, Tsankov N (2007). Temporary henna tattoos. *Clin Dermatol* **25**:383–7.

7 Kazandjieva J, Tsankov N (2007). Tattoos and piercings. *Clin Dermatol* **25**:361.

8 Parry A (1933). *Tattoo; secrets of a strange art as practised among the natives of the United States*. Simon and Schuster, New York, xii, 171 pp.

9 Geist RF (1988). Sexually related trauma. *Emerg Med Clin North Am* **6**:439–66.

10 Dingwall EJ (1925). *Studies in the Sexual Life of Ancient and Mediæval Peoples*. John Bale, Sons & Danielsson, London.

11 Waugh M (2007). Body piercing: where and how. *Clin Dermatol* **25**:407–11.

12 Mattelaer JJ (2004). Decoration et mutilation: etuis peniens, infibulation, corconcision, et castration chez l'homme. Livre Timperman, Bruxelles, 240 pp.

13 Summers JA (2003). A complication of an unusual sexual practice. *South Med J* **96**:716–17.

14 Armstrong ML, Koch JR, Saunders JC, *et al.* (2007). The hole picture: risks, decision making, purpose, regulations, and the future of body piercing. *Clin Dermatol* **25**:398–406.

15 Worp J, Boonstra A, Coutinho RA, *et al.* (2006). Tattooing, permanent make up and piercing in Amsterdam; guidelines, legislation, and monitoring. *Euro Surveill* **11**:34–6.

16 Armstrong ML, Caliendo C, Roberts AE (2006). Genital piercings: what is known and what people with genital piercings tell us. *Urol Nurs* **26**:173–80.

17 Kazandjieva J, Tsankov N (2007). Tattoos: dermatological complications. *Clin Dermatol* **25**:375–82.

18 Kazandjieva J, Grozdev I, Tsankov N (2007). Temporary henna tattoos. *Clin Dermatol* **25**:383–7.

CHAPTER 25 FEMALE GENITAL MUTILATION

1 http://www.who.int/mediacentre/factsheets/fs241/en/. Accessed 06/07/2010.
2 American Academy of Pediatrics Committee on Bioethics (1998). Female genital mutilation. *Pediatrics* **102**:153–6.
3 Monjok E, Essien EJ, Holmes L (2007). Female genital mutilation: potential for HIV transmission in sub-Saharan Africa and prospect for epidemiologic investigation and intervention. *Afr J Reprod Health* **11**:33–42.
4 Skaine R (2005). *Female Genital Mutilation: Legal, Cultural and Medical Issues*. McFarland, Jefferson, North Carolina, p. 205.
5 Mboto CI, Fielder M, Davies-Russell A, Jewell AP (2009). Prevalence of HIV-1, HIV-2, hepatitis C, and co-infection in The Gambia. *West Afr J Med* **28**: 16–19.
6 Maslovskaya O, Brown JJ, Padmadas SS (2009). Disentangling the complex association between female genital cutting and HIV among Kenyan women. *J Biosoc Sci* **41**:815–30.
7 Brewer DD, Potterat JJ, Roberts JM, Brody S (2007). Male and female circumcision associated with prevalent HIV infection in virgins and adolescents in Kenya, Lesotho, and Tanzania. *Ann Epidemiol* **17**:217–26.
8 Stallings RY, Karugendo E (2005). Female circumcision and HIV infection in Tanzania: for better or for worse? In: Proceedings of the 3rd International AIDS Society conference on HIV pathogenesis and treatment, 24–27 July, Rio de Janiero, Brazil.
9 Brady M (1999). Female genital mutilation: complications and risk of HIV transmission. *AIDS Patient Care STDS* **13**:709–16.
10 Nyindo M (2005). Complementary factors contributing to the rapid spread of HIV-I in sub-Saharan Africa: a review. *East Afr Med J* **82**:40–6.
11 Kapiga SH, Bang H, Spiegelman D, *et al.* (2002). Correlates of plasma HIV-1 RNA viral load among HIV-1-seropositive women in Dar es Salaam, Tanzania. *J Acquir Immune Defic Syndr* **30**: 316–23.
12 Amy J, Richard F (2009). Mutilations genitals féminines: les reconnaître, les prendre en charge. In: Amy J (ed). *GUNAIKEIA* **14**:98–102.
13 Ellaithi M, Nilsson T, Gisselsson D, *et al.* (2006). Female genital mutilation of a karyotypic male presenting as a female with delayed puberty. *BMC Women's Health* **6**:6.
14 Utz-Billing I, Kentenich H (2008). Female genital mutilation: an injury, physical and mental harm. *J Psychosom Obstet Gynaecol* **29**:225–9.

CHAPTER 26 GENITAL AND PERIANAL DISEASES OF PSYCHOGENIC ORIGIN

1 Harth W, Gieler U, Kusnir D, Tausk FA (2009). *Clinical Management in Psychodermatology*. Springer Verlag, Berlin, Heidelberg.
2 Lynch PJ, Moyal-Barracco M, Bogliatto F, Micheletti L, Scurry J (2007). 2006 ISSVD classification of vulvar dermatoses: pathologic subsets and their clinical correlates. *J Reprod Med* **52**:3–9.
3 Reed BD (2006). Vulvodynia: diagnosis and management. *Am Fam Physician* **73**:1231–8.
4 Arnold LD, Bachmann GA, Rosen R, Rhoads GG (2007). Assessment of vulvodynia symptoms in a sample of US women: a prevalence survey with a nested case control study. *Am J Obstet Gynecol* **196**:128.e1–6.
5 Sutton JT, Bachmann GA, Arnold LD, Rhoads GG, Rosen RC (2008). Assessment of vulvodynia symptoms in a sample of US women: a follow-up national incidence survey. *J Womens Health* (Larchmt) **17**:1285–92.
6 Arnold LD, Bachmann GA, Rosen R, Kelly S, Rhoads GG (2006). Vulvodynia: characteristics and associations with comorbidities and quality of life. *Obstet Gynecol* **107**: 617–24.
7 Foster DC, Kotok MB, Huang LS, *et al.* (2009). The tampon test for vulvodynia treatment outcomes research: reliability, construct validity, and responsiveness. *Obstet Gynecol* **113**:825–32.
8 Brown CS, Wan J, Bachmann G, Rosen R (2009). Self-management, amitriptyline, and amitripyline plus triamcinolone in the management of vulvodynia. *J Womens Health* (Larchmt) **18**:163–9.
9 Siddiqi S, Vijay V, Ward M, Mahendran R, Warren S (2008). Pruritus ani. *Ann R Coll Surg Engl* **90**:457–63.
10 Kuehn HG, Gebbensleben O, Hilger Y, Rohde H (2009). Relationship between anal symptoms and anal findings. *Int J Med Sci* **6**:77–84.
11 Harrington CI, Lewis FM, McDonagh AJ, Gawkrodger DJ (1992). Dermatological causes of pruritus ani. *Br Med J* **305**:955.
12 Pfenninger JL, Zainea GG (2001). Common anorectal conditions: Part I. Symptoms and complaints. *Am Fam Physician* **63**:2391–8.
13 MacLean J, Russell D (2010). Pruritus ani. *Aust Fam Phys* **39**:366–70.
14 Heard S (2004). Pruritus ani. *Aust Fam Phys* **33**:511–13.
15 Craven SA (2005). Pruritus ani. *S Afr Med J* **95**:75.

Index